Baillière's
CLINICAL
IMMUNOLOGY
AND
ALLERGY
INTERNATIONAL PRACTICE AND RESEARCH

Baillière's

CLINICAL IMMUNOLOGY AND ALLERGY

INTERNATIONAL PRACTICE AND RESEARCH

Volume 2/Number 3
October 1988

Immunological Disease in Pregnancy

P. M. JOHNSON MA, PhD, MRCPath
Guest Editor

Baillière Tindall
London Philadelphia Sydney Tokyo Toronto

Baillière Tindall   24–28 Oval Road
W.B. Saunders   London NW1 7DX, UK

The Curtis Center, Independence Square West,
Philadelphia, PA 19106–3399, USA

1 Goldthorne Avenue
Toronto, Ontario M8Z 5T9, Canada

Harcourt Brace Jovanovich Group (Australia) Pty Ltd
32–52 Smidmore Street, Marrickville, NSW 2204, Australia

Exclusive Agent in Japan:
Maruzen Co. Ltd. (Journals Division)
3–10 Nihonbashi 2-chome, Chuo-ku, Tokyo 103, Japan

ISSN 0950-3544

ISBN 0–7020–1300–5 (single copy)

Baillière's Clinical Immunology and Allergy is published three times each year by Baillière
Tindall. Annual subscription prices are:

TERRITORY	ANNUAL SUBSCRIPTION	SINGLE ISSUE
1. UK & Republic of Ireland	£29.50 post free	£17.50 post free
2. USA & Canada	US$58.00 post free	US$28.00 post free
3. All other countries	£37.50 post free	£19.50 post free

The editor of this publication is Tim McMonagle, Baillière Tindall,
24–28 Oval Road, London NW1 7DX, UK.

Baillière's Clinical Immunology and Allergy was published from 1982 to 1986 as *Clinics in
Immunology and Allergy*.

Typeset by Phoenix Photosetting, Chatham.
Printed and bound in Great Britain by Mackays of Chatham PLC, Chatham, Kent.

Contributors to this issue

MATTEO ADINOLFI MD, PhD, Professor of Developmental Immunology, Paediatric Research Unit, United Medical and Dental Schools of Guy's and St. Thomas's Hospitals, London Bridge, London SE1 9RT, UK.

DEBORAH J. ANDERSON PhD, Fearing Research Laboratory, Department of Obstetrics, Gynecology and Reproductive Biology, Brigham and Women's Hospital, Harvard Medical School, 250 Longwood Avenue, Boston, MA 02115, USA.

A. BASTEN AO, FTS, MBBS, DPhil(Oxon), FRCP, FRACP, FRCPA, Professor of Immunology, University of Sydney, Sydney 2006, Australia; Director, Clinical Immunology Research Centre, University of Sydney, Sydney 2006, Australia; Head, Department of Clinical Immunology, Royal Prince Alfred Hospital, Camperdown 2050, Australia.

ROSS S. BERKOWITZ MD, Associate Professor of Obstetrics and Gynaecology, Harvard Medical School; Associate Director of New England Trophoblastic Disease Center, Division of Gynecologic Oncology, Brigham and Women's Hospital, Department of Obstetrics and Gynecology, Harvard Medical School, 250 Longwood Avenue, Boston, MA 02115, USA.

W. D. BILLINGTON MA, BSc, PhD, Reader in Reproductive Immunology, University of Bristol, Department of Pathology, The Medical School, University Walk, Bristol BS8 1TC, UK.

JUDITH N. BULMER MB ChB, PhD, Lecturer in Pathology, University of Leeds, Leeds LS2 9JT, UK.

DONALD P. GOLDSTEIN MD, Associate Clinical Professor of Obstetrics and Gynecology, Harvard Medical School, Director of New England Trophoblastic Disease Center, Division of Gynecologic Oncology, Brigham and Women's Hospital, Department of Obstetrics and Gynecology, Harvard Medical School, 250 Longwood Avenue, Boston, MA 02115, USA.

C. ANTHONY HART MBBS, BSc, PhD, MRCPath, Professor of Medical Microbiology, University of Liverpool; Honorary Consultant Medical Microbiologist to the Royal Liverpool and Royal Liverpool Children's Hospitals, University of Liverpool, PO Box 147, Liverpool L69 3BX, UK.

JOSEPH A. HILL MD, Fearing Research Laboratory, Department of Obstetrics, Gynecology and Reproductive Biology, Brigham and Women's Hospital, Harvard Medical School, 250 Longwood Avenue, Boston, MA 02115, USA.

DAVID M. JENKINS MD, FRCOG, Professor of Obstetrics and Gynaecology, University College Cork, Wilton, Cork, Ireland.

PETER M. JOHNSON MA, PhD, MRCPath, Professor of Immunology, Department of Immunology, University of Liverpool, PO Box 147, Liverpool L69 3BX, UK.

WARREN R. JONES MD, PhD, FRCOG, FRACOG, Professor of Obstetrics and Gynaecology, Flinders Medical Centre, Bedford Park, SA 5042, Australia.

JILLIAN A. NEED MD, FRCOG, FRACOG, Senior Lecturer in Obstetrics and Gynaecology, Flinders Medical Centre, Bedford Park, SA 5042, Australia.

G. H. RAMSDEN MB, ChB, MRCOG, Birthright Clinical Research Fellow, Department of Immunology, University of Liverpool, PO Box 147, Liverpool L69 3BX, UK.

PAMELA V. TAYLOR BSc, PhD, Lecturer, Department of Obstetrics and Gynaecology, University of Leeds, Clarendon Wing, Belmont Grove, Leeds LS2 9NS, UK.

Table of contents

RECENT ISSUES

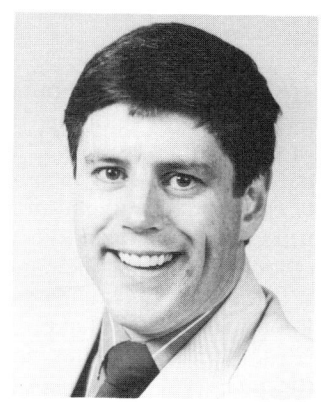

Foreword

The uniqueness of the conceptus as an allograft was recognized in the scientific literature in the 1920s following earlier landmarks by Charles Darwin in 1871 relating reduced fertility to profligacy in women and the successful transfer of allogeneic blastocysts to surrogate mother rabbits by Heape in 1890. In the early 1950s, P. B. Medawar, F. W. R. Brambell and their respective colleagues persuasively focussed attention by questioning in immunological terms how the pregnant mother succeeds in tolerating and nourishing a fetus in utero. Since that time, and particularly during the early 1980s, developments in our understanding of the immunobiology of pregnancy have been prominent. Along this road, isoimmunization against rhesus disease of the newborn became firmly established and represents one of the few true major therapeutic advances not based on surgery or pharmaceuticals.

The basic immunobiological model posed by pregnancy is one of the most obvious and fascinating, yet not fully explored, areas of research within the wider spectrum of immunology. As illustrated by careful reading of the chapters in this volume, there is much promise that both current and future research will offer further practical insight into five broader areas. Firstly, the specialized maternal immunoregulatory cognate responses to particular fetal antigens expressed in extraembryonic tissues, and our understanding of abnormal responses in certain cases of recurrent miscarriage, may prove to have application in clinical organ transplantation. Secondly, the anatomy of implantation and extraembryonic tissue development has several analogies with tumour growth and, indeed, there are many examples of specific biochemical and biological similarity; further research into pregnancy and its disorders now also holds promise for better understanding of host cellular responses in oncology. Thirdly, selective transfer of IgG immunity from mother to fetus in utero, as well as host resistance to infection within uteroplacental tissues, provide important mechanistic models in emergent clinical topics including the vertical transmission of AIDS. Fourthly, our understanding of natural and induced immune responsiveness in pregnancy has significant implications in the interrelation between maternal disease, particularly autoimmune disease, and fetal well-being. Finally, there is the exciting possibility of development of birth control vaccine of limited effective duration without further immunization. Large numbers of women in numerous developing countries shun available methods of contraception for practical or cultural reasons. Vaccination may yet prove to be a reliable and acceptable approach to relieve the dramatic population escalation and its concomitant social and economic problems in these areas, as well as providing an alternative contraception choice for women which avoids endocrinological, mechanical or surgical intervention.

The tremendous explosion in the available technology of modern immunology and molecular biology for detailed study of antigen expression in extraembryonic tissues and immunological interactions at feto–maternal interfaces has now given rise to many attractive concepts to explain the immunological protection normally afforded to the feto–placental unit. If all are contributory, it may be that the immunobiological alterations in pregnancy have now been identified and, even if the orchestrators remain shrouded, the success of the fetal allograft need not remain an immunological paradox. However, further advances can be confidently anticipated with the intense modern emphasis on reproductive biotechnology directed towards improvements in fecundity, prenatal diagnosis of genetic disorders and the establishment of reproductive models as bizarre as interspecies chimeras. Despite rhesus isoimmunization, the clinical impact of immunology in the detection and management of pregnancy disorders may not yet have reached full maturity. The chapters in this volume, each contributed by experienced investigators to whom I am indebted for their enthusiasm and application, present important stepping stones both detailing the past development and, to mix a metaphor, signposting future advances. These are intended to lead the reader through basic concepts, selected clinical events, immunopathological sequelae and, finally, more recent medical applications. I hope that inquiring minds will be stimulated by this volume and that the real advances of the past forty years will be mirrored in further practical progress in the coming years.

PETER M. JOHNSON

1

Maternal–fetal interactions in normal human pregnancy

W. D. BILLINGTON

It is of great importance to determine the extent to which the pregnant female is immunologically aware of her genetically alien conceptus. Only then is it possible to assess fully the relevance of any maternal immune responses to the establishment and maintenance of normal pregnancy and also of any causal relationship between maternal immunological perturbations and pregnancy disorders. It is stated or implied commonly in the literature that maternal immune recognition of the allogeneic embryo is actually essential for the success of pregnancy. As transplanted allogeneic tissues normally invoke an immunological rejection response in the host, it is necessary not only to determine the reasons why this manifestly does not occur in the pregnant female but also to question how immune recognition of the embryo could conceivably be beneficial. Almost all studies directed towards elucidation of the mechanisms responsible for the survival of the conceptus as an intrauterine allograft have been carried out within the context of an assumed involvement of the classically defined histocompatibility antigen system. This is understandable in view of the historical development of the analysis of the phenomenon of tissue transplantation rejection since its first definition by Medawar and his colleagues more than thirty years ago. More recent evidence, however, has implicated other cell surface molecular structures in host recognition and response, and it is possible that these may be of greater relevance in maternal–fetal interactions.

CENTRAL FEATURES OF PREGNANCY

There are certain features of the maternal–fetal relationship that are central to a consideration of the apparent immunological paradox of fetal allograft survival (Medawas, 1953). These may be summarized as follows:

Vascular isolation of the fetus

There is no vascular continuity between mother and fetus. The circulatory systems of the two individuals remain independent throughout gestation. This sets the fetus apart from any surgically constructed graft and renders inappropriate any direct comparison between them. In this sense it is not a useful concept to consider the fetus as an allograft.

Existence of a trophoblastic barrier

At the tissue level, contact between mother and conceptus is through fetal trophoblast. From the time of first attachment of the blastocyst to the uterine epithelium, the trophectoderm and its cellular descendants (the cytotrophoblast and syncytiotrophoblast) are the only fetal tissues in direct and continuous contact with the maternal environment. Fetal blood cells, and possibly solubilized fetal antigenic material, may cross the placenta to some degree at certain stages of gestation, but this is a separate issue not directly relevant to the question of transplantation immunity of the fetus. It is trophoblast that provides the fetal interface with the mother. It does so in a variety of biological forms at different anatomical sites in the pregnant uterus. The main areas of feto–maternal interface in a fully established pregnancy are: (i) at the chorionic villous surface of the placenta, where syncytiotrophoblast is bathed by maternal blood, (ii) in the placental bed, where cytotrophoblast populations are in direct contact with maternal uterine cells and blood, and (iii) at the level of the amniochorionic membrane around the non-placental region of the implantation site, where there is a layer of cytotrophoblast two to ten cells thick in intimate association with the maternal decidua.

Prevention of maternal cell passage to the fetus

The absence of a direct vascular pathway, and the presence of an intact trophoblastic barrier, prevents any significant traffic of maternal immunocompetent cells into the fetus in normal pregnancy. Maternal lymphocytes have not been convincingly demonstrated in cord blood samples in man or in fetal tissues in experimental animals (Hunziker et al, 1984). It is possible that the techniques which have been used are of insufficient sensitivity to detect very small numbers of cells or that the fetal immune system, through cytotoxic antibody, cytotoxic cells or suppressor cells, is able to eliminate rapidly any maternal lymphocytes that succeed in breaching the barrier. In either case, however, no threat would be posed to fetal survival. The fact that a graft-versus-host (GVH) reaction is elicited following experimental inoculation of immunocompetent cells into neonatal rodents, and that a clinically comparable condition occurs in rare instances where maternal cells can be identified in human neonates, is clear evidence that significant transplacental traffic of maternal cells does not normally occur. The picture of clinical GVH disease may be complicated by the existence of fetal immunodeficiency, which could possibly itself be responsible for the onset of the disease (Ammann, 1986).

Resistance to immune attack

The integrity of the maternal–fetal relationship cannot be prejudiced by the experimental introduction of the immune effector elements of a transplant-ation rejection reaction. Immunization of females of a number of different species with skin grafts or spleen cells from their eventual mate has not led to any detectable effect on a subsequent pregnancy. The conceptus is clearly resistant to immune attack specifically directed against its paternally-inherited alloantigens. The implications of this and the possible reasons for it are explored in some detail later in this review. It is, however, possible to induce abortion in mice by maternal immunization with tumour cells (Tarta-kovsky, 1987). The assumption is that this is produced by immunity against cross-reacting fetal (oncofetal) antigens.

TRANSMISSION OF IMMUNOGLOBULINS TO THE FETUS

Aside from considerations of transplantation immunity, there is one other extremely important aspect of maternal–fetal immunological interaction—namely the transmission of passive immunity. The human neonate does not develop full immune competence until several months after birth. For protection against a wide spectrum of environmental pathogens, the young child has a substantial dependence upon maternal immunoglobulins that are acquired either in utero, by transplacental transmission, or from the colostrum during suckling. In the former case, the antibodies are restricted to the IgG class, whilst in the latter they are mainly IgA. The IgG antibodies are transmitted across the placenta by virtue of the presence of Fc_γ receptors on the syncytiotrophoblast cell surface. It is, therefore, an active process and the placenta is not simply a molecular sieve. All four subclasses of IgG are transferred, some at differing relative rates and times in gestation. The precise cellular mechanisms involved in this selective IgG transfer are not known. For details of current theories and experimental evidence the reader is referred to the extensive review by Wild (1983).

An unfortunate consequence of the possession of Fc_γ receptors by the placental trophoblast is that the fetus is exposed to any deleterious maternal IgG antibodies (Scott, 1976). Isoimmune reactions of the mother to fetal blood cells leaking across the placenta, normally at or near the time of parturition but occasionally earlier in gestation, are well known clinical conditions (see Chapter 3). Antibodies to the Rh(D) antigen of fetal erythrocytes, leading to rhesus haemolytic disease, are by far the most common. Isoimmunization to other red cell antigens can occur, but much less frequently and with less severe effects. Isoimmunity to fetal platelets can lead to thrombocytopaenia of the newborn, usually in a transient form, although death from bleeding can occur. Maternal antibodies to fetal leukocytes are relatively common, as evidenced by the anti-paternal HLA specificities identified in a proportion of primiparous and multiparous females. This is of interest from the viewpoint of the transplantation immunology of pregnancy but has no apparent pathological consequences, although it may occasionally cause transient neonatal neutropaenia (Halvorsen, 1965).

Limited information is available on the timing of immunoglobulin trans-mission to the fetus. Anti-Rh(D) antibodies have been demonstrated in rhesus-negative fetuses at 10 weeks of gestation (Mollison, 1972). Determination of IgG concentrations indicates that active transport may begin by 6 weeks and remain at a fairly steady low rate until 16–22 weeks (Gitlin, 1974). By 26 weeks, however, the fetal concentrations reach those in the maternal circulation. Although the fetus is apparently capable of synthesizing IgG from about 12 weeks of gestation, as indicated by in vitro cultures of fetal tissues (van Furth et al, 1965), there is good evidence that the majority of the fetal immunoglobulins are derived from the mother. Human IgG molecules possess allotypic antigenic sites called Gm (genetic marker) groups. Analysis of paired serum samples from mothers and cord blood showed Gm type concordance irrespective of the fetal genotype (Grubb, 1970). Infants begin to replace the maternal IgG molecules during the first few months of life and by about 1 year all IgG molecules express only the child's own Gm markers. Surprisingly, over 75% of children between 1 and 10 years of age possess anti-Gm antibodies against the maternal Gm specificities (Adinolfi and Wood, 1969). Although the maternal IgG molecules are transmitted to the fetus some time before birth, their foreign antigenic determinants clearly do not induce any form of tolerance. This is not the case in mice, where tolerance has been demonstrated following exposure to maternal immunoglobulins of different allotypes (Warner and Herzenberg, 1970). Some further appraisal of the situation in human pregnancy appears warranted. Conversely, fetal IgG molecules bearing paternally-encoded Gm specificities can sometimes cross the placenta and induce the formation of maternal anti-Gm antibodies. How this 'reverse' transplacental transmission of IgG occurs is not known. It may simply result from leakage following physical disruption of the placental barrier towards the end of gestation as there is little likelihood that it could be via an Fc_γ receptor-mediated mechanism operating from the fetal aspect of the syncytiotrophoblast.

There is other evidence for a maternal modification of the fetal or neonatal immune response (see Billington and Wild, 1979). A number of studies in rodents have shown that immunization of the female before or during pregnancy can result in a diminished ability of the offspring to respond to the antigens involved. Varying the protocols employed, particularly the form of the antigen and the timing of immunization, can lead to an enhanced rather than a suppressed antibody response. Further understanding of the mechanisms involved in the manipulation of the fetal immune response could lead to clinical application with prophylactic immunization for children.

EXTENT OF MATERNAL IMMUNOLOGICAL CHANGES IN PREGNANCY

Largely on the basis of an increased production of certain hormones, notably corticosteroids, progesterone and oestrogens, which have known or assumed immunosuppressive properties in vivo, it is frequently stated that pregnant women suffer an impairment of immune responsiveness. If this were so, it would have two important implications—a deleterious lowering of natural resistance to disease and a beneficial inability to mount an effective rejection reaction against the alien conceptus (see Chapter 9). However desirable the latter might be in relation to the female's responsibility for the preservation of the species, it would hardly be a viable evolutionary policy to do so under an increased threat of morbidity or even mortality. In fact, there is evidence only for a very modest weakening of immune defences against infection in pregnancy (Larsen and Galask, 1978) and for factors other than generalized immunosuppression being responsible for non-rejection of the embryo.

Maternal anti-fetal antibody responses

Anti-HLA antibodies

Antibodies against paternally-encoded HLA antigens of the fetus have been recognized in pregnancy sera for many years (van Rood et al, 1958) and have proved valuable as reagents for tissue-typing in clinical transplantation. They are not, however, a consistent feature of human pregnancy. Only about 15% of primiparous and less than 60% of multiparous women have demonstrable antibodies (Ahrons, 1971; Doughty and Gelsthorpe, 1976). Although the kinetics of their production have not been documented in great detail it is clear that they appear by 12 weeks, and possibly as early as 6 weeks of gestation (van der Werf, 1971), decline during the third trimester and increase again post-partum (Vives et al, 1976; Koenig and Müller, 1983). The question is whether these anti-HLA antibodies have any vital role in pregnancy. To attempt to answer this, it is necessary to consider their precise kinetics, specificity and biological activities. They clearly cannot be essential for the establishment or maintenance of pregnancy since they occur in the minority of pregnant women. It should, however, be noted that almost all studies have employed a lymphocytotoxicity assay for their detection and therefore would not have detected any non-complement-fixing immuno-globulin subclasses or antibodies directed against widely spaced cell surface epitopes. Although anti-HLA antibodies could thus occur in a higher proportion of pregnant women than presently recognized, a considerable body of evidence from experimental animal studies indicates that cytotoxic or non-cytotoxic alloantibodies against fetal histocompatibility antigens are not ubiquitous in pregnancy, arguing against any essential function (Bell and Billington, 1983).

The cytotoxic anti-HLA antibody in maternal serum appears not to enter the fetus, as demonstrated by a lack of specificity for the extant fetus in cord serum samples (Tongio et al, 1975). The placenta has the ability to act as an immunoabsorbent (Swinburne, 1970) and specific anti-fetal HLA antibodies can be eluted from placental tissues (Doughty and Gelsthorpe, 1976). As anti-fetal cytotoxic antibody has been shown to enter the fetus without demonstrable harm in a number of other species (Bell and Billington, 1983), it may be that placental immunoabsorption is not an essential protective system. It should also be noted that antibody cytotoxicity is normally demonstrable as an in vitro phenomenon dependent upon the addition of heterologous complement. Homologous complement in vivo may very well not be effective in allowing the expression of the cytotoxic potential of an immunoglobulin.

The specificity of maternal anti-HLA antibodies may be against HLA-A, -B, -C (class I MHC) or -DR (class II) antigens (Vives et al, 1976). These may develop together or independently (Borelli et al, 1982). The fact that there are no directly exposed fetal target molecules for these antibodies (see Chapter 8) again questions their biological relevance. Cytotoxic antibodies that are not HLA-related have been reported to constitute the major proportion of pregnancy-induced immunoglobulins. Koenig and Müller (1983) claim that 82% of multiparous women have cytotoxic antibodies, but that most of the reactivity is due to cold-reactive IgM antibodies.

The source of the immunogenic stimulus responsible for maternal anti-HLA antibody in pregnancy has not been definitively established. The widely held view that this is the fetal leukocyte, gaining access to the maternal circulation through ante-partum leakage across the placenta or through haemorrhage at delivery, is most likely correct but should be accepted with some degree of caution (see Adinolfi, 1982). Most studies relevant to this issue have attempted to determine the presence of 46XY fetal cells in the maternal circulation, either by cytogenetic analysis of PHA-stimulated lymphocytes or by Y-chromosome fluorescence staining of interphase nuclei by quinacrine mustard. Both are subject to methodological errors, however, and can give not only false negatives but also positive results on blood samples taken from women who subsequently deliver a female child! The contention that the latter may result from long-term persistence of cells derived from a previous pregnancy with a male fetus is unlikely on the basis of almost certain maternal immune elimination of any such cells in the circulation after this time. False positives have also been recorded in primigravidae bearing female fetuses. The use of the fluorescence-activated cell sorter (FACS) has provided more reliable evidence of fetal cell presence in maternal blood (Herzenberg et al, 1979). Samples enriched for cells reacting with an anti-serum specific for paternal HLA antigens absent from the mother were shown to contain Y-chromatin positive cells by quinacrine staining. These were detectable from the 15th week of gestation and showed complete concordance with fetal sex. This has potential for a non-invasive approach to prenatal diagnosis (see also Chapter 11).

It may be concluded that fetal white cell traffic into the maternal circulation does occur but the frequency, timing and extent remain to be established. Adinolfi (1975) has estimated that, on the basis of an assumed leakage of 0.1–3.0 ml of fetal blood during gestation, and with a similar rate of transfer of lymphocytes as for red cells, there should be a fetal to maternal lymphocyte ratio of 1:1500 in maternal blood. When it is added that leakage is unlikely to occur continuously throughout gestation, and that immune elimination may be a continuous process, it is hardly surprising that fetal cell detection is so difficult. The development of new techniques for enrichment and identification may reveal a more consistent transfer. Although fetal lymphocytes are likely stimulators of the anti-HLA antibody in pregnancy, and the responsiveness of an individual may prove to correlate with the occurrence and extent of placental leakage, the possible contribution of certain cyto-trophoblast cell populations or of soluble HLA antigen (Charlton and Zmijewski, 1970) cannot be dismissed. Experimental animal studies have provided evidence both for maternal sensitization by trophoblast (Bell and Billington, 1986) and for release of soluble fetal antigen (paternal class I MHC) into the mother (Smith et al, 1987). It should also be noted that molar pregnancies, with no fetal circulation, can elicit maternal anti-HLA antibody (Lawler et al, 1974). The immunogen in these cases must be soluble or cellular antigen from the molar placenta itself. This could be a class II (HLA-DR) molecule on certain placental villous stromal cells, as suggested for the immunogenic stimulus from the normal placenta (Redman et al, 1987).

Non-HLA antibodies

Maternal antibody may be directed against fetal antigens other than those encoded by the major histocompatibility complex. Catto and his colleagues have reported the consistent presence in maternal serum of non-cytotoxic Fc receptor-blocking antibodies directed against paternal B lymphocytes (Power et al, 1983; Stewart et al, 1984). The authors suggest that the antibodies are directed against a novel, currently undefined, HLA-linked alloantigen system. An independent study has confirmed the existence of Fc receptor-blocking activity in maternal serum, but only in a minority of the pregnant and post-partum women examined (Carter et al, 1986). The assay employed is a rather capricious EA (erythrocyte–antibody) rosette inhibition technique which appears to be difficult to standardize in different laboratories.

There is also evidence for maternal antibody against syncytiotrophoblast antigens. Using a recently developed ELISA technique with immobilized syncytiotrophoblastic plasma membrane vesicles, Davies and Browne (1985a) identified both IgM and IgG anti-trophoblast antibodies in primiparous and multiparous women. Antibody levels were maximal in the first trimester with a gradual decline throughout the second and third trimesters, a phenomenon seen also with anti-HLA antibody titres (Vives et al, 1976). The possibility that this reflects an increasing rate of antibody transmission to the developing fetus, or the immunoabsorptive activities of the placenta, is unlikely since maternal total serum IgG concentrations remain relatively constant (Gusdon, 1969) or decrease only slightly (Maroulis et al, 1971) throughout gestation. The decline in anti-trophoblast antibody levels might also be explained by the development of a regulatory network based on auto-anti-idiotypic antibodies. Autoantibodies to the paternal HLA antigen receptor idiotype have been reported to be present in normal pregnancy serum (Suciu-Foca et al, 1983; Singal et al, 1984). However, there is more direct evidence demonstrating that immune complexes are formed between the antibody and antigens of the trophoblast, thus leading to a reduction of detectable free antibody (Davies, 1985a). Dissociation of the complexes has enabled quantitation of the bound antibody and the biochemical characterization of the antigens involved (Davies, 1985b). Five major proteins were identified that reacted with affinity-purified anti-trophoblast antibody and had a similar relative mass (M_r) to the proteins demonstrated following solubilization and subsequent fractionation of syncytiotrophoblast plasma membranes (Davies and Browne, 1985b). The antigens appear to be tissue-

534 W. D. BILLINGTON

specific, since the antibodies bind to trophoblast vesicles prepared from many unrelated placentae (Davies and Browne, 1985c). The kinetics of anti-trophoblast antibody production and immune complex formation accord well with the observation that trophoblast antigens are shed into the maternal circulation in increasing quantities as pregnancy progresses (O'Sullivan et al, 1982).

The nature of the maternal humoral immune response against trophoblast cell surface antigens is, in fact, controversial. Some investigators have been unable to demonstrate consistent anti-trophoblast antibody activity in any group of normal pregnancy or post-partum sera (Hole et al, 1987) whilst others, using a different assay, have suggested that the activity in the serum may be due to a macroglobulin (Nickson and Sutcliffe, 1986). The conditions under which the assays are performed appear to be a critical factor in the detection of anti-trophoblast antibody (Billington and Davies, 1987), which currently precludes their use for clinical evaluation.

Faulk and his colleagues (1978) have proposed a further form of maternal response to trophoblast. Human trophoblast antigens that elicited antibodies in rabbits to cross-reacting antigens on lymphocytes were termed trophoblast–lymphocyte cross-reactive (TLX) antigens. Absorption of the heterologous anti-TLX sera with trophoblast membranes from different human placentae has indicated that these antigens exhibit limited allotypy (McIntyre et al, 1984). This antigen system is presently undefined. It may be encoded within, or exist in linkage disequilibrium with, the major histocompatibility gene complex. A possible monomorphic determinant of TLX antigens has recently been identified using a murine monoclonal antibody (H316) against trophoblast plasma membranes (Stern et al, 1986).

It has long been hypothesized that TLX antigens induce an antibody response of importance in the maintenance of normal pregnancy but direct evidence has been lacking. The anti-trophoblast antibodies detected by Davies and Browne cannot be directed against TLX antigens as they are not absorbed out by incubation with pooled peripheral blood lymphocytes. It has recently been reported, however, that the removal of specific maternal anti-idiotype may allow the recognition of anti-paternal TLX antibodies in primiparous women (Faulk and McIntyre, 1986). Whether anti-idiotype reactions are a consistent and necessary feature of pregnancy, in relation to the control of maternal immune responses against the defined HLA or the other, ill-defined antigen systems, is still a matter of speculation. If they were to be involved in the prevention of the generation of maternal allogeneic rejection reactions, presumably at the T cell receptor level, they would need to be elicited in every pregnancy and at an early post-implantation stage.

It may be concluded that maternal recognition of a variety of fetal antigens is a relatively common but far from ubiquitous phenomenon. Whether the lack of antibody in many pregnancies is due to absence of exposure to antigen, maternal immune response gene variation (as in rodents, Bell, 1984; Smith et al, 1987), immunoregulatory control by such mechanisms as anti-idiotype antibodies or suppressor cell activities, or simply insensitive and/or inappropriate detection techniques, remains to be determined. It is difficult to construct a satisfactory hypothesis to explain the success of normal pregnancy in terms of essential maternal antibody production against any of the presently known fetal antigen systems. This has frequently been attempted in terms of a proposed role in the inhibition or 'blocking' of potentially deleterious cell-mediated immune rejection reactions, but the conceptual basis of this can be questioned.

Maternal cell-mediated immunity to the fetus

It is widely accepted that allograft rejection is brought about principally by host cell-mediated immune reactions to foreign antigens displayed on the surface of the cells of the grafted tissue. The generation of cytotoxic T lymphocytes (CTL) in the host is a prime factor in the rejection mechanism. Classical transplantation immunity is also an MHC-restricted process, whereby the foreign transplantation antigens are recognized only in the context of the MHC of the cells, of graft or host origin, that present them to the immune system. A full appraisal of current evidence on the nature and role of these antigen-presenting cells (APC) is outside the scope of this chapter but, as this has direct relevance to the theories of immunoregulation in normal and pathological pregnancy, some aspects of their activity will be considered in the appropriate section below. There is clear experimental evidence that in situations of MHC incompatibility (which, owing to the high degree of genetic polymorphism, is the case in very nearly all human fetal–maternal associations) extremely small numbers of APC are required for sensitization. They may therefore have a crucial role in pregnancy and be particularly sensitive to environmental changes, which could in turn produce a profound effect on the helper T lymphocyte (T_H) population which has a pivotal role in the regulation of the immune response.

Since the conceptus has the genetic status of an allograft, it is essential to determine whether its presence leads to the expected generation of maternal cell-mediated immunity. In particular, whether anti-fetal cytotoxic lymphocytes are induced in normal pregnancy. If they are, it is necessary to establish the reason why they have no deleterious effects. If they are absent, it would very likely be the major, if not the sole, reason for the paradoxical survival of the allogeneic conceptus, although it would be important to identify the mechanisms responsible for the failure of their induction.

The literature is replete with reports of studies aimed at providing evidence for maternal cell-mediated immunity in pregnancy. Much of the data is conflicting and confusing. Many of the studies have employed assays that give only general indications of maternal cell-mediated immune status, such as mitogen-induced lymphocyte transformation, rather than evidence of specific immune response to fetal antigens. They have also been carried out under such heterogeneous conditions that it is impossible to compare results effectively in many cases. Little of scientific value and no clinical benefit has accrued from these approaches.

There is some evidence for maternal sensitization to fetal HLA antigens from studies measuring lymphokine release following incubation of maternal lymphocytes with neonatal and paternal lymphocytes (Rocklin et al, 1982).

However, not all women, either primigravidae or multigravidae, show such responses and other workers have been unable to confirm the findings (Sargent et al, 1982).

The mixed lymphocyte reaction (MLR) has frequently been used to assess maternal sensitization. Unfortunately, as pointed out by Sargent and Redman (1985), few investigators have appreciated the need to perform time-course studies in order to detect the early and elevated peak of a secondary response. A primary response in the MLR measured after 6 days of culture largely reflects histocompatibility differences between the lymphocytes involved. Appropriate one-way MLR assays between maternal and neonatal or paternal lymphocytes have been carried out in a few instances, and these reports are in agreement that there is no secondary maternal response such as would be seen if specific sensitization to fetal HLA had occurred in pregnancy (e.g. Moen et al, 1982; Genetet et al, 1980; Moore et al, 1983). There is no intrinsic lack of responsiveness in the lymphocytes during pregnancy, as demonstrated by their ability to undergo in vitro priming to these antigens. It could, however, be argued that conditions in vivo, such as the presence of one or more of the pregnancy-associated serum molecules (steroids, proteins, glycoproteins, or even antibodies) might inhibit the potential for priming. Attempts to identify the presence of maternal cells exhibiting direct cytotoxic activity in vitro against neonatal or paternal cells have produced conflicting data and few positive findings.

Current evidence from studies on primiparous and multiparous women supports the conclusion that generation of cytotoxic cells against fetal HLA antigens is not a common occurrence (Sargent et al, 1987). In the few women possessing such cytotoxic cells, pregnancy outcome is unaffected. This concurs with the well established fact that pregnancy in a number of laboratory animal species cannot be prejudiced by the experimental induction of high levels of cytotoxic T cell activity directed specifically against the paternal histocompatibility antigens (see Bell and Billington, 1983). This may be an indication that maternal immunization against fetal HLA antigens is not an important issue in relation to the survival of the human conceptus.

INSUSCEPTIBILITY OF TROPHOBLAST TO LYSIS

As pointed out earlier, fetal trophoblast is the allografted tissue of pregnancy and it is this that must face the consequences of any maternal immunity. The HLA antigenic status of trophoblast presents a complex picture which is central to this problem (see next section). There are a few reports on the use of trophoblast as the target in cultures with maternal lymphocytes. Little conclusive information has been obtained owing to the lack of adequate specificity controls and the fact that it is not possible to obtain trophoblast uncontaminated with other fetal material, especially stromal mesenchymal cells (Loke, 1983). The available evidence indicates that trophoblast is, in fact, highly resistant to lysis by either immune effector cells or antibody. Only by pre-treatment with neuraminidase and incubation with experimentally sensitized cells, such as interferon-boosted natural killer (NK) cells, has trophoblast been shown to exhibit any significant degree of susceptibility (Paul and Jailkhani, 1982; Pross et al, 1985).

It appears likely that there is no consistent generation of maternal cells with cytotoxic activity directed towards trophoblast. This applies to cytotoxic T cells, which are antigen-specific, and MHC-restricted. Their presence in a small number of women could possibly be correlated with ante-partum placental bleeds, the concomitant induction of anti-HLA antibody, and the need to eliminate the invading allogeneic fetal lymphocytes. The reason for their failure to destroy the fetal trophoblast is discussed below. The other major type of maternal cell with cytotoxic potential, the NK cell, which is present as part of the normal unsensitized individual's armamentarium, is not MHC-restricted and recognizes targets via an as yet unidentified structure. These cells should, therefore, be able to recognize foreign determinants other than HLA on the surface of the trophoblastic barrier. However, unless endogenous interferon were present locally at levels capable of boosting their activity to at least that observed under experimental conditions, it is not likely that the NK cells would be capable of producing trophoblast lysis. In vitro studies on NK cell activity in pregnancy have, in fact, shown that this is significantly depressed in the second and third trimesters (Alanen and Lassila, 1982). More importantly, although the target binding capacity of maternal NK cells is unimpaired in the first trimester, their post-binding lytic potential is significantly reduced and there is loss of the more mature NK cell subpopulations (Lee et al, 1987). The reason for the lowered NK cell activity in pregnancy is not known, but some investigators believe that polypeptide (but not steroid) hormones and/or pregnancy-associated serum glycoproteins exert a regulatory influence. It is also possible that there could be a suppressor cell involvement in NK cell down-regulation in vivo.

MHC ANTIGEN EXPRESSION ON THE FETAL TROPHOBLAST

It is clear that a major question is whether the fetal trophoblast, in its different forms and locations at the maternal–fetal interface, expresses cell surface antigens capable of being recognized and reacted against by the maternal immune system. In addition to the potentially important, but as yet undefined, non-HLA systems previously referred to (TLX and trophoblast-specific antigens), the MHC antigenic status of trophoblast is of particular relevance. It is firmly established that the syncytiotrophoblast and underlying cytotrophoblast of the placental chorionic villus is devoid of class I MHC antigens. The initial reports of Faulk and Temple (1976) and Goodfellow et al (1976) have been confirmed repeatedly using monoclonal antibodies (mAbs) in immunofluorescence or immunoperoxidase labelling studies on cryostat sections of term placentae (see Faulk and McIntyre, 1983). This lack of antigen has been shown to have a genetic basis. There is little detectable transcription of class I heavy-chain genes in trophoblast (Kawata et al, 1984), very likely due to hypermethylation of the DNA of the genes for HLA (Alberti and Herzenberg, 1986). These data appear to preclude any further consideration of the idea that there may be modulation of the antigens by maternal antibody (Underwood et al, 1985). The major trophoblastic interface at the placental intervillous space is undoubtedly antigenically inert in this respect. This led to the belief that non-expression of class I antigens could alone explain the survival of the allogeneic conceptus (Barnstable and Bodmer, 1978). However, it was subsequently reported that the proliferating extravillous cytotrophoblast of the 6-week chorionic sac displayed HLA-A, -B and -C antigens (Sunderland et al, 1981). Examination of the non-villous cytotrophoblast cell populations in such diverse sites as the developing placenta, the placental bed, spiral arteries and the amniochorionic membrane has now similarly demonstrated the expression of an HLA antigen (see Bulmer and Johnson, 1985). The definitive identification of many of these trophoblastic cells, often in intimate association with maternal tissues, has been facilitated by the use in immunohistology of mAbs raised against syncytiotrophoblastic plasma membranes (Bulmer et al, 1984; Loke and Butterworth, 1987; see also Chapter 8).

The precise nature of the HLA antigen(s) expressed on the various cytotrophoblast cells is unclear. The positive labelling in immunohistology was obtained with mAbs directed only against the monomorphic (common framework) determinant of the class I MHC molecule. In addition, not all mAbs to the monomorphic region have proved to be reactive with cytotrophoblast (Hsi et al, 1984; Wells et al, 1984). There is also a report that four different mAbs directed against polymorphic determinants of the class I molecule specific for the fetal (paternal) allotype showed no reactivity with trophoblast (Redman et al, 1984). The HLA antigen recognized by certain mAbs (mainly W6/32) may, therefore, not be a classical class I MHC molecule but rather an incomplete or aberrant class I structure. Evidence that this may be a novel antigen has come from a biochemical study of the molecule isolated from trophoblast cells of the amniochorion (Ellis et al, 1986). This has identified a non-polymorphic glycoprotein with a heavy chain of 40 kD associated with β_2-microglobulin. It is assumed, but not yet proven, that the same molecular structure is present on the placental cytotrophoblast cells. This may well be a trophoblast-specific class I MHC differentiation antigen, but confirmation will only be obtained by gene sequencing and mapping. It is worth noting that there is increasing evidence for the presence of unusual class I antigens produced by splicing off an extracellular portion of the molecule (Transy et al, 1984).

The lack of class I MHC antigens on syncytiotrophoblast, taken together with the apparently atypical nature of the HLA antigen expressed on cytotrophoblast and the complete absence of class II MHC (HLA-DR, -DP, -DQ) antigens on any form of trophoblast (see Redman, 1983), makes it difficult to accept that this fetal tissue can be involved in currently recognized types of allogeneic immune reactions either as an immunogen for maternal sensitization or a target for any specific cellular immunity. If the phenomenon of MHC restriction applies to trophoblast, then absence of classically defined class I MHC antigens should prevent the co-recognition of any cell surface antigen by maternal cytotoxic T cells. It should, however, be mentioned that the dogma of MHC-associated recognition has recently been challenged (Werdelin, 1987).

Processing and presentation to the maternal immune system of other forms of foreign antigen on the trophoblast by maternal class II positive cells in the decidua has been suggested to be a possible pathway of sensitization (Oksenberg et al, 1986; Dorman and Searle, 1988). In experimental animal systems, it is usually only in MHC-compatible situations that *host* antigen-presenting cells (APC) are responsible for the processing of foreign trans-plantation antigens for the induction of an immune response (Silvers et al, 1987). There is recent evidence, however, for a second important mechanism in allosensitization whereby graft MHC antigens can be presented by host APC (Sherwood et al, 1987). In organ allografting, recognition of 'passenger' class II positive cells plays a major role in determining host sensitization and hence graft outcome. Although there are significant numbers of class II positive cells, mainly macrophages, in the placental villous stroma (Sutton et al, 1983; Redman et al, 1987) there is no evidence to suggest that these are able to breach the overlying trophoblastic barrier and gain access to the maternal circulation during the course of pregnancy. They could, however, be at least partly responsible for the immunogenic stimulus leading to maternal anti-HLA-DR antibody production following disruption of the barrier at parturition.

IMMUNOREGULATION IN PREGNANCY

Much of what is known about host recognition and rejection of transplanted human allogeneic tissues is related to the involvement of class I and II MHC antigens. On this basis, the evidence presented above could lead to the reasonable conclusion that the unique MHC antigenic characteristics of the fetal trophoblast are alone sufficient to explain the survival of the allogeneic conceptus. Whilst this may ultimately prove to be the case, it is necessary for the present to consider also the possible involvement of the other antigenic moieties identified on the surface of the various trophoblast populations. There is accumulating evidence for a contributory role of non-HLA related organ-specific and tissue-specific molecules in allograft rejection reactions (Lalezari, 1980). 'Full-house' tissue-type matching of donor and host HLA antigens does not guarantee successful organ transplantation. Although, for practical reasons, such matches do not usually include HLA-C or HLA-DP and -DQ, the rejection could in part be due to host recognition of non-HLA antigens. There is direct evidence for this from studies on rejection of HLA-identical sibling transplants (Hildeman, 1983).

It must be emphasized that none of the trophoblast-associated antigenic systems has yet been sufficiently well characterized nor any maternal immune responses to them adequately documented for a clear statement to be made concerning their importance in the establishment and maintenance of pregnancy. To this must be added the previously noted fact that anti-fetal HLA responses, especially those of a cellular nature, are only a sporadic feature of pregnancy and, when they do occur, have no demonstrable ill-effects. It follows, therefore, that the main issues needing to be addressed are those relating to the possible contribution of the non-histocompatibility antigen systems. The popular concept that active immunoregulatory processes are essential for fetal survival (see Gill and Wegmann, 1987) must be viewed in this light. It is thus necessary to question the relevance of the many studies and hypotheses centred upon the premise that there must be some form of inhibition or blocking of the generation of a potentially deleterious anti-fetal HLA reaction, of a classically defined type, in the pregnant female.

Efferent blocking mechanisms

The first formulated hypotheses on maternal immunoregulation in pregnancy considered the necessity of suppressing the effector activity of cell-mediated immunity. This was deemed to operate through the action of serum 'blocking' factors, in the form of either an antibody or a non-specific pregnancy serum molecule. A variety of substances, ranging from anti-HLA-DR antibody to steroids, proteins and glycoproteins associated with pregnancy, were shown to be capable of inhibiting in vitro reactivities of lymphocytes (see Rocklin et al, 1979; Cooper, 1980; Davies, 1986). Apart from the obvious difficulty of relating these in vitro findings to any comparable in vivo function of the various substances, there is now the serious objection that in most pregnancies there is no cell-mediated response present to require any blocking action. It could, however, be argued that these efferent blocking processes are necessary as a secondary mechanism in those individuals in whom cellular sensitization has occurred. This is of course still based on the unfounded assumption that trophoblast is susceptible to immune lysis.

Afferent blocking mechanisms

Maternal blocking activity may be more relevant at the afferent level, in the prevention of the generation of any cell-mediated immunity. Current hypotheses are based upon the belief that maternal induction of a deleterious anti-fetal immunity is inhibited by local factors operating within the decidual tissues and/or elaborated by the fetal trophoblast itself.

Regulation by decidual factors

Clark and his colleagues have carried out a series of studies, largely in mice but also on human material, that have led to the proposal that maternal lymphocytic populations in the decidua suppress the induction of a maternal immune response (Clark et al, 1986a,b; Daya et al, 1987). These suppressor cells are non-T lymphocytes that are able to prevent the generation (and expression) of anti-paternal cytotoxic T lymphocytes (CTL) by the release of a soluble factor that blocks the response of T cells to interleukin-2, a T cell growth factor. There is evidence for the existence of two types of suppressor cell. The first is small in size, Fc receptor-bearing, dependent upon the

presence of trophoblast for its recruitment and/or activation and is associated with the IL-2 blocking effect. A second, larger, one that is phenotypically different, occurs earlier in pregnancy and is hormonally-activated
and trophoblast-independent. The former type is believed to be the more
important and to correlate with pregnancy outcome. Preliminary data
suggest that deficient suppressor cell activity in the decidua is associated with
missed abortions (Daya et al, 1985) and with miscarriage (Clark et al,
1987a). These potentially important clinical observations require independent confirmation. It will also be necessary to establish whether a reduction
in the number of such suppressor cells is a cause or an effect of pregnancy
failure.

Trophoblastic regulatory factors

A variety of in vitro and in vivo techniques has been employed to demonstrate that mouse placental extracts and culture supernatants are able to
exert immunoregulatory influences (Chaouat et al, 1985; Chaouat, 1987;
Duc et al, 1985). Among the more important of these are the recruitment of
suppressor cells and the inhibition of CTL and NK cell activity, with
deviation of antibody isotype and blocking of antibody and complement-
dependent lysis perhaps of less significance. Although it has not yet been
formally established that these mouse placental factors are of trophoblastic
origin, or that they have an active role in pregnancy, the recent finding that
soluble extracts of human placental syncytiotrophoblast plasma membranes
can block CTL generation against allogeneic target cells in vitro, as well as
inhibit CTL and NK cell effector activity (Bardos et al, 1987), provides firm
support for this thesis.

These proposed decidual and trophoblastic stimulated blocking systems,
both of which are able to operate at the afferent and efferent level in the
experimental models and involve control of the two major cytotoxic cell
populations commonly implicated in graft destruction, could therefore act
independently or in concert to protect the developing embryo (Figure 1).
Again the assumption must be made that the trophoblast is potentially
susceptible or that cytotoxic cells, despite any supporting evidence, are able
to gain access to the fetal environment. There are further speculations that
trophoblast may be more susceptible to antibody-mediated damage and that
'para-immunological' mechanisms (involving activated macrophages and
NK cells and their associated toxins) are the more important elements to be
controlled by maternal immunoregulation (Clark et al, 1987b). Any
regulatory system dependent upon maternal antibody cannot be regarded as
essential in view of the finding that pregnancy occurs normally in mice with
functional B cell depletion (Rodger, 1985).

A different form of pregnancy immunoregulatory process has been
proposed (Athanassakis and Wegmann, 1986). This contends that
maternal–fetal histoincompatibility triggers the release of T cell-derived
lymphokines that exert a stimulatory effect on the growth of placental
tissues. A deficiency of such immunotrophic T cell growth factors might then
lead to reduced placental development and function, and subsequently to

AFFERENT INHIBITION

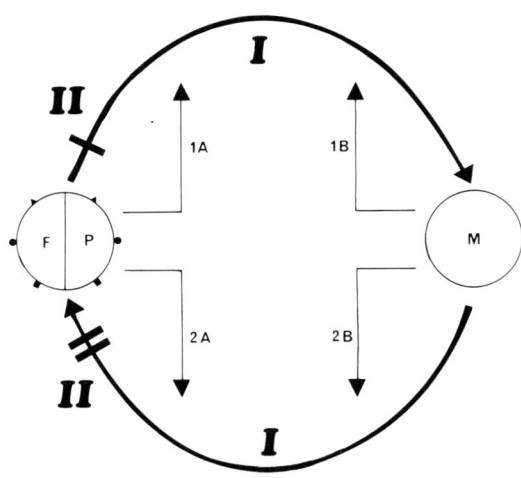

EFFERENT BLOCKING

Figure 1. Possible mechanisms for the survival of the allogeneic conceptus in normal pregnancy. *Mechanism I: active immunoregulatory control.* Regulatory factors of placental (trophoblastic) (1A) and/or maternal (decidua-associated suppressor lymphocytes) (1B) origin prevent the generation of anti-fetal rejection reactions—an afferent inhibition process. A secondary back-up system is brought into operation in the occasional event of maternal cytotoxic cell induction—the efferent blocking being mediated by factors (2A, 2B) which are identical to those responsible for primary inhibition, but may be supplemented by others present in the form of pregnancy-associated serum molecules. *Mechanism II: trophoblastic barrier and insusceptibility to lysis.* Trophoblast prevents the passage of maternal immunocompetent cells to the fetus and is itself insusceptible to antibody or immune cell lysis. No immunoregulatory mechanisms involved. Absence of classically defined class I and class II MHC antigens from all trophoblast populations renders them non-immunogenic in this respect and also lacking in these target molecules for immune attack. Role of any non-HLA antigen systems, which may or may not require immunoregulatory control, not yet established. M, Mother; F, Fetus; P, Placenta.

pregnancy loss (Clark et al, 1987b). Some support for this has been provided by the recent finding that spontaneous abortion in mice can result from epidermal growth factor deficiency (Tsutsumi and Oka, 1987).

IMPLICATIONS OF MATERNAL IMMUNOREGULATION FOR PREGNANCY FAILURE

It is clear from the foregoing discussion that there is a persistent belief that maternal recognition of the implanting embryo and the generation of a protective immune response is an absolute requirement for normal pregnancy. Notwithstanding the lack of convincing evidence, this has been elevated to the status of a dogma by many workers in the field of reproductive immunology. It has also provided the conceptual basis for the assessment and treatment of patients with certain pregnancy disorders that are purported to have an immunological aetiology residing in maternal regulatory failure, especially recurrent miscarriage (Taylor and Faulk, 1981). Whilst this has proved a valuable approach to clinical problems that have not yielded to other forms of investigation, it is necessary to establish a clear understanding of the processes involved. This is particularly important in order to determine whether any immunological changes observed are the prime cause or simply the consequence of the pregnancy loss, a point that not all investigators appear to have appreciated.

The evidence available could lead to the minimal interpretation that immunoregulation is not required. Such a reductionist view would be based on only two assumptions; that trophoblast in vivo is insusceptible to any form of cellular or humoral immune attack, and that it provides an effective barrier to the passage of any potentially destructive maternal cells to the fetus (Figure 1). This would appear to be true as far as classical transplantation immunity involving class I and II MHC antigen systems is concerned. This implies that immunogenetic analyses of normal or pathological pregnancies with respect only to HLA incompatibility are of themselves of little value. However, the possibility exists that other antigen systems, perhaps linked to HLA, may be involved in maternal recognition and immunoregulatory control mechanisms. These would include TLX and trophoblast-specific antigens; it is these that are deserving of further study. Some inconsistencies in the logic of approach in immunotherapy of recurrent miscarriage, especially in relation to different patient selection criteria and the use of paternal or third-party leukocytes, or of trophoblast membrane or seminal plasma preparations (see Chapter 4), should be resolved by such information. It would then be possible to establish the relative roles of immunoregulation and genetic factors in human fetal wastage. It has been suggested that the prime requirement is for genetic compatibility between the mating partners, having no recessive lethal genes able to act alone or epistatically with similar genes and not producing any severe chromosomal abnormalities, and that under these conditions immunoregulatory mechanisms are brought into operation to ensure successful pregnancy (Gill et al, 1987).

SUMMARY

Maternal–fetal immunological interactions have been studied largely within the context of disparity of classically-defined major histocompatibility complex (MHC) antigens. There is accumulating evidence that this may be of little or no importance in relation to an understanding of the reasons for the successful implantation and development of the genetically foreign embryo. Anti-HLA antibody production and generation of anti-fetal cytotoxic T cell activity is not a consistent feature of normal pregnancy. The commonly held concept of the fetus as an intrauterine allograft is not valid since there is no vascular continuity with the maternal host nor any evidence of cell traffic into the fetal circulation. The fetal interface is provided by the trophoblastic tissue, which in its diverse forms presents an unbroken barrier at the level of the placenta and the amniochorionic membrane. Trophoblast is either totally lacking in class I MHC antigens (syncytiotrophoblast) or expresses only an aberrant non-polymorphic form yet to be defined (some, if not all, cytotrophoblast). All populations of trophoblast lack class II MHC antigen expression. Attention is now being directed towards analysis of the molecular structures on the trophoblastic plasma membranes and evaluation of any maternal immune responses to them.

It is not known whether trophoblast is susceptible to any form of cellular or humoral immune attack in vivo. Resistance to immune lysis through absence of appropriate target antigens, or possibly the local secretion of substances capable of inhibiting cytolytic interactions, could alone explain the survival of the allogeneic conceptus. Current theories, however, hold that maternal recognition of the implanting embryo and the generation of a complex immunoregulatory protective system is essential for the success of pregnancy. This is no longer viewed as a generalized systemic immunosuppressive effect but a more subtle locally-acting regulation of immune responses that normally prevents the induction of any potentially deleterious anti-fetal effector cells, but can also function to block the activity of any such cells that may occasionally arise. These proposed regulatory factors derive from the trophoblast and/or a population of decidua-associated maternal suppressor lymphocytes. In the light of the apparently unique but ill-defined antigenic status of the trophoblast and the lack of evidence of cytotoxic cell passage into the fetus, it is not yet clear how or even why these local regulatory systems are required to operate.

Failure of the proposed immunoregulatory mechanisms is considered by some investigators to be associated with certain pregnancy disorders, especially recurrent miscarriage. It remains to be established whether the reported differences in various immunological parameters between those women with normal pregnancy and those with unsuccessful pregnancy reflect the underlying cause or merely the consequence of the fetal loss. The validity of immunotherapeutic approaches to pregnancy failure depends upon the resolution of this point.

There is a wealth of intriguing hypotheses but a dearth of established facts in this important area of reproductive medicine.

REFERENCES

Adinolfi M (1975) The human placenta as a filter for cells and plasma proteins. In Edwards RG, Howe CWS & Johnson MH (eds) *Immunobiology of Trophoblast*, pp 193–215. Cambridge: Cambridge University Press.

Adinolfi M (1982) The immunosuppressive role of alpha-fetoprotein and the transfer of lymphocytes across the placenta: two controversial issues in the materno–fetal relationship. In Adinolfi M, Benson P, Gianelli F & Seller M (eds) *Paediatric Research: A Genetic Approach*, pp 183–196. London: Heinemann.

Adinolfi M & Wood CBS (1969) Ontogenesis of immunoglobulins and components of complement in man. In Adinolfi M (ed.) *Immunology and Development*, pp 27–61. London: Spastics International Medical Publications.

Ahrons S (1971) Leucocyte antibodies: occurrence in primigravidae. *Tissue Antigens* **1:** 178–182.

Alanen A & Lassila O (1982) Deficient natural killer cell function in pre-eclampsia. *Obstetrics and Gynaecology* **60:** 631–634.

Alberti S & Herzenberg LA (1986) Transfection of DNA from choriocarcinoma cell lines and sperm cells: DNA methylation prevents the expression of genes for the major histocompatibility complex (HLA) Class I and the T cell differentiation antigen, Leu-2. In Clark DA & Croy BA (eds) *Reproductive Immunology 1986*, pp 60–66. Amsterdam: Elsevier Science Publishers.

Ammann AJ (1986) Fetal and neonatal graft vs host and immunodeficiency diseases. In Clark DA & Croy BA (eds) *Reproductive Immunology 1986*, pp 19–26. Amsterdam: Elsevier Science Publishers.

Athanassakis I & Wegmann TG (1986) The immunotrophic interaction between maternal T cells and fetal trophoblast/macrophages during gestation. In Clark DA & Croy BA (eds) *Reproductive Immunology 1986*, pp 99–105. Amsterdam: Elsevier Science Publishers.

Bardos P, Canepa S, Degenne D, Guillaumin JM & Khalfoun B (1987) Biochemical and functional properties of syncytiotrophoblastic plasma membranes from term human placenta. In Chaouat G (ed.) *Reproductive Immunology: Materno–Fetal Relationship*, pp 365–380. Paris: INSERM.

Barnstable CJ & Bodmer WF (1978) Immunology and the fetus. *Lancet* **i:** 326.

Bell SC (1984) Humoral immune responses in murine pregnancy. IV Strain dependency and alloantibody specificity. *Journal of Immunogenetics* **11:** 21–31.

Bell SC & Billington WD (1983) Anti-fetal alloantibody in the pregnant female. *Immunological Reviews* **75:** 5–30.

Bell SC & Billington WD (1986) Humoral immune responses in murine pregnancy. V. Relationship to the differential immunogenicity of placental and fetal tissues. *Journal of Reproductive Immunology* **9:** 289–302.

Billington WD & Davies M (1987) Maternal antibody to placental syncytiotrophoblast during pregnancy. In Gill TJ & Wegmann TG (eds) *Immunoregulation and Fetal Survival*, pp 15–26. New York: Oxford University Press.

Billington WD & Wild AE (1979) Maternal immunological factors in embryonic and post-natal development. In Newth DR & Balls M (eds) *Maternal Effects in Development*, pp 321–350. Cambridge: Cambridge University Press.

Borelli I, Amoroso A, Richiardi P & Curtoni ES (1982) Evaluation of different technical approaches for the research of human anti-Ia alloantisera. *Tissue Antigens* **19:** 380–387.

Bulmer JN & Johnson PM (1985) Antigen expression by trophoblast populations in the human placenta and their possible immunobiological relevance. *Placenta* **6:** 127–140.

Bulmer JN, Billington WD & Johnson PM (1984) Immunohistologic identification of trophoblast populations in early human pregnancy with the use of monoclonal antibodies. *American Journal of Obstetrics and Gynecology* **148:** 19–26.

Carter J, Sargent IL & Redman CWG (1986) Antibodies in human pregnancy. *Journal of Reproductive Immunology* **Supplement:** 105.

Chaouat G (1987) Placental immunoregulatory factors. *Journal of Reproductive Immunology* **10:** 179–188.

Chaouat G, Kolb JP, Rivière M & Chaffaux S (1985) Local and systemic regulation of maternal antifetal cytotoxicity during murine pregnancy. In Toder V & Beer AE (eds) *Contributions to Gynecology and Obstetrics*, pp 54–65. Basel: S. Karger.

Charlton RK & Zmijewski CM (1970) Soluble HL-A7 antigen: localization in β-lipoprotein fraction of human serum. *Science* **170:** 636–637.

Clark DA, Slapsys R, Chaput A, Walker C, Brierley J, Daya S & Rosenthal K (1986a) Immunoregulatory molecules of trophoblast and decidual suppressor cell origin at the materno–fetal interface. *American Journal of Reproductive Immunology and Microbiology* **10:** 100–104.

Clark DA, Damji N, Chaput A, Daya S, Rosenthal KL & Brierley J (1986b) Decidua-associated suppressor cells and suppressor factors regulating interleukin-2: their role in the survival of the 'fetal allograft'. In Cinader B & Miller RG (eds) *Progress in Immunology*, vol. VI, pp 1089–1099. New York: Academic Press.

Clark DA, Mowbray J, Underwood J & Lidell H (1987a) Histopathologic alterations in the decidua in human spontaneous abortion: loss of cells with large cytoplasmic granules. *American Journal of Reproductive Immunology and Microbiology* **13:** 19–22.

Clark DA, Croy BA, Wegmann TG & Chaouat G (1987b) Immunological and para-immunological mechanisms in spontaneous abortion: recent insights and future directions. *Journal of Reproductive Immunology* **12**: 1–12.

Cooper DW (1980) Immunological relationships between mother and conceptus in man. In Hearn JP (ed.) *Immunological Aspects of Reproduction and Fertility Control*, pp 33–61. Lancaster: MTP Press.

Davies M (1985a) The formation of immune complexes in primiparous and multiparous human pregnancies. *Immunology Letters* **10**: 199–205.

Davies M (1985b) Antigenic analysis of immune complexes formed in normal human pregnancy. *Clinical and Experimental Immunology* **61**: 406–415.

Davies M (1986) Blocking factors and human pregnancy: an alternative explanation for the success of lymphocyte transfusion therapy in abortion-prone women. *American Journal of Reproductive Immunology and Microbiology* **10**: 58–63.

Davies M & Browne CM (1985a) Anti-trophoblast antibody responses during normal human pregnancy. *Journal of Reproductive Immunology* **7**: 285–297.

Davies M & Browne CM (1985b) Identification of selectively solubilized syncytiotrophoblast plasma membrane proteins as potential antigenic targets during normal human pregnancy. *Journal of Reproductive Immunology* **8**: 33–44.

Davies M & Browne CM (1985c) The partial characterization of maternal anti-trophoblast antibody responses generated during normal human pregnancy. *Journal of Developmental Physiology* **7**: 269–280.

Daya S, Clark DA, Devlin C & Jarrell J (1985) Preliminary characterization of two types of suppressor cells in the human uterus. *Fertility and Sterility* **44**: 778–785.

Daya S, Rosenthal KL & Clark DA (1987) Immunosuppressor factor(s) produced by decidua-associated suppressor cells: a proposed mechanism for fetal allograft survival. *American Journal of Obstetrics and Gynecology* **156**: 344–350.

Dorman PJ & Searle RF (1988) Alloantigen presenting capacity of human decidual tissue. *Journal of Reproductive Immunology* **13**: (in press).

Doughty RW & Gelsthorpe K (1976) Some parameters of lymphocyte antibody activity through pregnancy and from eluates of placental material. *Tissue Antigens* **8**: 43–48.

Duc HT, Massé A, Bobé P, Kinsky RG & Voisin GA (1985) Deviation of humoral and cellular alloimmune reactions by placental extracts. *Journal of Reproductive Immunology* **7**: 27–39.

Ellis SA, Sargent IL, Redman CWG & McMichael AJ (1986) Evidence for a novel HLA antigen found on human extra-villous trophoblast and a choriocarcinoma cell line. *Immunology* **59**: 595–601.

Faulk WP & McIntyre JA (1983) Immunological studies of human trophoblast: markers, subsets and functions. *Immunological Reviews* **75**: 139–175.

Faulk WP & McIntyre JA (1986) Role of anti-TLX antibody in human pregnancy. In Clark DA & Croy BA (eds) *Reproductive Immunology 1986*, pp 106–114. Amsterdam: Elsevier Science Publishers.

Faulk WP & Temple A (1976) Distribution of β_2 microglobulin and HLA in chorionic villi of human placentae. *Nature* (London) **262**: 799–802.

Faulk WP, Temple A, Lovins RE & Smith NC (1978) Antigens of human trophoblast: a working hypothesis for their role in normal and abnormal pregnancies. *Proceedings of the National Academy of Sciences, USA* **75**: 1947–1951.

Genetet N, Genetet B, Amice V & Fauchet R (1982) Allogeneic responses in vitro induced by fetomaternal alloimmunization. *American Journal of Reproductive Immunology* **2**: 90–96.

Gill TJ & Wegmann TG (1987) *Immunoregulation and Fetal Survival*. New York: Oxford University Press.

Gill TJ, MacPherson TA, Ho HN, Kunz HW, Hassett AC, Stranick KS & Locker J (1987) Immunological and genetic factors affecting implantation and development in the rat and in the human. In Gill TJ & Wegmann TG (eds) *Immunoregulation and Fetal Survival*, pp 137–155. New York: Oxford University Press.

Gitlin D (1974) Protein transport across the placenta and protein turnover between amniotic fluid, maternal and fetal circulations. In Moghissi KS & Hatze ESE (eds) *The Placenta: Biological and Clinical Aspects*, pp 151–191. Illinois: CC Thomas.

Goodfellow PN, Barnstable CJ, Bodmer WF, Snary D & Crumpton MJ (1976) Expression of HLA system antigens on placenta. *Transplantation* **22**: 595–603.

Grubb R (1970) *The Genetic Markers of Human Immunoglobulins*. London: Chapman and Hall.

Gusdon JP (1969) Fetal and maternal immunoglobulin levels during pregnancy. *American Journal of Obstetrics and Gynecology* 103: 895–900.

Halvorsen K (1965) Neonatal leucopenia due to feto–maternal leucocyte incompatibility. *Acta Paediatrica* (Uppsala) 54: 86–90.

Herzenberg LA, Bianchi DW, Schroder J, Cann HM & Iverson GM (1979) Fetal cells in the blood of pregnant women: detection and enrichment by fluorescence-activated cell sorting. *Proceedings of the National Academy of Sciences USA* 76: 1453–1455.

Hildeman WH (1983) HLA typing: exaggerated and misdirected emphasis? *Tissue Antigens* 22: 1–6.

Hole N, Cheng HM & Johnson PM (1987) Antibody reactivity against human trophoblast membrane antigens in the context of normal pregnancy and unexplained recurrent miscarriage? In Chaouat G (ed.) *Reproductive Immunology: Materno–Fetal Relationship*, pp 213–223. Paris: INSERM.

Hsi B-L, Yeh CJH & Faulk WP (1984) Class I antigens of the major histocompatibility complex on cytotrophoblast of human chorion laeve. *Immunology* 52: 621–629.

Hunziker RD, Gambel P & Wegmann TG (1984) Placenta as a selective barrier to cellular traffic. *Journal of Immunology* 133: 667–671.

Kawata M, Parnes JR & Herzenberg LA (1984) Transcriptional control of HLA-A, B, C antigens in human placental cytotrophoblast isolated using trophoblast- and HLA-specific monoclonal antibodies and the fluorescence-activated cell sorter. *Journal of Experimental Medicine* 160: 633–651.

Koenig UD & Müller N (1983) Occurrence and characterization of different types of cytotoxic antibodies in pregnant women in relation to parity and gestational age. *American Journal of Obstetrics and Gynecology* 147: 671–675.

Lalezari P (1980) Organ-specific and systemic alloantigens: interrelationships and biologic implications. *Transplantation Proceedings* 12: 12–21.

Larsen B & Galask RP (1978) Host–parasite interactions during pregnancy. *Obstetrical and Gynaecological Survey* 33: 297–318.

Lawler SD, Klouda PT & Bagshawe KD (1974) Immunogenicity of molar pregnancies in the HLA system. *American Journal of Obstetrics and Gynecology* 120: 857–861.

Lee H, Gregory CD, Rees GB, Scott IV & Golding PR (1987) Cytotoxic activity and phenotypic analysis of natural killer cells in early normal human pregnancy. *Journal of Reproductive Immunology* 12: 35–47.

Loke YW (1983) Human trophoblast in culture. In Loke YW & Whyte A (eds) *Biology of Trophoblast*, pp 663–701. Amsterdam: Elsevier/North Holland.

Loke YW & Butterworth BH (1987) Heterogeneity of human trophoblast populations. In Gill TJ & Wegmann TG (eds) *Immunoregulation and Fetal Survival*, pp 197–209. New York: Oxford University Press.

Maroulis GB, Buckley RH & Younger JB (1971) Serum immunoglobulin concentrations during normal pregnancy. *American Journal of Obstetrics and Gynecology* 109: 971–976.

McIntyre JA, Faulk WP, Verhulst SJ & Colliver JA (1984) Human trophoblast-lymphocyte cross-reactive (TLX) antigens define a new alloantigen system. *Science* 222: 1135–1137.

Medawas PB (1953) Some immunological and endocrinological problems raised by the evolution of viviparity in vertebrates. *Symposium of the Society for Experimental Biology* VII: 320–338.

Moen T, Moen M, Palbo V & Thorsby E (1980) In vitro foeto–maternal lymphocyte responses at delivery: no gross changes in MLC and PLT responsiveness. *Journal of Reproductive Immunology* 2: 213–224.

Mollison PL (1972) *Blood Transfusion in Clinical Medicine* 5th edn. Oxford: Blackwell Scientific Publications.

Moore MP, Sargent IL, Ting A & Redman CWG (1983) Maternal cell-mediated immunity in pregnancy: lymphocyte responses of mothers and their non-pregnant HLA-identical sisters to paternal HLA. *Clinical and Experimental Immunology* 54: 91–94.

Nickson DA & Sutcliffe RG (1986) A search for antibodies in term maternal sera to solubilised syncytiotrophoblast surface components. A passive haemagglutination assay yields negative evidence. *Journal of Reproductive Immunology* 9: 303–312.

Oksenberg JR, Mor-Yosef S, Persitz E, Schenker Y, Mozes E & Brautbar C (1986) Antigen presenting cells in human decidual tissue. *American Journal of Reproductive Immunology and Microbiology* **11:** 82–88.

O'Sullivan MJ, McIntyre JA, Prior M, Warriner GA & Faulk WP (1982) Identification of trophoblast membrane antigens in maternal blood during human pregnancy. *Clinical and Experimental Immunology* **48:** 279–285.

Paul S & Jailkhani BL (1982) Lysis of placental syncytiotrophoblast by allogeneic leukocytes in vitro: effects of neuraminidase and chorionic gonadotrophins. *American Journal of Reproductive Immunology* **2:** 204–207.

Power DA, Catto GRD, Mason RJ, MacLeod AM, Stewart GM, Stewart KN & Shewan WG (1983) The fetus as an allograft: evidence for protective antibodies to HLA-linked paternal antigens. *Lancet* **ii:** 701–704.

Pross H, Mitchell H & Werkmeister J (1985) The sensitivity of placental trophoblast cells to intraplacental and allogeneic cytotoxic lymphocytes. *American Journal of Reproductive Immunology and Microbiology* **8:** 1–9.

Redman CWG (1983) HLA-DR antigen on human trophoblast: a review. *American Journal of Reproductive Immunology* **3:** 175–177.

Redman CWG, McMichael AJ, Stirrat GM, Sunderland CA & Ting A (1984) Class I major histocompatibility complex antigens on human extra-villous trophoblast. *Immunology* **52:** 457–468.

Redman CWG, Arenas J, Mason DY, Sargent IL & Sutton L (1987) Maternal alloimmune recognition of the fetus in human pregnancy. In Gill TJ & Wegmann TG (eds) *Immunoregulation and Fetal Survival*, pp 210–229. New York: Oxford University Press.

Rocklin RE, Kitzmiller JL & Kaye MD (1979) Immunobiology of the maternal–fetal relationship. *Annual Review of Medicine* **30:** 375–404.

Rocklin RE, Kitzmiller J & Garovoy MR (1982) Maternal–fetal relation. II. Further characterization of an immunologic blocking factor that develops during pregnancy. *Clinical Immunology and Immunopathology* **22:** 305–315.

Rodger JC (1985) Lack of a requirement for a maternal humoral immune response to establish or maintain successful allogeneic pregnancy. *Transplantation* **40:** 372–375.

Sargent IL & Redman CWG (1985) Maternal cell-mediated immunity to the fetus in human pregnancy. *Journal of Reproductive Immunology* **7:** 95–104.

Sargent IL, Redman CWG & Stirrat GM (1982) Maternal cell-mediated immunity in normal and pre-eclamptic pregnancy. *Clinical and Experimental Immunology* **50:** 601–609.

Sargent IL, Arenas J & Redman CWG (1987) Maternal cell-mediated sensitization to paternal HLA may occur, but is not a regular event in normal human pregnancy. *Journal of Reproductive Immunology* **10:** 111–120.

Scott JS (1976) Immunological diseases in pregnancy. In Scott JS & Jones WR (eds) *Immunology of Human Reproduction*, pp 229–295. London: Academic Press.

Sherwood RA, Brent L & Rayfield LS (1987) Major histocompatibility complex antigens are presented by murine host accessory cells. *Transplantation Proceedings* **19:** 239–241.

Silvers WK, Kimura H, Desquenne-Clark L & Miyamoto M (1987) Some new perspectives on transplantation immunity and tolerance. *Immunology Today* **8:** 185–190.

Singal DP, Butler L, Liao S-K & Joseph S (1984) The fetus as an allograft: evidence for anti-idiotypic antibodies induced by pregnancy. *American Journal of Reproductive Immunology* **6:** 145–151.

Smith RN, Amsden A & Chirakalwasan N (1987) Paternal antigen and the pregnancy induced alloantibody response. In Chaouat G (ed.) *Reproductive Immunology: Materno–Fetal Relationship*, pp 33–40. Paris: INSERM.

Stern PL, Beresford N, Thompson S, Johnson PM, Webb PD & Hole N (1986) Characterization of the human trophoblast-leukocyte antigenic molecules defined by a monoclonal antibody. *Journal of Immunology* **137:** 1604–1609.

Stewart GM, Mason RJ, Thomson MAR, MacLeod AM & Catto GRD (1984) Non-cytotoxic antibodies to paternal antigens in maternal sera and placental eluates. *Transplantation* **38:** 111–115.

Suciu-Foca N, Reed E, Rohowsky C, Kung P & King DW (1983) Anti-idiotypic antibodies to anti-HLA receptors induced by pregnancy. *Proceedings of the National Academy of Sciences USA* **80:** 830–834.

Sunderland CA, Redman CWG & Stirrat GM (1981) HLA-A, B, C antigens are expressed on non-villous trophoblast of the early human placenta. *Journal of Immunology* **127:** 2614–2615.

Sutton L, Mason DY & Redman CWG (1983) HLA-DR positive cells in the human placenta. *Immunology* **49**: 103–112.

Swinburne LM (1970) Leukocyte antigens and placental sponge. *Lancet* **ii**: 592–594.

Tartakovsky B (1987) Immune disruption of gestation. In Gill TJ & Wegmann TG (eds) *Immunoregulation and Fetal Survival*, pp 233–238. New York: Oxford University Press.

Taylor C & Faulk WP (1981) Prevention of recurrent abortion with leucocyte transfusions. *Lancet* **ii**: 68–70.

Tongio MM, Mayer S & Lebec A (1975) Transfer of HLA antibodies from the mother to the child. *Transplantation* **20**: 163–166.

Transy C, Lalanne J-L & Kourilsky P (1984) Alternative splicing in the 5′ moiety of the H-2K^d gene transcript. *EMBO Journal* **3**: 2383–2386.

Tsutsumi O & Oka T (1987) Epidermal growth factor deficiency during pregnancy causes abortion in mice. *American Journal of Obstetrics and Gynecology* **156**: 241–244.

Underwood JL, Ruszkiewicz M, Barnden KL, Beard RW, Mowbray JF & Sanderson AR (1985) Does antigenic modulation cause the absence of major histocompatibility complex antigens on the syncytiotrophoblast? *Transplantation Proceedings* **17**: 921–924.

van der Werf AJM (1971) Are lymphocytotoxic iso-antibodies induced by the early human trophoblast? *Lancet* **i**: 595.

van Furth R, Schuit HRE & Hijmans W (1965) The immunological development of the human fetus. *Journal of Experimental Medicine* **122**: 1173–1188.

van Rood JJ, Eernisse JG & van Leeuwen A (1958) Leucocyte anti-bodies in sera from pregnant women. *Nature* (London) **181**: 1735–1736.

Vives J, Gelabert A & Castillo R (1976) HLA antibodies and period of gestation: decline in frequency of positive sera during last trimester. *Tissue Antigens* **7**: 209–212.

Warner NL & Herzenberg LA (1970) Tolerance and immunity to maternally derived incompatible IgG$_{2a}$-globulin in mice. *Journal of Experimental Medicine* **132**: 440–447.

Wells M, Hsi B-L & Faulk WP (1984) The expression of Class I antigens of the major histocompatibility complex on cytotrophoblast of the human placental basal plate. *American Journal of Reproductive Immunology* **6**: 167–174.

Werdelin O (1987) T cells recognize antigen alone and not MHC molecules. *Immunology Today* **8**: 80–84.

Wild AE (1983) Trophoblast cell surface receptors. In Loke YW & Whyte A (eds) *Biology of Trophoblast*, pp 471–512. Amsterdam: Elsevier.

2

Immunological mechanisms of female infertility

JOSEPH A. HILL
DEBORAH J. ANDERSON

Approximately 15% of couples desiring children in the United States are infertile. For about 10% of these couples the cause of infertility is unknown, and may be attributable to gamete dysfunction, fertilization failure or to failure of post-fertilization events in early embryonic development and implantation. Infertility secondary to immunological factors has been estimated to occur in up to 20% of couples with unexplained infertility—approximately 100 000 couples in the United States alone (Mosher, 1982).

The female reproductive tract, like other mucosal organs, must withstand the onslaught of a myriad of foreign antigens while maintaining tissue integrity. Female reproductive tissues are unique in being exposed to at least four classes of antigens: (i) chronic exposure to microorganisms, (ii) episodic exposure to sperm, which express auto- and alloantigens, and to soluble antigens of seminal plasma, (iii) exposure to reproductive tissue antigens, such as certain endometrial and ovarian antigens, which are expressed as a result of differentiation at puberty, and may be novel antigens capable of eliciting autoimmune responses, and (iv) episodic exposure to products of conception, tissue allografts expressing their own differentiation and paternal transplantation antigens (Hill and Anderson, 1988a). Immunization to these antigens may occur in several components of the female reproductive tract, as lymphocytes and macrophages are present throughout (Plentl and Friedman, 1971). It appears, however, that immunological infertility is normally prevented from occurring by immunological barriers, immunosuppressive factors, and unique immunoregulatory mechanisms in the female reproductive tissues (Head and Billingham, 1986).

This chapter provides evidence that the normal female reproductive tract is immunologically dynamic and that both humoral and cellular immune responses can occur locally in reproductive tissues. Furthermore, evidence will be presented that humoral and cellular mediators (antibodies and cytokines) can affect reproductive processes in several ways to cause reproductive failure.

IMMUNOLOGY OF THE FEMALE REPRODUCTIVE TRACT

Vagina

The vagina is lined with stratified squamous epithelium that undergoes cyclical changes in response to ovarian hormones (Rakoff, 1961). Vaginal secretions are apparently a transudate of peripheral plasma (Wagner and Levin, 1978). Leukocytes (lymphoid and myeloid cells) are infrequently found in vaginal lavages from normal healthy women (usually $< 10^4$); however, approximately 20% of healthy women attending an infertility clinic had $> 10^5$ leukocytes in vaginal secretions (Hill and Anderson, 1988b). Subepithelial plasma cells have been localized along the lamina propria of the normal human vagina (Kutteh et al, 1988). Vaginal secretions do not affect leukocyte viability, surface antigen expression or phagocytic function. However, the ability of T lymphocytes to proliferate in response to mitogenic stimulation was significantly suppressed by vaginal secretions in some women, suggesting that lymphocyte activation and immune defence mechanisms may at times be inhibited in this location (Hill and Anderson, 1988b).

Cervix

The cervix acts as a barrier preventing the spread of organisms that colonize the vagina into the normally sterile uterus (Ansbacher et al, 1967; Larson and Galask, 1982; Hill et al, 1986). Cervical cell morphology and secretions, are also influenced by cyclic hormonal variations (Rakoff, 1961). Serum-type immunoglobulins are abundant in cervical secretions, as is the mucosal-associated dimeric secretory IgA (Rebello et al, 1975). Numerous antibody-secreting plasma cells are detectable in cervical biopsies. Approximately two thirds of these cells contain IgA and J-chain, indicating that they produce polymeric IgA locally in the reproductive tract (Kutteh et al, 1988). This may represent a mechanism for maintaining sterility higher in the reproductive tract, yet at the same time permitting the normal cervico–vaginal flora. Cervicitis and vaginitis, however, can occur and among other things are characterized by an abundance of leukocytes in secretions (Monif, 1982). It has been demonstrated in rabbits (Phillips and Mahler, 1977), and recently in humans (Pandya and Cohen, 1985), that semen contains factors that are chemotactic for cervico–vaginal leukocytes. It is not known whether the function of these cells extends beyond simply providing a 'clean-up' mechanism for introduced bacteria and sperm. The cells attracted to the insemination site have not been adequately characterized; one group has proposed that seminal plasma locally activates suppressor cells that inhibit sensitization to sperm antigens in women (Witkin, 1984).

Endometrium

The human endometrium under hormonal stimulation, cyclically prepares to receive a fertilized ovum in a process known as the menstrual cycle (Healy and Hodgen, 1983). Since the classic histological description of Noyes et al (1950) on cyclical changes in the normal human endometrium, investigators have questioned the nature and activity of lymphoid, myeloid and other antigen-presenting cells that migrate to the human endometrium and decidua (Sen and Fox, 1967; Kearns and Lala, 1982; Bulmer and Sunderland, 1984). Endometrial leukocyte populations are similar to those found in other mucosal lymphoid tissues in the body; however, they are located primarily in the stratum functionalis which is cyclically shed during menstruation (Morris et al, 1985). The numbers of leukocytes appear to increase in late secretory endometrium. The major leukocyte populations are T lymphocytes, macrophages, and lymphoid cells expressing the NKH-1 marker (possibly analogous to natural killer cells) (Kamat and Isaacson, 1987; Xu et al, 1987). A premenstrual increase in neutrophils has been reported (Morris et al, 1985). We have noted that T-helper/inducer lymphocyte populations outnumber T-suppressor/cytotoxic lymphocyte populations throughout the menstrual cycle (Xu et al, 1987). All the major immunoglobulin classes, including IgG, IgM and IgA, appear to be present in uterine fluid (Lint, 1980). The secretory component of IgA has been identified in epithelial cells of the endometrial glands (Rebello et al, 1975). Complement activity in uterine fluid, however, has been reported to be only 3% that of serum levels (Lint, 1980).

Decidua

Decidualization is the endometrial response to the hormonal changes in the luteal phase and pregnancy. At implantation, there is a dramatic influx of lymphoid and myeloid cells to the endometrium/decidua (Bulmer and Sunderland, 1984; Kabawat et al, 1985). As trophoblast cells proliferate outwards from the cytotrophoblast columns of some chorionic villi to infiltrate the decidua, they expose themselves to immunologically relevant response cells located in the endometrial stroma, glands and blood sinusoids. There is considerable evidence to indicate, however, that decidual lymphoid and myeloid cells do not function normally. Potent immunosuppressive factors have been identified in decidual and trophoblast extracts (Golander et al, 1981; Clark and McDermott, 1981; Slapsys and Clark, 1983; Vlasselaer and Vandeputte, 1984; Daya et al, 1985), and in supernatants from embryo cultures (Daya and Clark, 1986). In normal decidua, T lymphocytes do not express detectable levels of IL-2 receptor (Bulmer and Johnson, 1986; Hill et al, 1988a). Fetal resorption in mice has been associated with a lack of decidual suppressor cells (Slapsys and Clark, 1985), giving rise to the concept that such cells could locally regulate maternal immune responses directed against fetal tissues and play a critical role in the maintenance of early pregnancy.

Limited immunohistology studies have demonstrated that T lymphocytes may be scarce at the normal implantation site, and that macrophages are abundant (Bulmer and Sunderland, 1984; Kabawat et al, 1985). This indicates that T cell responses are not evident at the fetal–maternal interface. Non-T cells, possibly monocytes or natural killer cells, have been associated with the immunosuppressive activity (Slapsys and Clark, 1985). The endometrial glands in early pregnancy contain macrophages and T lymphocytes, indicating that in early human pregnancy the endometrial glands may mediate immunological activity possibly through hormonally regulated secretions (Bulmer and Sunderland, 1984). Successful implantation requires synchronization between embryonic and endometrial development. Prostaglandins produced by endometrial macrophages have been proposed to play a key role in implantation and decidualization by increasing endometrial vascular permeability at the initiation of implantation (Kennedy, 1977) and by stimulating the proliferation and differentiation of decidual cells (Kennedy, 1985). Prostaglandins may also act as immunosuppressive agents and may down-regulate IL-2 receptor expression on T lymphocytes (Lala et al, 1986), thus preventing immune activation. Studies from our laboratory have indicated that cells positive to interleukin-2 receptor are present in normal human decidua only in very low numbers (confirming studies of Bulmer and Johnson (1986)), but are present in significant numbers in the decidua from many women with recurrent miscarriage (Hill et al, 1988a). These IL-2 receptor positive cells may be activated T lymphocytes or natural killer cells (Clark et al, 1987; Herberman et al, 1987).

Fallopian tube

Fluid within the fallopian tube is derived from a combination of selected transudation from the blood, active secretion from its hormonally influenced epithelial tissues, and contributions from both peritoneal fluid and follicular fluid. Macrophages have been detected in the fallopian tube and are believed to originate from the peritoneal cavity (Haney et al, 1983a). Peritoneal macrophages may have leuteotropic effects on cumulus cells while the oocyte resides in the fallopian tube (Halme et al, 1985). The concentration of immunoglobulins within oviductal fluid is reported to be approximately one tenth the concentration of serum (Oliphant et al, 1977). Immunoglobulin-producing plasma cells have been found beneath the fallopian tube epithelium in humans (Lippes et al, 1970). The concentration of complement in oviducts of rhesus monkeys is reported to be less than 10% that of serum (Yang et al, 1983).

Ovary

Immunological mechanisms may regulate human ovarian physiology. Evidence has been provided that T lymphocyte and macrophage products stimulate gonadotrophin and steroid production and promote normal folliculargenesis (Bukovsky et al, 1981; Presl and Bukovsky, 1986). Evidence has also been provided that macrophages infiltrating into the developing corpus luteum modulate granulosa–luteal cell progesterone production (Halme et al, 1985). A predominance of T-cytotoxic/suppressor lymphocytes are detected in ovarian follicular fluid and may be involved in the suppression of autoimmune responses directed against ovarian antigens (Hill et al, 1987a).

Follicular fluid appears to be an ultrafiltrate of plasma. The follicular fluid levels of the immunoglobulins IgA and IgG, and complement, are reported to be similar to peripheral plasma. The follicular fluid concentration of IgM, however, is only 10% that of peripheral blood levels (Clarke et al, 1984). There is no evidence for local antibody production in the ovary (Ingerslev, 1981). Follicular fluid also contains all of the components necessary to support the complement cascade (Schumacher, 1980).

Peritoneal cavity

The female peritoneal cavity is an immunologically dynamic environment. Peritoneal fluid leukocyte subpopulation concentrations in fertile women consist of a 2:1 ratio of macrophages to lymphocytes. The majority of lymphocytes are T lymphocytes. The ratio of T-helper to T-suppressor/cytotoxic lymphocytes is approximately 3.5:1. Natural killer cells comprise approximately 10% of all leukocytes found in normal peritoneal fluid from fertile women (Hill et al, 1988b). Leukocyte activation and proliferation is stimulated in the presence of normal peritoneal fluid (Hill and Anderson, 1988c).

MECHANISMS OF IMMUNOLOGICAL INFERTILITY: BASIC RESEARCH

The introduction of seminal, microbial or embryonic and trophoblast antigens into the female genital tract, or the occurrence of endometriosis on peritoneal surfaces, can evoke immune responses. Immune responses to these antigens may be humoral or cellular, local or systemic. Their effects may be interruption of oocyte development; inhibition of ovulation; immobilization, agglutination or cytolysis of spermatozoa; interference with sperm–ovum contact and transport; and early embryonic mortality.

Humoral mechanisms

Antibody production has long been the central theme of discussions in reproductive immunology. Antibodies directed against gamete, ovarian, endometrial and embryo/trophoblast antigens have all been implicated in the pathogenesis of reproductive failure.

Antibodies to spermatozoa may inhibit fertility before, during or after fertilization. Anti-sperm antibodies could interfere with sperm transport, gamete interaction, embryo development, implantation, or trophoblast outgrowth. Binding of anti-sperm antibodies to the sperm surface can impair their ability to penetrate cervical mucus (Menge et al, 1982), thus inhibiting sperm access to the site of fertilization. Sperm-reactive antibodies may also subject spermatozoa to complement-mediated lysis (Beer and Neaves, 1978). Tail-directed antibodies that fix complement (IgM and IgG but usually not IgA) may render sperm immotile (Bronson et al, 1982a). Binding of complement components (C3) to antibody-coated spermatozoa could also cause opsonization, increasing sperm phagocytosis by macrophages residing in female reproductive tissues (London et al, 1985). Head-directed antibodies could interfere with the acrosome reaction or other enzyme-dependent mechanisms of sperm penetration of the oocyte (Bronson et al, 1982b), or could occlude binding sites for the zona pellucida or ovum thereby preventing sperm–oocyte attachment.

In addition to affecting pre-fertilization events, anti-sperm antibodies may be a cause of early embryonic mortality. The zona pellucida is permeable to both antibody and complement (Shivers and Dunbar, 1977), and sperm antigens are present on the fertilized egg and early embryo since at fertilization the sperm plasma membrane fuses with that of the egg (Menge and Fleming, 1978; Gaunt, 1983; Anderson and Madrigal, 1985). Cross-reactive antigens on sperm and trophoblast have also been documented (Anderson et al, 1987), and provide a further mechanism whereby anti-sperm antibodies may disrupt implantation events or trophoblast outgrowth and function.

Anti-ovarian antibodies have recently been described (Mathur et al, 1982). These antibodies may interfere with ovum maturation, ovulation and oocyte viability. Antibodies directed against zona pellucida antigens could cause infertility by inhibiting sperm–egg interactions, inhibiting blastocyst hatching prior to implantation, or by exerting complement-mediated cytotoxicity effects on unfertilized and fertilized eggs (Hill and Anderson, 1988a).

Embryonic antigens are differentiation antigens expressed by the developing conceptus from the time of fertilization through the immediate post-implantation phase of development (Jacob, 1977). These antigens are specialized stage-specific molecules that serve as recognition and adhesion structures underlying early embryonic development (Hill and Anderson, 1988a). They are also potential immunological targets for reproductive failure. Animal studies indicate that embryonic antigens can elicit immune responses culminating in infertility (Hamilton et al, 1979; Webb, 1980). These antigens, however, have not been thoroughly explored as targets of immunological infertility in humans.

Extra-embryonic (trophoblast and amnion) tissues also express unique antigens that could be targets for tissue-specific antibodies (Johnson et al, 1981). In addition to trophoblast-specific antigens, paternally acquired polymorphic antigens, such as trophoblast–lymphocyte crossreactive (TLX) antigens and placental-type alkaline phosphatase, may be expressed on the developing trophoblast at the fetal–maternal interface (McIntyre et al, 1983; Johnson, 1984). Although not as yet conclusively documented as immunogenic in humans, these polymorphic antigens could serve as immunologic targets for reproductive failure. Expression of paternal major histocompatibility (MHC) antigens by the early conceptus and fetal membranes is limited and may be in altered (non-immunogenic) forms (Ozato et al, 1985; Head et al, 1987; see also Chapter 8).

Antibodies directed against endometrial antigens have been described (Mathur et al, 1982; Wild and Shivers, 1985). Such antibodies could theoretically interfere with the normal events surrounding implantation and trophoblast proliferation by disrupting deciduagenesis. It is possible that hormonal synchronization between the implanting conceptus and the decidual bed, which is critical for successful gestation, is inhibited by antibodies specific for endometrial antigens.

Cellular mechanisms

Recent technological advances in the field of cellular immunology have enabled advanced studies on the cellular and soluble mediators of cell-mediated immune responses and their interactions with reproductive processes. Cell-mediated immunity is achieved both through cell–cell interactions and by the effects of soluble factors produced by the cell types involved (Tables 1 and 2). The predominant cell types participating in these responses are as follows:

1. Macrophages, which process and present foreign antigens to T lymphocytes. These cells carry out microbiocidal and cytocidal functions either directly by cell–cell contact or indirectly by the release of monokines (i.e. interleukin-1 (IL-1) and tumour necrosis factor (TNF)), free oxygen radicals, hydrogen peroxide and other enzymes.
2. T lymphocytes, which home to the site of a foreign antigenic stimulus and perform many effector and immunoregulatory functions. T lymphocyte subpopulations do this primarily through the release of lymphokines, such as interleukin-2 (IL-2), granulocyte/macrophage-colony stimulating factor (GM-CSF), lymphotoxin (LTN) and γ-interferon (γ-IFN).
3. Antibody-dependent killer (K) and natural killer (NK) cells, which achieve cytolysis primarily through cell–cell contact.
4. Granulocytes (neutrophils, eosinophils and basophils), which often use antibodies to recognize and process foreign antigens, and release soluble factors causing inflammation and tissue cell destruction.
5. Plasma cells, which produce cytophilic antibodies enabling neutrophils, macrophages, and K cells to participate in antibody-dependent cellular cytotoxic (ADCC) immune responses (Anderson and Hill, 1988).

The secreted soluble products of cell-mediated immune reactions are important inducers and regulators of immunological responses. The effects of these substances, however, are not restricted only to immune cells. Evidence is accumulating that many of these factors can adversely affect reproductive cells and their functions.

A specialized role in immune regulation for the T-helper lymphocyte product, γ-IFN, has been proposed because of its ability to increase the surface expression of class I, and induce the surface expression of class II, MHC antigens. The aberrant expression of class II MHC antigens induced by γ-IFN has been proposed as a potential mechanism for a variety of autoimmune endocrinopathies (Bottazzo et al, 1983). Gamma-IFN has been shown to induce HLA-DR antigen expression in human endometrial epithelial cells (Tabidzadeh et al, 1986). Uterine glandular epithelial cells have also been noted to express class II MHC antigens (Bulmer and Johnson, 1985). The role of HLA-DR antigen expression in endometrial epithelium remains to be clarified, although these molecules could be

Table 1. Cells and soluble mediators of cell-mediated immune responses. From Anderson and Hill (1988).

Cell type	Characteristics	Principal relevant soluble factors
T lymphocytes	Found primarily in circulation and lymphoid tissues; will home to site of foreign antigenic stimulus in response to bacterial and leukocytic chemotactic factors; may also be responsive to hormonal influences; recognize foreign antigens when presented with class I or class II MHC membrane antigens; long-lived memory cells rapidly respond to specific foreign antigens to mount rapid effective secondary immune response; subsets with a variety of effector and immunoregulatory functions.	Lymphokines (IL-2, IL-3, IL-4, IL-5, γ-IFN, CSF, LT); PGE_2; diamine oxidase; perforins.
Monocytes, macrophages	High phagocytic and pinocytotic capacity; long life in tissue, capacity to differentiate locally; ability to interact specifically with lymphocytes to promote antigen-specific response; usually become prominent in inflammatory lesions after 8 to 12 hours; have Fc receptors for IgG antibodies, use IgG to identify foreign antigens (ADCC, opsonization mechanisms).	Monokines (IL-1, TNF, CSF); complement components (C1, C2, C3, C4, C5, factor B, properdin); PGE_2, PGF_2, leukotrienes B and C; peroxidase; superoxide, hydrogen peroxide, hydroxyl radicals; monohydroxy, eicosatetraenoic acids; prostacyclin; elastase, collagenase, plasminogen activator, lysozyme, procoagulant activity (PCA) factor; fibrinectin.
Neutrophils	Rapid migration; availability in large numbers; short life-span in tissues; high phagocytic capacity; rapid burst of oxidative metabolism following stimulation; potent repertoire of oxidative metabolites and digestive enzymes; major element in acute inflammation; have Fc receptors for IgG subclass antibodies (IgG_1 and IgG_3 in humans) and participate in ADCC responses.	Peroxidase, PMN elastase, collagenase, lysozyme, myeloperoxidase, lactoferrin, alkaline phosphatase, β-glucuronidase, acid glycerophosphatase, cathepsins, α-fucosidase, 5'nucleotidase, β-galactosidase, arylsulfatase, N-acetyl-β-glucosaminidase, mucopolysaccharides, trypsin-like proteases, histamine-release inhibitors, histaminase, PGE_2, superoxide, hydrogen peroxide, hydroxyl radicals.
Eosinophils	Frequently found in tissues infected with parasites or with high levels of IgE; cytotoxic activity directed towards parasites; surface receptors for IgG, IgE and complement components (providing recognition sites for cell activation and release of granule contents).	Peroxidase, superoxide, hydrogen peroxide, PGE_2, leukotrienes B and C, diamine oxidase, kinase, lysophospholipase, arylsulfatase B, phospholipase D, lysophospholipase.

Cell	Description	Products
Basophils	High affinity receptors for IgE; degranulation triggered by IgE receptor cross-linking, and also by some lymphokines; circulating cells, localize in tissue only under special circumstances; cutaneous basophil hypersensitivity reactions in response to soluble antigens, parasites, tumour cells or allogeneic cells; activated by soluble products of lymphocytes, PMNs, macrophages.	Histamine, serotonin, dopamine, plasminogen activator, PGD$_2$, heparin, diverse proteolytic enzymes, acidic proteoglycans, chemotactic factors for neutrophils, limited amount of classical lysosomal enzymes listed for neutrophils, peroxidase, superoxide, hydrogen peroxide.
Mast cells	High affinity receptors for IgE; sessile cells, located primarily in blood vessels, lymphatics and connective tissues; especially abundant in skin and mucosal tissues.	Essentially the same as those produced by basophils.
Platelets	Circulating non-replicating cells derived from megakaryocytes; may undergo activation during immune reactions; activated platelets become sticky and aggregate, trapping leukocytes in areas of inflammation and CMI reactions; secrete clotting and growth factors, vasoactive amines and lipids, neutral and acid hydrolases which contribute to inflammatory responses.	Platelet derived growth factor, serotonin, catecholamines, fibrinogen, cathepsin, alkaline phosphatase, β-glucuronidase.
Plasma cells	Cells of B lymphoid lineage which reside primarily in lymphoid tissues and at mucosal surfaces; their presence in reproductive tissues may be hormonally controlled; are directed by specific antigens and lymphokines to produce a variety of immunoglobulins, many of which bind to immunoglobulin Fc receptors on macrophages, NK cells and neutrophils, and allow them to participate in ADCC CMI responses.	Immunoglobulins (IgG, IgA, IgE, IgM).
Natural killer cell	Human cells with NK activity may possess a combination of B-cell, macrophage (CD11) and T-cell markers (CD2, CD3, CD7, CD8, CD25 and OKT10), although the major human NK effector cell is a non-T/non-B CD3$^-$, CD16$^+$, Leu 19$^+$ lymphoid cell. NK activity defines a function rather than a cell type.	A variety of cytokines with immunoregulatory properties and cytocidal capabilities.

Table 2. Properties and activities of principal lymphokines and monokines. From Anderson and Hill (1988).

Abbreviation	Name	Producing the factor	Principal activities
IL-1	Interleukin 1	Activated macrophages	Activates resting T cells; induces IL-2 secretion by T cells; stimulates B cell proliferation and secretion of antibody; fibroblast and endothelial cell growth factor activity; stimulates bone resorption; endogenous pyrogen.
IL-2	Interleukin 2 T cell growth factor	Activated T lymphocytes (T_H1)	Autocrine T cell growth factor; induces synthesis of other lymphokines; activates macrophages, B cells, natural killer and other cytotoxic cells.
IL-3	Interleukin 3 Mast cell growth factor	Activated T lymphocytes (T_H1 and T_H2)	Supports the growth of pluripotent bone marrow stem cells; growth factor for mast cells.
IL-4	Interleukin 4 B cell growth factor B cell stimulating factor 1	Activated T lymphocytes (T_H2)	Growth factor for B cells; synergizes with IL-3 in promoting mast cell growth; enhances IgE and IgG production; stimulates expression of HLA-DR (Ia) on B cells and macrophages; enhances cytolytic activity of cytotoxic T cells; stimulates resting T cells.
IL-5	Interleukin 5 T-cell replacing factor B-cell growth factor 2 IgA enhancing factor Eosinophil differentiation factor	Activated T lymphocytes (T_H2)	Co-stimulates B-cell proliferation; isotype specific stimulation of IgA synthesis; induces eosinophil differentiation.

α-IFN	Alpha-interferon	Activated leukocytes	
γ-IFN	Gamma-interferon	Activated T lymphocytes (T_H1, T_C)	Inhibits viral replication; induces MHC class I (HLA-A, -B, -C) and class II (HLA-DR) antigen expression on a variety of cell types; stimulates NK, basophil and mast cell activity; cytolytic factor for virally infected neoplastic and reproductive cells in vitro.
TNF	Tumour necrosis factor	Activated macrophages	Direct cytolysis of tumour cells in vitro and in vivo; toxic to spermatozoa, embryonic and trophoblastic cell lines; stimulates granulocyte ADCC functions; induction of class II MHC antigens on a variety of cell types; stimulates osteoclasts to resorb bone tissue.
LT	Lymphotoxin Tumour necrosis factor	Activated T lymphocytes (T_H1, T_C)	Same as TNF
CSF	Colony stimulating factors		
GM-CSF	Granulocytes, Macrophage	Activated T lymphocytes (T_H1 and T_H2)	Stimulates granulocytic and monocytic bone marrow colonies; activates mature granulocytes; affects some reproductive processes in vitro.
M-CSF	Macrophage	Activated macrophages	Stimulates monocytic bone marrow colonies.

involved in antigen presentation by the uterine epithelium to T cells. Auto-immunity to endometrial antigens or adjacent tissues may be invoked subsequent to HLA-DR expression leading to reproductive failure by dysynchronous decidualization and disruption of implantation events.

Immunofluorescence and radioimmunoassay techniques used to detect and quantitate class I and class II MHC antigen expression in human ovarian granulosa cell cultures have revealed that class II MHC expression is induced and class I MHC expression is enhanced in granulosa cells by γ-IFN (Hill and Anderson, 1988d). These results provide evidence that class I and class II MHC antigen enhancement and induction in human granulosa cells by γ-IFN may be mechanisms contributing to autoimmune ovarian failure due to presentation of ovarian antigens to helper and cytotoxic T cells. These mechanisms could also be involved in anovulatory and ovum maturational disturbances which can be a cause of reproductive failure.

Soluble products of cell-mediated immunity have recently been shown to impair human sperm function. Supernatants from activated leukocyte cultures and highly purified recombinant preparations of the lymphokine, γ-IFN and the monokine, TNF, decreased both human sperm motility (Hill et al, 1987b) and fertilization ability as measured by the hamster egg penetration test (Hill et al, 1988c).

A variety of lymphokines and monokines have been studied for effects on early embryonic development. Gamma-IFN has been reported to adversely affect development of early mouse embryos (Hill et al, 1987c) and fetal cells at later stages of gestation (Drasner et al, 1979). GM-CSF may also adversely affect early embryo development (Hill et al, 1987c). The effects of the monokine, IL-1, on embryo development are controversial (Fakih et al, 1987; Schneider et al, 1987); in our studies, adverse effects were observed only at high concentrations (Hill et al, 1987c). Effects seen only at high concentrations, however, can not be summarily dismissed as the local levels achieved at the site of in vivo development are not known. Cell–cell contact may ensure that high levels are delivered to potential target cells, although adverse effects observed over a wide concentration range in vitro may be more indicative of adverse effects in vivo.

Lymphocyte and macrophage products may also affect the immunogenicity and viability of trophoblast cells. A number of laboratories have reported enhancement or induction of class I MHC antigens on cells of trophoblastic lineage in the presence of γ-IFN (recently reviewed by Head et al, 1987). Induction of MHC antigens on trophoblast by lymphokines could be a significant mechanism in cell-mediated immunity (CMI) culminating in spontaneous abortion since paternal MHC antigens could serve as targets of maternal cytotoxic T cells as well as humoral immunological responses. Studies from our laboratory have recently provided evidence that γ-interferon and GM-CSF also inhibit the proliferation of human choriocarcinoma cells in vitro (Berkowitz et al, 1988). Such lymphokines may be produced at the fetal–maternal interface in some women in response to gestational or microbial antigens and could be a cause of reproductive failure.

EVIDENCE OF IMMUNOLOGICAL MECHANISMS IN FEMALE REPRODUCTIVE FAILURE

Female infertility can be classified according to abnormalities occurring within various anatomical compartments of the reproductive tract. Thus, infertility can be discussed in terms of vaginal/cervical factor, endometrial/ tubal factor, ovarian and peritoneal factor. Immunological responses culminating in reproductive failure may either be restricted to discrete anatomical regions or be more generalized, as is possibly the case in endometriosis or systemic humoral immunity to sperm or gestational antigens.

Vaginal/cervical factor

Over the course of her reproductive life (approximately 30 years) the average women, assuming coitus three times weekly and an average sperm count of 100×10^6 sperm/ejaculate, is exposed to over 500 billion (5×10^{11}) spermatozoa. Despite repeated antigenic exposure, intravaginal insemination does not usually lead to sperm immunity resulting in infertility. Amount of sperm exposure may be a factor, as prostitutes are reported to have an increased frequency of sperm immunity compared with controls (Schwimmer et al, 1967). Lesions in the female reproductive tract may also be a cofactor in the development of anti-sperm antibodies (Boettcher, 1974). A higher incidence of sperm immunity has also been reported in women with cervical cancer compared with women with other reproductive cancers (Jones et al, 1973). The immunosuppressive properties of seminal plasma (reviewed in Alexander and Anderson, 1987) and vaginal secretions (Hill and Anderson, 1988b) may account for the lack of anti-sperm immune reactivity in normal women. There is also evidence to suggest that women whose sexual partners have anti-sperm antibodies are more likely to be anti-sperm antibody-positive than women whose partners do not have immunity to sperm (Mathur et al, 1981a). Although rare, IgE-mediated allergic reactions to seminal components have been demonstrated and increases in the total level of circulating IgE has been associated with infertility (Mathur et al, 1981b).

Anti-sperm immunity may be either humorally or cellularly mediated. Fertility prognosis for women with systemic immunity to sperm is less than in women without evidence of systemic anti-sperm immunity (Menge, 1980). Humoral immunity to sperm antigens can be determined by detecting circulating anti-sperm antibodies, which occur in approximately 13% of infertile women (Moghissi et al, 1980). Cervical mucus or cervico-vaginal secretions in infertile women may contain IgA- or IgG-specific antibodies directed against seminal components (Menge, 1980). Anti-sperm antibodies are detected in the cervical mucus of approximately 8% of infertile women (Moghissi et al, 1980). Anti-sperm antibodies attached to the sperm surface may cause infertility by (i) promoting the phagocytosis of sperm along the reproductive tract, (ii) limiting their ability to traverse the reproductive tract, or (iii) causing sperm membrane damage and cytolysis by activating complement either through classical or alternate complement pathways

(Adams, 1983; Haas and Beer, 1986). Anti-sperm antibodies have also been noted in human ovarian follicular fluid (Clarke et al, 1984; Anderson et al, 1985) and may cause infertility if transported with the ovum into the fallopian tube after ovulation. Sperm autoantibodies of several immuno-globulin classes have been shown to interfere with human fertilization in vitro (Clarke et al, 1985a). Women with humoral immunity to spermatozoa are more likely to fail in vitro fertilization if their embryos are cultured in the presence of their anti-sperm antibody-rich serum (Clarke et al, 1985b).

Cell-mediated immunity to sperm, as detected by the in vitro macrophage migration inhibition or lymphocyte transformation tests, has been documented in a significant number of infertile women with and without anti-sperm antibodies (Marcus et al, 1973; Mettler and Schirwami, 1975; McShane et al, 1985). Cellular immunity to seminal antigens has been more difficult to measure than humoral immunity. Due to recent advances in immunology, however, sensitive and specific RIA and ELISA methods to measure cellular immune mediators may be forthcoming.

Endometrial/tubal factor

The histological diagnosis of acute and chronic endometritis and salpingitis is based on the finding of either polymorphonuclear leukocytes (acute) or plasma cells and lymphocytes (chronic) in endometrial or fallopian tube sections (Wheeler, 1982; Blaustein, 1985). Both endometritis and salpingitis have been associated with human infertility (Monif, 1982). Uterine leuko-cytosis and infection have also been associated with infertility in experi-mental animals (Ogra et al, 1981). Inflammation can promote adhesion formation and physical blockages which are obvious causes of infertility. Endometrial/tubal factor infertility without anatomical distortion is poorly understood. It is possible in such cases that reproductive processes are interrupted by leukocyte products as described above, resulting from leuko-cyte activation by microbial/viral antigens or reproductive antigens. Com-pared with fertile controls, many women with unexplained infertility have high levels of T-helper lymphocytes in their endometrial tissues (Lint, 1980). This may have important implications regarding potential mechanisms of immunological infertility since activated T-helper lymphocytes produce several lymphokines, including γ-IFN, which may directly affect repro-ductive processes and also potentiate other immune responses in the local tissue area. Uterine inflammation in intrauterine device (IUD) users is believed to underlie the contraceptive effectiveness of the device (Parr et al, 1967). Women who use this method for contraception also have a statistic-ally higher incidence of asymptomatic (Hill et al, 1986) and clinically overt pelvic infections (Burkman, 1981), which may predispose them to infertility even after the device is discontinued.

Ovarian factor

Ovarian granulosa cells in women experiencing autoimmune ovarian failure may express high levels of class II MHC (HLA-DR) antigens (Hill and

Anderson, 1988d). Because this class of molecules is involved in antigen presentation, and because aberrant expression of HLA-DR in tissues such as the thyroid and pancreas is associated with autoimmune disorders, γ-IFN induced expression of HLA-DR in the ovary may be a mechanism for reproductive failure. Whether subtle alterations in ratios of T-lymphocyte subpopulations within ovarian follicles could be responsible for ovulation disorders is not known, although an imbalance of T-lymphocyte subpopulations in experimental animals is associated with autoimmune destruction of ovarian follicles (Taguchi and Nishizuka, 1985). Similarly, it is not known what effect anti-ovarian antibodies have on reproductive function, although they have been associated with ovarian autoimmunity (Vallotton and Forbes, 1966).

Antibodies reactive with zona pellucida have been reported to occur in 15% of women with otherwise unexplained infertility and in 25% of women with recurrent spontaneous abortion (Urry et al, 1985). Anti-zona pellucida antibodies have been detected in human ovarian follicular fluid and can apparently coat the ovum in situ. Titres of such anti-zona pellucida antibodies greater than 1:4 were also demonstrated to inhibit human in vitro fertilization. In these studies, the presence of antibodies to the zona pellucida did not correlate with the production of other autoimmune antibodies (Urry et al, 1985). This area is still controversial. The zona pellucida is a matrix which non-specifically traps proteins including immunoglobulins (Mori et al, 1985). Other investigators, using isolated zona pellucida antigens and strict experimental conditions, have failed to detect anti-zona pellucida antibodies in a large panel of sera from women with ovarian disorders, and question the concept of anti-zona pellucida antibodies in infertility (Mori et al, 1985).

Peritoneal factor

Peritoneal factor infertility is usually attributed to either pelvic inflammatory disease (PID), or to endometriosis, which is the occurrence of endometrium in ectopic locations, usually on peritoneal surfaces.

Peritoneal fluid of women with PID contains increased concentrations of macrophages, T-helper lymphocytes and natural killer cells compared with peritoneal fluid from fertile women (Hill, unpublished data). This may have important clinical implications regarding potential mechanisms for reproductive failure in these women since macrophages may themselves mediate reproductive failure by phagocytosing sperm or secreting cytotoxic oxygen free-radicals, hydrogen peroxide, monokines and enzymes which could adversely affect reproductive cells (Anderson and Hill, 1988). Also, activated T-helper lymphocytes secrete γ-interferon, which has been shown to interfere with many reproductive processes as discussed earlier. Natural killer cells are cytotoxic effector cells which could also interfere with normal reproduction. Both peritoneal fluid and supernatants of peritoneal fluid leukocytes from women with PID interfere with blastocyst development and trophoblast proliferation in vitro, further suggesting that soluble factors released by peritoneal leukocytes are responsible for reproductive failure in these women (Hill et al, unpublished data). The gametes or developing conceptus could be killed inadvertently by the immune effectors and/or their products which have been mobilized against offending pathogens in women with PID.

IMMUNOLOGICAL MECHANISMS OF REPRODUCTIVE FAILURE IN ENDOMETRIOSIS

Endometriosis is one of the most enigmatic and challenging problems affecting the reproductive health of women. The pathogenesis of endometriosis is poorly understood, although retrograde menstruation with subsequent implantation of ectopic endometrium over visceral and parietal surfaces has long been proposed (Sampson, 1927). In one study, retrograde menstruation was observed in 76% of infertile women having laparoscopy at the time of menses, yet only 54% of these women had visible evidence of endometriosis (Liu and Hitchcock, 1986). Alterations in immunity have been proposed to explain why some women develop the disease while others do not (Weed and Arquembourg, 1980; Damouski et al, 1981; Badaway et al, 1984a; Bartosik, 1985). It has been hypothesized that endometrial cells translocated from their normal location implant only in women with specific alterations in cell-mediated immunity (Damouski et al, 1981). Peripheral blood leukocyte profiles in women with endometriosis have been investigated with conflicting results. One study indicated deficient peripheral blood lymphocyte reactivity in both women and animals with endometriosis (Damouski et al, 1981). Another study determined an increased T-helper to T-suppressor lymphocyte ratio in the peripheral blood of women with endometriosis (Badaway et al, 1987). A third study, however, found no significant difference in peripheral blood leukocyte subpopulation profiles in women with endometriosis, unexplained infertility and fertile controls (Gleicher et al, 1984). Recent data from our laboratory have concurred with the third study, providing further evidence that systemic white blood cell profiles are not markedly affected in endometriosis patients (Hill et al, 1988b).

Data are also controversial concerning significantly altered peritoneal fluid volumes, as well as hormonal and prostaglandin levels, in endometriosis (Maathius et al, 1978; Drake et al, 1980; Donnez et al, 1982; Sgarlata et al, 1983; Dawood et al, 1984; Drake et al, 1984; Ylikorkala et al, 1984; Berger and Rock, 1985; DeLeon et al, 1986). There is, however, compelling evidence for increased cellularity in the peritoneal fluid of women with endometriosis (Halme et al, 1957; Halme et al, 1983; Haney et al, 1983a,b; Badaway et al, 1984b; Badaway et al, 1987; Hill et al, 1988b). Previous reports have stated, based on morphologic assessment, that 80–90% of peritoneal fluid leukocytes are macrophages (Halme et al, 1957; Haney et al, 1983; Badaway et al, 1984b). Using monoclonal antibodies to leukocyte phenotypic markers, we reported that macrophages predominate in peritoneal fluid, but that a significant number of T lymphocytes are also recovered. The ratio of macrophages to lymphocytes was between 1 : 1 and 3 : 1 for peritoneal fluid samples of women with endometriosis, unexplained infertility and fertile controls (Hill et al, 1988b). Our results also demonstrated an increased T-helper to

T-suppressor lymphocyte ratio in peritoneal fluid from women with endometriosis. This finding, which was also observed in a previous study using an immune rosette technique (Badaway et al, 1987a), suggests immunological activity in the peritoneal environment of women with endometriosis.

T-helper lymphocytes can promote humoral immune responses, and anti-endometrial and anti-ovarian antibodies have been reported in women with endometriosis (Mathur et al, 1982; Wild and Shivers, 1985). It is unknown whether these autoantibodies contribute to reproductive failure. In our study, B lymphocytes and plasma cells were extremely scarce in peritoneal fluid (Hill et al, 1988b), suggesting that peritoneal T-helper lymphocytes probably do not promote a significant local humoral immune response. Another report (Badaway et al, 1984a), which indicated that peritoneal fluid concentrations of IgG and IgA were not significantly different between samples from women with and without endometriosis, provides further evidence that local humoral immunity is not markedly elevated in women with endometriosis. As discussed above, T-helper lymphocytes also produce a number of biologically active soluble mediators such as interleukin-2 (IL-2) and γ-IFN, which promote cell-mediated immunological responses and may adversely affect reproductive processes. Natural killer cells are also found in abundance in peritoneal fluid of women with endometriosis (Hill et al, 1988b). These cells can be activated by IL-2 (Reynolds and Ortaldo, 1987). Evidence of elevated numbers of helper T lymphocytes and natural killer cells in peritoneal fluid from women with endometriosis may indicate that cellular immune responses are a component of this disease. We have noted similar peritoneal fluid leukocyte profiles in women with unexplained infertility and those with endometriosis (Hill et al, 1988b). Electron microscopic studies which have detected microscopic endometrial implants in the peritoneum of women with unexplained infertility indicate that endometriosis may not be a discrete disease entity, but represents a spectrum of morphologically different lesions accounting for the widely differing clinical presentations seen in this disease (Schweppe et al, 1984). Endometriosis-like peritoneal leukocyte profiles in a significant number of women with unexplained infertility could indicate a local response to microscopic endometrial implants, as have been detected in electron microscopic studies on visually normal peritoneum (Brosens et al, 1984; Murphy et al, 1986). Alternatively, peritoneal fluid leukocytosis could also reflect an inflammatory or immunological response incited by factors other than endometriosis (Schumacher, 1980).

Human endometrial explants reportedly produce soluble non-specific immunosuppressive factors (Wang et al, 1987). However, we have recently found that in contrast to expected immunosuppressive effects, peritoneal fluids from endometriosis patients enhance cell-mediated immunological responses (Hill and Anderson, 1988c). Peritoneal fluid samples from women with unexplained infertility and fertile controls also significantly enhanced lymphocyte proliferation in both mitogen-stimulated and unstimulated cultures as compared with serum controls. Lymphocyte proliferation was further enhanced without mitogen in the presence of peritoneal fluid from women with unexplained infertility. Increased levels of interleukin-2 (IL-2) were found in the peritoneal fluid of women with unexplained infertility and may account for the lymphocyte proliferation enhancement. Lymphocyte proliferation was most significantly increased in the presence of mitogen and peritoneal fluid from women with stage III endometriosis (Hill and Anderson, 1988c).

Peritoneal fluid factors thought to be produced either by or in response to endometriosis have also been reported to interfere with in vitro reproductive processes (Halme and Hall, 1982; Burke, 1986; Chacho et al, 1986; Hahn et al, 1986). Peritoneal washings from women with endometriosis have been shown to have detrimental effects on human sperm velocity in vitro (Burke, 1986). Supernatants from activated peritoneal macrophages from women with endometriosis have been shown to interfere with sperm–oocyte interaction as assessed in the zona-free hamster egg sperm penetration assay (Chacho et al, 1986). In another study using peritoneal fluid from women with endometriosis, a heat-labile factor was found to be responsible for interfering with human sperm penetration of hamster oocytes (Halme and Hall, 1982). Peritoneal fluid from women with endometriosis has also been reported to interfere with implantation in experimental animals (Hahn et al, 1986). Experimental evidence suggests that the lymphokine, γ-IFN, and the monokine, TNF, may be factors in peritoneal fluid of women with endometriosis responsible for the adverse effects seen in vitro (Hill et al, 1987b; 1987c). This is further supported by the fact that the activity of γ-IFN is heat-labile (Trinchieri and Persussia, 1985) and the detrimental effects seen with this lymphokine on fertilization are abrogated by heat-inactivation and neutralizing antibody (Hill et al, 1987c).

Further evidence that endometriosis-associated reproductive failure may have a leukocyte-product aetiology comes from studies on the effects of peritoneal fluid leukocyte supernatants from women with endometriosis on embryo development and trophoblast proliferation in vitro (Hill et al, 1989). The percentage of two-cell mouse embryos grown in the presence of peritoneal fluid leukocyte supernatants developing to the blastocyst stage was significantly less in samples from women with endometriosis compared with fertile controls. Similarly, trophoblast proliferation, as assessed with a tritiated thymidine incorporation assay, is significantly inhibited in the presence of peritoneal fluid leukocyte supernatants from women with endometriosis compared with fertile controls (Hill et al, 1989). This is interesting in light of the clinical association of endometriosis with spontaneous abortion (Haydon, 1942; Naples et al, 1981; Wheeler et al, 1983).

Peritoneal fluid is immunologically dynamic containing many diverse cells and cell products. In the presence of antigenic stimulation (i.e. endometriosis) the proliferation of recruited lymphocytes and macrophages may be enhanced. These cells upon activation may then release bioactive products that could locally affect the occurrence and progression of disease or reproductive potential, thus providing a mechanism for endometriosis-associated infertility. The finding that danazol, the isoxazol derivative of the synthetic steroid 17α-ethinyl testosterone used in the medical management of endometriosis, is immunosuppressive in vitro provides an additional mechanism how this treatment could be efficacious in ameliorating adverse reproductive sequelae attributable to endometriosis through direct suppressive effects on peritoneal leukocyte populations (Hill et al, 1987d).

SUMMARY

Achievement of successful reproduction is an immunological paradox because spermatozoa and the conceptus express allogeneic and differentiation antigens that are foreign to the female host. Interactions between the immune system and female reproductive tissues are complex, and recent evidence indicates that immunological reproductive failure may result not only from antibody-mediated responses but, perhaps more importantly, from cell-mediated immune responses. The ubiquity of immune cells in female reproductive tissues, coupled with the fact that a number of auto- and allo-antigens associated with microbial and reproductive tissues can potentially stimulate immune responses in these tissues, suggest that soluble cell products produced by immune activation may play a role in mechanisms of female infertility. Spermatozoa and/or the conceptus may be killed as a result of leukocyte activation triggered by microbial, viral or endometrial antigens, or specifically as a result of immune responses directed against seminal, embryonic or trophoblast antigens in women with immunologic infertility.

Acknowledgements

The authors would like to acknowledge the other members of the Fearing Laboratory Drs R. Berkowitz, F. Haimovici, H. Wolff, C. Xu and W. Zhang, and Ms H. Faris and A. Martinez for their research contributions and Ms D. Meehan for her assistance in the preparation of the manuscript. Supported by grants CA42738, HD00815, and HD23547, from the United States Public Health Service, Bethesda, MD, the 1987–88 American Fertility Society—Ortho Distinguished Fellowship Award, and by the Fearing Laboratory Endowment.

REFERENCES

Adams DD (1983) Autoimmune mechanisms. In Davies TF (ed.) *Autoimmune Endocrine Diseases*, p 124. New York: John Wiley and Sons.

Alexander NJ & Anderson DJ (1987) Immunology of semen. *Fertility and Sterility* **47**: 192–205.

Anderson DJ & Hill JA (1988) Cell-mediated immunity in infertility. *American Journal of Reproductive Immunology and Microbiology* **17**: 22–30.

Anderson DJ & Madrigal JA (1985) Variability in antisperm and antiembryonic humoral immune responses. In Runnebaum B, Rabe T & Kiesel L (eds) *Future Aspects in Contraception*, p 305. Boston: MTP Press.

Anderson DJ, Boyer S, DeCherny A & Haeltine F (1985) Antisperm antibodies in sera and follicular fluid of in vitro fertilization patients with poor prognosis. *Fertility and Sterility* (Supplement, abstract).

Anderson DJ, Johnson PM, Alexander NJ, Jones WR & Griffin PD (1987) Monoclonal antibodies to human trophoblast and sperm antigens: Report of two WHO-sponsored workshops. *Journal of Reproductive Immunology* **10**: 231–257.

Ansbacher R, Boyson WA, Morris JA (1967) Sterility of the uterine cavity. *American Journal of Obstetrics and Gynecology* **99**: 394–396.

Badaway SZA, Cuenca V, Stitzel A, Jacobs RB & Tomar RH (1984a) Autoimmune phenomena in infertile patients with endometriosis. *Obstetrics and Gynecology* **63**: 271–275.

Badaway SZA, Cuenca V, Marshall L, Muncchback R, Rinos AC & Coble DA (1984b) Cellular components in peritoneal fluid in infertile patients with and without endometriosis. *Fertility and Sterility* **42**: 704–708.

Badaway SZA, Cuenca V, Stitzel A & Tice D (1987) Immune rosettes of T and B lymphocytes in infertile women with endometriosis. *Journal of Reproductive Medicine* **32**: 194–197.

Bartosik DK (1985) Immunological aspects of endometriosis. *Seminars in Reproductive Endocrinology* **3**: 329–337.

Beer AE & Neaves WB (1978) Antigenic status of semen from the viewpoints of the female and male. *Fertility and Sterility* **29**: 322.

Berger NG & Rock JA (1985) Peritoneal fluid environment in endometriosis. *Seminars in Reproductive Endocrinology* **3**: 313–318.

Berkowitz RS, Hill JA, Kurtz CB & Anderson DJ (1988) Effects of products of activated leukocytes (lymphokines and monokines) on the growth of malignant trophoblast cells in vitro. *American Journal of Obstetrics and Gynecology* **158**: 199–203.

Blaustein A (1985) Interpretation of endometrial biopsies, 2nd edn, p 88. New York: Raven Press.

Boettcher B (1974) The molecular nature of spermagglutinins and sperm antibodies in human sera. *Journal of Reproduction and Fertility* **21** (supplement): 151–167.

Bottazzo GF, Pujol-Borrell R, Hanafusa T & Feldman M (1983) Role of aberrant HLA-Dr expression and antigen presentation in induction of endocrine autoimmunity. *Lancet* **ii**: 1115–1119.

Bronson RA, Cooper GW & Rosenfeld DL (1982a) Correlation between regional specificity of antisperm antibodies to the spermatozoa surface and complement-mediated sperm immunobilization. *American Journal of Reproductive Immunology* **2**: 222–224.

Bronson RA, Cooper GW & Rosenfeld DL (1982b) Sperm-specific isoantibodies and autoantibodies inhibit the binding of human sperm to the human zona pellucida. *Fertility and Sterility* **38**: 724–729.

Brosens I, Vasquez G & Gordts S (1984) Scanning electron microscopy study of pelvic peritoneum and unexplained infertility in endometriosis. *Fertility and Sterility* **41**: 21–25.

Bukovsky A, Presl J & Holub M (1981) The role of the immune system in ovarian function control. *Allergo et Immunopathologie* **9**: 447–456.

Bulmer JN & Johnson PM (1985) Immunological characterization of the decidual leukocytic infiltrate related to endometrial gland epithelium in early human pregnancy. *Immunology* **55**: 35–44.

Bulmer JN & Johnson PM (1986) The T lymphocyte population in first trimester human decidua does not express the interleukin-2 receptor. *Immunology* **58**: 685–687.

Bulmer JN & Sunderland CA (1984) Immunohistological characterization of lymphoid cell populations in the early human placental bed. *Immunology* **52**: 349–357.

Burke RR (1986) Effect of peritoneal washings from women with endometriosis on sperm velocity. *34th Annual Clinical Meeting of the American College of Obstetricians and Gynecologists* May 1986, New Orleans (abstract).

Burkman RT (1981) Association between intrauterine device and pelvic inflammatory disease. *Obstetrics and Gynecology* **57**: 269–272.

Chacho KJ, Chacho MS, Andresen PF & Scommegna A (1986) Peritoneal fluid in patients with and without endometriosis: Prostanoids and macrophages and their effect on the spermatozoa penetration assay. *American Journal of Obstetrics and Gynecology* **154**: 1290–1299.

Clark DA & McDermott M (1981) Active suppression of host vs. graft reaction in pregnant mice. III. Developmental kinetics, properties and mechanisms of induction of suppressor cells during first pregnancy. *Journal of Immunology* **127**: 1267–1271.

Clark DA, Mowbray J, Underwood L & Lidell H (1987) Histopathologic alterations in the decidua in human spontaneous abortion: loss of cells with large cytoplasmic granules. *American Journal of Reproductive Immunology and Microbiology* **13**: 19–22.

Clarke GN, Hsieh C, Koh SH & Cauchi MN (1984) Sperm antibodies, immunoglobulins, and complement in human follicular fluid. *American Journal of Reproductive Immunology* **5**: 179–181.

Clarke GN, Lopata A, McBain JC, Baker HWG & Johnston WIH (1985a) Effect of sperm antibodies in males on human in vitro fertilization. *American Journal of Reproductive Immunology and Microbiology* **8:** 62–66.

Clarke GN, McBain JC, Lopata A & Johnston WIH (1985b) In vitro fertilization results for women with sperm antibodies in plasma and follicular fluid. *American Journal of Reproductive Immunology and Microbiology* **8:** 130–131.

Damowski WP, Steele RW & Baker GF (1981) Deficient cellular immunity in endometriosis. *American Journal of Obstetrics and Gynecology* **141:** 377–383.

Dawood MY, Khan-Dawood FS & Wilson L (1984) Peritoneal fluid prostaglandins and prostanoids in women with endometriosis, chronic pelvic inflammatory disease, and pelvic pain. *American Journal of Obstetrics and Gynecology* **148:** 391–395.

Daya S & Clark DA (1986) Production of immunosuppressive factors by preimplantation embryos. *American Journal of Reproductive Immunology and Microbiology* **11:** 98–101.

Daya S, Clark DA, Derlin C, Jarrett J & Chaput A (1985) Suppressor cells in human decidua. *American Journal of Obstetrics and Gynecology* **151:** 267–270.

DeLeon FD, Vijayakumar R, Brown M, Rao CHV, Yussman MA & Schultz G (1986) Peritoneal fluid volume, estrogen, progesterone, prostaglandin, and epidermal growth factor concentrations in patients with and without endometriosis. *Obstetrics and Gynecology* **68:** 189–194.

Donnez J & Langerock S (1982) Peritoneal fluid volume and 17β estradiol and progesterone concentration in ovulatory, anovulatory and postmenopausal women. *Obstetrics and Gynecology* **59:** 687–692.

Drake TS, Metz SA, Grunert GM & O'Brien WF (1980) Peritoneal fluid volume in endometriosis. *Fertility and Sterility* **34:** 280–281.

Drasner K, Epstein CJ & Epstein LB (1979) The antiproliferative effects of interferon on murine embryonic cells. *Proceedings of the Society of Experimental Biology and Medicine* **160:** 46–49.

Fakih H, Baggett B, Holtz G, Tsange KY, Lee JC & Williamson HO (1987) Interleukin-1: a possible role in the infertility associated with endometriosis. *Fertility and Sterility* **47:** 213–217.

Gaunt SJ (1983) Spreading of a sperm surface antigen within the plasma membrane of the egg fertilized in the rat. *Journal of Embryology and Experimental Morphology* **75:** 259–270.

Gleicher N, Damowski WP, Siegel I et al (1984) Lymphocyte subsets in endometriosis. *Obstetrics and Gynecology* **63:** 463–466.

Golander G, Zakuth V, Shechter A & Spirer Z (1981) Suppression of lymphocyte activity in vitro by a soluble factor secreted by explants of human decidua. *European Journal of Immunology* **1:** 849–851.

Haas GG Jr & Beer AE (1986) Immunologic influences on reproductive biology. Sperm gametogenesis and maturation in the male and female genital tracts. *Fertility and Sterility* **46:** 753–766.

Hahn DW, Carraher RP, Foldesy RG & McGuire JL (1986) Experimental evidence for failure to implant as a mechanism of infertility associated with endometriosis. *American Journal of Obstetrics and Gynecology* **155:** 1109–1113.

Halme J & Hall JL (1982) Effect of pelvic fluid from endometriosis patients on human sperm penetration of zona-free hamster ova. *Fertility and Sterility* **37:** 573–576.

Halme J, Becker S & Haskill S (1987) Altered maturation and function of peritoneal macrophages: Possible role in pathogenesis of endometriosis. *American Journal of Obstetrics and Gynecology* **156:** 783–789.

Halme J, Becker S, Hammond MG, Raj MHG & Raj S (1983) Increased activation of pelvic macrophages in infertile women with mild endometriosis. *American Journal of Obstetrics and Gynecology* **145:** 333–337.

Halme J, Hammond MG, Syrop CH & Talbert LM (1985) Peritoneal macrophages modulate human granulosa–luteal cell progesterone production. *Journal of Clinical and Endocrinological Metabolism* **61:** 912–916.

Hamilton MS, Beer AE, May RD & Vitetta ES (1979) The influence of immunization of female mice with F9 teratocarcinoma cells on their reproductive performance. *Transplantation Proceedings* **11:** 1069–1072.

Haney AF, Misukonis MA & Weinberg JB (1983a) Macrophages and infertility: oviductal macrophages as potential mediators of infertility. *Fertility and Sterility* **39:** 310–315.

Haney AF, Muscato JJ & Weinberg JB (1983b) Peritoneal fluid cell populations in infertility patients. *Fertility and Sterility* **39:** 310–315.

Haney AF, Hanewerger S & Weinberg JB (1984) Peritoneal fluid prolactin in infertile women with endometriosis: Lack of evidence of secretory activity by endometrial implants. *Fertility and Sterility* **42**: 935–938.

Haydon GB (1942) A study of 569 cases of endometriosis. *American Journal of Obstetrics and Gynecology* **43**: 704–709.

Head JR & Billingham RE (1986) Concerning the immunology of the uterus. *American Journal of Reproductive Immunology and Microbiology* **10**: 76–81.

Head JR, Drake BL & Zuckerman FA (1987) Major histocompatibility antigens on trophoblast and their regulation: implications in the maternal–fetal relationship. *American Journal of Reproductive Immunology* **15**: 12–18.

Healy DL & Hodgen GD (1983) The endocrinology of human endometrium. *Obstetrical and Gynecological Survey* **38**: 509–530.

Herberman RB, Hiserodt J, Vujanovic N et al (1987) Lymphokine-activated killer cell activity. *Immunology Today* **8**: 178–181.

Hill JA & Anderson DJ (1988a) The embryo as an immunologic target in recurrent abortion. In Mathur S & Fredericks CM (eds) *Perspectives in Immunoreproduction: Conception, Contraception*, pp 261–277. New York: Hemisphere Publishing Corporation.

Hill JA & Anderson DJ (1988b) Quantification of human vaginal leukocytes and effects of vaginal secretions on mechanisms of HIV transmission. 4th International Conference on AIDS, Stockholm, Sweden, June 13–16, Abstract 2551.

Hill JA & Anderson DJ (1988c) Lymphocyte reactivity in the presence of peritoneal fluid from women with endometriosis. *American Journal of Obstetrics and Gynecology* (in press).

Hill JA & Anderson DJ (1988d) Induction of Class II MHC antigen expression in human granulosa cells by gamma-interferon. 35th Annual Meeting of the Society for Gynecologic Investigation, Baltimore, Maryland, March 17–20, Abstract 78.

Hill JA, Talledo OE & Steele J (1986) Quantitative transcervical uterine cultures in asymptomatic women using an intrauterine contraceptive device. *Obstetrics and Gynecology* **68**: 700–704.

Hill JA, Barbieri RL & Anderson DJ (1987a) Detection of T8 (suppressor/cytotoxic) lymphocytes in human ovarian follicular fluid. *Fertility and Sterility* **47**: 114–117.

Hill JA, Haimovici F, Politch JA, Anderson DJ (1987b) Effects of soluble products of activated lymphocytes and macrophages (lymphokines and monokines) on human sperm motion parameters. *Fertility and Sterility* **47**: 460–465.

Hill JA, Haimovici F & Anderson DJ (1987c) Products of activated lymphocytes and macrophages inhibit mouse embryo development in vitro. *Journal of Immunology* **139**: 2250–2254.

Hill JA, Barbieri RL & Anderson DJ (1987d) Immunosuppressive effects of danazol in vitro. *Fertility and Sterility* **48**: 414–418.

Hill JA, Kern LL & Anderson DJ (1988a) Il-2 receptor positive cells in the decidua of woman with recurrent spontaneous and elective abortions. 35th Annual Meeting of the Society of Gynecologic Investigation, Baltimore, Maryland, March 17–20, Abstract 81.

Hill JA, Faris HMP, Schiff I & Anderson DJ (1988b) Characterization of leukocyte subpopulations in the peritoneal fluid of women with endometriosis. *Fertility and Sterility* **50**: 216–222.

Hill JA, Cohen J & Anderson DJ (1988c) The effects of lymphokines and monokines on human sperm fertilizing ability in the hamster egg penetration test. *American Journal of Obstetrics and Gynecology* (in press).

Hill JA, Haimovici F, Schiff I & Anderson DJ (1989) Peritoneal fluid and peritoneal fluid leukocyte supernatants from women with endometriosis inhibit mouse embryo development and human trophoblast proliferation in vitro: a possible mechanism for endometriosis-associated reproductive failure. 2nd International Symposium on Endometriosis, Houston, Texas, May 1–3.

Ingerslev HJ (1981) Antibodies against spermatozoal surface membrane antigens in female infertility. *Acta Obstetricia et Gynecologica Scandinavica* **100** (supplement). 1–52.

Jacob F (1977) Mouse teratocarcinoma and embryonic antigens. *Immunological Reviews* **33**: 3–32.

Johnson PM (1984) Immunobiology of human trophoblast. In Crighton DB (ed.) *Immunological Aspects of Reproduction in Animals*, pp 109–131. London: Butterworth Press.

Johnson PM, Cheng HM, Molloy CM, Stern CMM & Slade MB (1981) Human trophoblast-specific surface antigens identified using monoclonal antibodies. *American Journal of Reproductive Immunology* **1:** 246–254.

Jones WR, Kaye MD & Ing RMY (1973) Sperm microagglutinating activity in the serum of patients with carcinoma of the cervix. *American Journal of Obstetrics and Gynecology* **116:** 883–884.

Kabawat SE, Mostoufi-Zadeh M, Driscoll SG & Bhan AK (1985) Implantation site in normal pregnancy: A study with monoclonal antibodies. *American Journal of Pathology* **118:** 76–84.

Kamat BR & Isaacson PG (1987) The immunocytochemical distribution of leukocytic subpopulations in human endometrium. *American Journal of Pathology* **127:** 66–73.

Kearns M & Lala PK (1982) Bone marrow origin of decidual cell precursors in the pseudopregnant mouse uterus. *Journal of Experimental Medicine* **155:** 1537–1554.

Kennedy TG (1977) Evidence for a role for prostaglandins in the initiation of blastocyst implantation in the rat. *Biology of Reproduction* **16:** 286–291.

Kennedy TG (1985) Evidence for the involvement of prostaglandins throughout the decidual cell reaction in the rat. *Biology of Reproduction* **33:** 140–146.

Kutteh WH, Hatch KD, Blackwell RE & Mestecky J (1988) Secretory immune system of the female reproductive tract: I. Immunoglobulins and secretory component-containing cells. *Obstetrics and Gynecology* **71:** 56–60.

Lala PK, Parker RS, Kearns M, Johnson S & Scodras JM (1986) Immunologic aspects of the decidual response. In Clark DA & Cray BA (eds) *Reproductive Immunology 1986*, p 190. New York: Elsevier Science Publishers.

Larson B & Galask RP (1982) Vaginal microbial flora: Composition and influences of host physiology. *Annals of Internal Medicine* **96:** 926–930.

Lint TF (1980) Complement. In Dhindsa DS & Schumacher GFB (eds) *Immunological Aspects of Infertility and Fertility Regulation*, p 13. New York: Elsevier-North Holland.

Lippes J, Ogra S, Tomasi TB Jr & Tourville DR (1970) Immunohistological localization of G, A, M secretory piece and lactoferrin in the human female genital tract. *Contraception* **1:** 163–183.

Liu DTY & Hitchcock A (1986) Endometriosis: its association with retrograde menstruation, dysmenorrhea and tubal pathology. *British Journal of Obstetrics and Gynecology* **93:** 859–862.

London SN, Haney AF & Weinberg JB (1985) Macrophages and infertility enhancement of human macrophages mediated sperm killing by antisperm antibodies. *Fertility and Sterility* **43:** 274–278.

Maathius JB, Van Look PFA & Michie EA (1978) Changes in volume, total protein, ovarian steroid concentrations of peritoneal fluid throughout the menstrual cycle. *Journal of Endocrinology* **76:** 123–133.

McIntyre JA, Faulk WP, Verhulst SJ & Colliver J (1983) Human trophoblast–lymphocyte cross-reactive (TLX) antigens define an alloantigen system. *Science* **222:** 1135–1137.

McShane PM, Schiff I & Trentham D (1985) Cellular immunity to sperm in infertile women. *Journal of the American Medical Association* **253:** 3555–3559.

Marcus ZH, Soffer Y, Ben-David A, Peleg S & Nebel L (1973) Studies on sperm antigenicity. I. Delayed hypersensitivity to spermatozoa. *European Journal of Immunology* **3:** 75–78.

Mathur S, Baker WR, Williamson HO, Derrick F, Teaque KJ & Fudenberg HH (1981a) Clinical significance of sperm antibodies in infertility. *Fertility and Sterility* **136:** 486–495.

Mathur S, Williamson HO, Baker ER & Fudenberg HH (1981b) Immunoglobulin E levels and antisperm antibody titers in infertile couples. *American Journal of Obstetrics and Gynecology* **40:** 923–930.

Mathur S, Peress WR, Williamson HO et al (1982) Autoimmunity to endometrium and ovary in endometriosis. *Clinical and Experimental Immunology* **50:** 259–266.

Menge AC (1980) Clinical immunologic infertility. Diagnostic measures, incidence of antisperm antibodies, fertility and mechanisms. In Dhindsa DS & Schumacher GFB (eds) *Immunologic Aspects of Infertility and Fertility Regulation*, pp 205–224. New York: Elsevier Inc.

Menge AC & Fleming CH (1978) Detection of sperm antigen on mouse ova and early embryos. *Developmental Biology* **63:** 111–117.

Menge AC, Medley NE, Mangione CM & Dietrech JW (1982) The incidence and influence of antisperm antibodies in infertile human couples on sperm–cervical mucus interactions and subsequent fertility. *Fertility and Sterility* **38:** 439–446.

Mettler L & Schirwami D (1975) Macrophage migration inhibitory factor in female sterility. *American Journal of Obstetrics and Gynecology* **121:** 117–121.

Moghissi KS, Sacco AG & Borin K (1980) Immunologic infertility. I. Cervical mucus antibodies and postcoital test. *American Journal of Obstetrics and Gynecology* **136:** 941–950.

Monif GRG (1982) Infectious diseases in obstetrics and gynecology. Philadelphia: Harper and Row.

Mori T, Kamada M, Hasebe H et al (1985) Antibody reactivity with porcine zona pellucida. *Journal of Reproductive Immunology* **8:** 337–345.

Morris H, Edwards J, Tiltman A & Emms M (1985) Endometrial lymphoid tissue: an immunohistologic study. *Journal of Clinical Pathology* **38:** 644–652.

Mosher WD (1982) Infertility trends among US couples: 1965–1976. *Family Planning Perspective* **14:** 22–27.

Murphy A, Green R, Bobbie D, Delocruz Z & Rock JA (1986) Unsuspected endometriosis documented by scanning electron microscopy on visually normal peritoneum. *Fertility and Sterility* **46:** 522–527.

Naples JD, Batt RE & Sadigh H (1981) Spontaneous abortion rate in patients with endometriosis. *Obstetrics and Gynecology* **57:** 509–512.

Noyes RW, Hertig AT, Rock J (1950) Dating the endometrial biopsy *Fertility and Sterility* **1:** 3–25.

Ogra PL, Yamaraka T & Losonsky GA (1981) Local immunologic defenses in the genital tract. In *Reproductive Immunology*, p 381. New York: Alan R. Liss Inc.

Oliphant G, Randall P & Cabot CL (1977) Immunological components of rabbit fallopian tube fluid. *Biology of Reproduction* **16:** 463–469.

Ozato K, Wan YJ & Orrison BM (1985) Mouse major histocompatibility class I gene expression begins at midsomite stage and is inducible in earlier stage embryos by interferon. *Proceedings of the National Academy of Science USA* **82:** 2427–2431.

Pandya IJ & Cohen J (1985) The leukocytic reaction of the human uterine cervix to spermatozoa. *Fertility and Sterility* **43:** 417–421.

Parr EL, Schaedler RW & Hirsch JG (1967) The relationship of polymorphonuclear leukocytes to infertility in uteri containing foreign bodies. *Journal of Experimental Medicine* **126:** 523–538.

Phillips DM & Mahler S (1977) Leukocyte emigration and migration in the vagina following mating in the rabbit. *Anatomical Research* **189:** 45–59.

Plentl AA & Friedman EA (1971) Lymphatic system of the female genitalia: the morphologic basis of oncologic diagnosis and therapy. Philadelphia: WB Saunders.

Presl J & Bukovsky A (1986) Role of Thy−I+ and Ia+ cells in ovarian function. *Biology of Reproduction* **34:** 159–169.

Rakoff AE (1961) Hormonal cytology in gynecology. *Clinical Obstetrics and Gynecology* **4:** 1045–1061.

Rebello R, Green FHY & Fox H (1975) A study of the secretory immune system of the female genital tract. *British Journal of Obstetrics and Gynecology* **82:** 812–816.

Reynolds CW & Ortaldo JR (1987) Natural killer activity: the definition of a function rather than a cell type. *Immunology Today* **8:** 172–174.

Sampson JA (1927) Peritoneal endometriosis due to menstrual dissemination of endometrial tissue into peritoneal cavity. *American Journal of Obstetrics and Gynecology* **14:** 422–469.

Schneider EG, Danide AE & Polan ML (1987) Lymphokines (Interleukins-1 and 2) are not toxic to early mouse embryo development. *American Fertility Society*, 28–30 September. Reno, Nevada (abstract).

Schumacher GFB (1980) Humoral immune factors in the female reproductive tract and their changes during the cycle. In Dhindsa DS & Schumacher GFB (eds) *Immunological Aspects of Infertility and Fertility Regulation*, p 93. New York: Elsevier-North Holland.

Schweppe KW, Wyann RM & Baller FK (1984) Ultrastructural comparison of endometriotic implants and ectopic endometrium. *American Journal of Obstetrics and Gynecology* **148:** 1024–1039.

Schwimmer WB, Ustay KA & Behrman SJ (1967) Sperm-agglutinating antibodies and increased fertility in prostitutes. *Obstetrics and Gynecology* **30:** 192–195.

Sen DR & Fox H (1967) The lymphoid tissue of the endometrium. *Gynecologia* **163:** 371–378.

Sgarlata CS, Hertelendy F & Mikhail G (1983) The prostanoid content in peritoneal fluid and plasma of women with endometriosis. *American Journal of Obstetrics and Gynecology* **47**: 563–565.

Shivers CA & Dunbar BS (1977) Autoantibodies to zona pellucida: A possible cause for infertility in women. *Science* **197**: 1082–1084.

Slapsys R & Clark DA (1983) Active suppression of host versus graft rejection in pregnant mice. V. Kinetics, specificity and in vivo activity of non-T suppressor cells localized to the genital tract of mice during first pregnancy. *American Journal of Reproductive Immunology* **3**: 65–71.

Tabibzadeh SS, Gerber MA & Satyaswaroop PG (1986) Induction of HLA-Dr antigen expression in human endometrial epithelial cells in vitro by recombinant gamma-interferon. *American Journal of Pathology* **125**: 90–96.

Taguchi O & Nishizuka Y (1987) Self tolerance and localized autoimmunity. Mouse models of autoimmune disease that suggest tissue-specific suppressor T cells are involved in self tolerance. *Journal of Experimental Medicine* **165**: 146–156.

Trinchieri G & Persussia B (1985) Immune interferon: a pleiotropic lymphokine with multiple effects. *Immunology Today* **6**: 131–136.

Urry RL, Laudle MR & Rote NS (1985) Autoimmune infertility and recurrent abortion. In Scott JR & Rote NS (eds) *Immunology in Obstetrics and Gynecology*, p 77. Norwalk: Century Crafts.

Vallotton MB & Forbes AP (1966) Antibodies to cytoplasm of ova. *Lancet* **ii**: 264–265.

Vlasselaer VP & Vandeputte M (1984) Immunosuppressive properties of murine trophoblast. *Cellular Immunology* **83**: 422–432.

Wagner G & Levin RJ (1978) Vaginal fluid. In Hafez ESE & Evans TW (eds) *The Human Vagina*, pp 121–137. New York: Elsevier.

Wang HS, Kanazaki H, Yoshida M, Sato S, Tokushigem M & Mori T (1987) Suppression of lymphocyte reactivity in vitro by supernatants of explants of human endometrium. *American Journal of Obstetrics and Gynecology* **157**: 956–963.

Webb CG (1980) Decreased fertility in mice immunized with teratocarcinoma OTT 6050. *Biology of Reproduction* **22**: 695–704.

Weed JC & Arquembourg PC (1980) Endometriosis: Can it produce an autoimmune response resulting in infertility? *Clinical Obstetrics and Gynecology* **23**: 885–893.

Wheeler JE (1982) Pathology of the fallopian tube. In Blaustein A (ed.) *Pathology of the female genital tract*, pp 393–415. New York: Springer-Verlag.

Wheeler JM, Johnston BM & Madinek LR (1983) The relationship of endometriosis to spontaneous abortion. *Fertility and Sterility* **39**: 656–660.

Wild RA & Shivers CA (1985) Antiendometrial antibodies in patients with endometriosis. *American Journal of Reproductive Immunology and Microbiology* **8**: 84–86.

Witkin S (1984) Suppressor T cells in human semen. *AIDS Research* **1**: 339–345.

Xu C, Hill JA & Anderson DJ (1987) Identification of T-lymphocyte subpopulations in normal and abnormal human endometrial biopsies. *Society of Gynecological Investigation*, 18–21 March, Atlanta (abstract).

Yang S-L, Schumacher GFB, Broer KA & Holt JA (1983) Specific antibodies and immunoglobulins in the oviductal fluid of the rhesus monkey. *Fertility and Sterility* **39**: 359–369.

Ylikorkala O, Koskimies A, Laatkainen T, Tenhunen A & Vinikka L (1984) Peritoneal fluid prostaglandins in endometriosis, tubal disorders, and unexplained infertility. *Obstetrics and Gynecology* **63**: 616–620.

3

Maternal–fetal cell surface antigen incompatibilities

WARREN R. JONES
JILLIAN A. NEED

This chapter deals with maternal isoimmunization against cell surface antigens of erythrocytes, leukocytes and platelets. The term isoimmunization, by common usage, refers to a maternal immune response to paternal antigens expressed in the fetus. This departs from classical immunological nomenclature and replaces the term alloimmunization, which describes immunization against antigens in another member of the same species. The special feature inherent in maternal isoimmunization is that the immune recognition and response mechanisms are generated in an 'individual' who shares 50% of her genetic composition with her fetus.

Any antigens of fetal origin, be they cellular, particulate or soluble, that are capable of gaining access to the maternal circulation may theoretically provoke an isoimmune response. For practical purposes, the isoimmune states of clinical significance involve the passage of fetal cells across the placenta although, in some circumstances, maternal sensitization may follow blood transfusion. The situation with regard to leukocyte isoimmunization is also complicated by mechanisms involving exposure of the fetus to soluble human leukocyte antigens (HLA) and to antigens that are common to leukocytes, trophoblast and spermatozoal cells.

Whatever the nature of the immunizing event, should the fetal response involve the production of antibodies which subsequently complete the circle of 'two-way' traffic, they may exert deleterious effects on their target cells in the fetus and ultimately in the newborn. Clinical sequelae of isoimmunization involving cell surface antigens other than those of fetal erythrocytes are relatively rare and are restricted to isoimmune reactions to leucocytes and platelets.

THE MECHANISMS OF ISOIMMUNIZATION TO FETAL BLOOD CELLS

For a fetal antigen to cause an isoimmune reaction in the mother and to be subsequently associated with clinical effects in the fetus and neonate, it must: (i) be present on the fetal cell surface, (ii) be absent in the mother, (iii) be sufficiently immunogenic to provoke an antibody response, and (iv) stimulate antibodies of an immunoglobulin class (IgG) and subclass able to cross the placenta to the fetus. The nature of and factors influencing fetal–maternal cell traffic will be considered below in relation, particularly, to erythrocytes and leukocytes. The mechanisms whereby maternal antibodies gain access to the fetus, however, are common to all types of isoimmunity.

Immunoglobulin (antibody) transport from mother to fetus

The effector arm of any clinical sequelae of maternal isoimmunization depends on the transport of antibodies across the placenta from mother to fetus. This is dependent on immunoglobulin class rather than on molecular size. Thus, immunoglobulin G (IgG) crosses the placenta readily whereas smaller protein molecules and the other immunoglobulin classes (IgM, IgA, IgD and IgE) do not.

The placental transmission of IgG is active as well as selective, and is determined by the ability of its Fc portion to bind to receptors on coated micropinocytotic vesicles in the membrane of syncytiotrophoblast cells. The expression of Fc_γ receptors by human trophoblast, therefore, appears to be related to its function as a transport membrane for the selective transmission of immunoglobulins from mother to fetus (Johnson and Brown, 1981). These receptors may also have a role in protecting the placenta against maternal immunological attack. It has been proposed that Fc binding of maternal IgG leaves insufficient remaining IgG antibodies for specific F(ab')2 binding to fetal antigenic determinants on the trophoblast. Thus, the placenta is shielded from harmful (cytotoxic?) antibodies. There are other potential protective mechanisms involving the interaction of leukocyte antigen–antibody systems in the placenta, and these will be discussed below.

The active transport of IgG into the fetus commences at about 12 weeks' gestation. Fetal levels equal those in the mother by the third trimester, and at term they exceed them. Neonatal IgG concentrations are higher following vaginal delivery than after elective Caesarean section, suggesting that uterine contractions provide a final 'boost' to the acquisition of maternal antibodies by the fetus. All four subclasses of IgG are transferred, IgG2 less readily than the others.

RHESUS BLOOD GROUP ISOIMMUNIZATION

Isoimmunization against fetal erythrocytes exclusively involves cell surface blood group antigens. The prototype and best known example of erythrocyte isoimmunization involves the rhesus (Rh) antigens and will be considered in some detail.

The rhesus antigen system and its expression

The Rh blood group system, with its high degree of polymorphism, is second in complexity only to the HLA system. At least five major and numerous minor variants have been identified.

The nomenclature of the Rh system is confused. The major classifications are those of Fisher–Race (Race & Sanger, 1975) and Wiener (Wiener, 1944) (Table 1). The Fisher–Race classification assumes that three genes are responsible for the production of Rh antigens, each of which has at least two major alleles and some rare variants. The gene loci are closely linked on the

Table 1. Rhesus antigen nomenclature.

Fisher-Race		Wiener	
Genotype	Phenotype	Genotype	Phenotype
cde	ce	r	rh
Cde	Ce	r'	rh'
cdE	cE	r''	rh''
CdE	CE	r^y	rh^y
cDe	cDe	R_o	Rh_o
CDe	CDe	R_1	Rh_1
cDE	cDE	R_z	Rh_2
CDE	CDE	R_z	Rh_z

short arm of chromosome 1 and have been designated C (alleles C, c), D (alleles D,d) and E (alleles E,e) which are probably linked in the sequence CDE. The designation d signifies absence of D, whereas antigenic cell surface structures have been identified for all other alleles (D,c,C, e,E). D is a moderately potent immunogen compared with E and C, which are immunogenically weak so that differences at the D locus are clinically the most important. Wiener's scheme assumes a single gene locus with various alleles at this one locus.

In white populations, 85% are Rh-positive and carry the Rh(D) antigen, while 15% do not and are designated Rh-negative. Of the Rh-positive phenotypes, some are much more prevalent than others. For example, more than 50% of whites are CcDe or CDe, with the most prevalent genotypes being CDe/cde and CDe/CDe. Some haplotypes (genetic material from a single chromosome) are rare (CdE), some are of intermediate frequency (cDe, cdE, Cde, CDE) while others are common (cDe, cde, cDE) (Table 2).

Table 2. Approximate frequencies of Rh alleles and genotypes in European populations. From Davey (1979).

Allele	Frequency
CDe	0.41
cde	0.39
cDE	0.15
Others with D	0.03
Others without D	0.02

By the 6th week of gestation the Rh antigen is fully expressed on the human red cell. It is a small protein of 7–10 kD with multiple antigenic epitopes, i.e. it is a protein mosaic with multiple variable antigenic determinants distributed in non-random clusters on the cell surface.

The variations of D antigen expression may be conceptualized as follows. Absence of antigen is typed as Rh-negative, strong expression of antigen as Rh-positive, and variable expression gives rise to the D^u phenotypes. In some D-positive blood, parts of the D antigen complex are missing and when exposed to the complete D-positive cells, the incomplete D antigen is capable of making allo-anti-D antibody against the portion it lacks. Such blood is called D variant (when the red cells react promptly with commercial anti-D) or D^u variant (when the cells react only by the indirect antiglobulin technique). It seems that blood which lacks part of the D mosaic is capable of producing antibodies against the missing pieces. Thus D^u variant may represent expression of only a portion of the determinants which make up the complete D antigen. There is no specific D^u antigen, so that Rh-negative blood stimulated by D^u cells produces anti-D and not anti-D^u antibody. Thus, the production of allo-anti-D antibody in D- and D^u-positive blood may lead to transfusion reactions and haemolytic disease of newborn. Blood containing D^u cells has been considered to be weakly D- or Rh-positive. Rh-negative women who complete a pregnancy with a D^u infant are therefore rightful candidates for Rh-immune globulin; however, mothers with D^u blood are not generally considered for prophylaxis if the infants are D- or D^u-positive.

Rhesus antigen expression appears to be controlled by several factors, including the number of antigenic sites (Table 3), the presence of other antigens (C/E) and the relative position of the loci on the same or the opposite chromosome. The presence of D seems to have a suppressive effect on the expression of C, E and e antigens, but these antigens in turn also control the expression of D.

The frequency of the D^u phenotype is around 0.2% (0.6% in Caucasians), and about 1.5% of all Rh-negative gravid women. Some individuals do not express any Rh antigens, and are designated as Rh_{null} phenotype.

Table 3. Gene dosage – number of antigenic sites. From Hughes-Jones (1975).

Antigen	Phenotype	Number of sites per red cell
c	cc	70 000–85 000
C	cC	37 000–53 000
D	R_1r	10 000–15 000
D	R_2R_2	25 000–35 000
E	Various	450–25 600
e	ee	18 200–24 400
e	Ee	13 400–14 500

The mechanism of Rh haemolytic disease of the fetus and newborn

Maternal isoimmunization

Apart from the immunogenic capacity of the antigen(s) described above, three other major factors are required for the production of maternal antibodies: Rh incompatibility, feto–maternal haemorrhage, and the maternal capacity to respond to the antigen with antibody production. Not all Rh-negative individuals become sensitized by even large volumes of ABO-compatible Rh-positive blood on repeated exposure. Such individuals are designated 'non-responders'. In the two-thirds of Rh-negative individuals who are capable of responding to Rh(D), the sensitizing fetal haemorrhage usually occurs at delivery, although it may occur antenatally. While the minimum dose of fetal red cells required to cause maternal antibody formation is unknown, it is generally regarded as 0.1–0.25 ml.

Fetal haemolysis

The transfer of anti-Rh(D) antibody from the maternal circulation to the fetus occurs freely across the placenta by a process of active transport. It then acts as a powerful opsonin by facilitating phagocytosis and intracellular lysis of the fetal red blood cells, resulting in their eventual destruction either intravascularly or extravascularly. Most anti-Rh(D) antibody is IgG, in subclasses 1 and 3 which are complement-fixing. For these antibodies to cause haemolysis, the complement cascade must be activated by two antibody molecules being bound to the cell surface in close proximity. The IgG-coated red blood cells then undergo extravascular haemolysis primarily through reticuloendothelial phagocytosis in the spleen. Other blood group antibodies, such as anti-A, anti-B and anti-Le^a, are of the IgM class and are therefore capable of directly fixing complement and mediating haemolysis.

Another mechanism which may contribute to Rh-positive red cell haemolysis is antibody-dependent cell-mediated cytotoxicity (ADCC). Mononuclear phagocytes and lymphoid 'killer' (K) cells have Fc receptors. These receptors are capable of interacting in vitro with the Fc portion of an IgG molecule on the surface of the cell, with subsequent target cell lysis. The role of ADCC reactions in Rh-positive red cell haemolysis, in vivo, is uncertain.

The pathology of haemolytic disease of the fetus and newborn (HDFN)

The clinico-pathological manifestations of HDFN range through neonatal anaemia and jaundice to hydrops fetalis.

Neonatal anaemia and jaundice

In the mildest form of HDFN, the neonate is pale with minimal hepatosplenomegaly. Mild anaemia will be present with polychromasia and anisocytosis. The increased intrauterine haemolysis results in elevated bilirubin levels in the amniotic fluid and cord blood. Such haemoglobin breakdown products readily cross the placenta to be conjugated to albumin in the maternal liver. After delivery, however, the bilirubin must then be conjugated in the relatively immature neonatal liver. Thus, low levels of glucuronyl transferase limit the amount of bilirubin which can be conjugated and neonatal hyperbilirubinaemia develops. If excessive, this may lead to kernicterus where bilirubin complexes are deposited in the basal ganglia of the central nervous system. In severe cases of kernicterus, lethargy, hypotonia, opisthotonia and spasticity may develop and ultimately respiratory failure and death may result. The critical level of serum bilirubin is 18 mg/100 ml (18 ml/dl) but, if complicated by sepsis, dehydration, acidosis or prematurity, levels below this may predispose the infant to kernicterus. Levels greater than 30 mg/100 ml (30 mg/dl) will be associated with kernicterus in 75% of infants.

Hydrops fetalis

When anaemia is very severe, hydrops fetalis develops usually prior to 34 weeks' gestation, but it may occur as early as 22 weeks and perinatal mortality is high. The criteria for the diagnosis of hydrops are oedema, anaemia, hepatosplenomegaly, elevated serum bilirubin and placental enlargement. The pathogenesis of the syndrome is uncertain, but heart failure, increased capillary permeability from the chronic tissue hypoxia of severe anaemia, portal and umbilical venous hypertension caused by distortion of the liver parenchyma with erythropoietic tissue, and the decreased colloidal osmotic pressure of hypoproteinaemia resulting from liver dysfunction have all been implicated. Most likely, it is the severe anaemia which leads to tissue hypoxia and acidosis, as shown in fetal cord blood samples (collected at fetoscopy) where a haemoglobin level of greater than 4 g/dl differentiates an hydropic from a non-hydropic fetus.

The anaemia is chronic and, apart from causing tissue hypoxia and acidosis, also stimulates erythrocytosis in the bone marrow to compensate for the severe loss of red cells. The bone marrow becomes hyperplastic and filled with immature erythroid cells; the granulocytic precursors are depressed. Further progression of the anaemia is associated with failure of medullary erythropoiesis to compensate for the red cell loss. Consequently, extramedullary sites will be activated, e.g. in the spleen leading to severe splenomegaly with associated lymphoid hypoplasia; the kidney, adrenals, placenta and liver may also be involved.

Placental enlargement occurs secondary to hypoxia and erythropoiesis, inducing umbilical venous hypertension with placental oedema and trophoblastic hypertrophy. The weight relationships of the fetus and placenta are altered so that the fetal/placental weight ratio may approach one instead of the normal 5–7. This decreased ratio occurs in spite of the grossly oedematous fetus that may be twice its normal weight. The altered placental morphology decreases placental transfer of nutrients with chronic fetal malnutrition and potentially retarded brain growth.

Extreme hepatomegaly reflects extensive erythropoiesis in the liver with compression and degeneration of the surrounding tissues and gross distortion of the hepatic parenchyma. Hepatic blood flow is decreased and then increased portal hypertension further reduces hepatic metabolic activity. The production of vitamin K-dependent coagulation factors is markedly decreased and, in the most severely affected infants, there will be transient defibrination and/or coagulation failure due to deficiencies in multiple coagulation factors.

Platelet numbers may be moderately to severely depressed, secondary to the splenomegaly. Defibrination may be produced by depressed fibrin clearance in the reticuloendothelial system, together with thromboplastin release from haemolysed red cells with tissue acidosis acting as a promoting factor. Ascites may develop due to the combination of hypoxia and low values of plasma total protein and albumin, as demonstrated in fetal blood samples collected by fetoscopy in non-hydropic fetuses prior to intrauterine transfusion. The total protein concentration in the ascitic fluid of hydropic fetuses is higher than would be expected in an ascitic transudate, such as occurs in isolated portal hypertension or cardiac failure, and suggests the presence of an endothelial defect secondary to hypoxic damage. The hypoproteinaemia, together with increasing portal hypertension, may lead to extreme generalized oedema and even the development of hydrothorax with associated compression and pulmonary hypoplasia. Pulmonary oedema and haemorrhage may also occur.

Management of Rh-isoimmunization

Rh-erythroblastosis fetalis is a unique problem in that there are effective screening procedures to identify the woman at risk for immunization (Rh type), and to predict the degree of severity of the affected fetus (Kochenour and Scott, 1985). The indirect antiglobulin (Coombs') test screens for sensitization. If there are no antibodies, there will be no disease. If antibodies are present, then erythroblastosis may occur provided the fetus is Rh-positive but not if the fetus is Rh-negative, as it does not then carry the relevant antigen(s).

Maternal antibody screening

At the first antenatal visit, the Rh type and indirect antiglobulin (Coombs') test identifies those women at risk or who are already sensitized. Furthermore, in all immunized pregnancies, the establishment of correct gestational age is critical, since intervention later in gestation is likely.

Antibody assays using the Coombs' test. In 1945, Coombs and colleagues (Coombs et al, 1945) described a method of testing serum to detect an antibody (direct test) and to determine whether the antigenic sites were coated or blocked (indirect test). In this latter case, Rh-positive cells in saline are added to the test serum; if there is no agglutination the cells are washed to remove all excess serum. To the washed cells, rabbit anti-human globulin (AHG) is added which will result in agglutination if the D sites are coated, thus demonstrating that there was incomplete anti-D antibody in the original serum (indirect Coombs' test). In the case of rhesus isoimmunization, the first part of the test will have been performed in utero since the fetal cells have been coated with the mother's antibodies, so that it is only necessary for the cells to be washed and put up against AHG to detect agglutination (direct Coombs' test). Subsequently, an enzyme (trypsin) test was developed which renders the antibody-coated cells agglutinable by incomplete antibody.

In Rh-negative women without antibodies at initial screening, the indirect globulin test should be repeated at 32 and 36 weeks' gestation and possibly also at 28 weeks. If the screening antiglobulin test is positive, then anti-D titres should be determined; 1:2 will suggest mild, and 1:512 severe, immunization. Low titres (1:16 or 1:32) correspond with mild disease of the fetus and a very low rate of intrauterine death.

In the first immunized pregnancy, serum titres correlate reasonably well with the severity of the disease. This is particularly true since the introduction of the British anti-D working standard which has standardized methods and reagents. Using this standard, it has been reported that women with rhesus antibody levels below 5 IU/ml delivered neonates with mild disease (moderate jaundice controlled by phototherapy), those whose values were above 5 IU/ml had a high incidence of exchange or top-up transfusions, and values greater than 50 IU/ml were associated with a severely affected fetus. Thus, maternal serum values may allow deferment of amniocentesis until maternal anti-D levels are greater than 5 IU/ml. If sensitization has occurred in a prior pregnancy, then the antibody titre has value only in determining the timing of amniocentesis and is poorly correlated with disease severity.

Antibody-dependent cell-mediated cytotoxicity (ADCC) assay. A more relevant predictor of the severity of disease may be the ADCC assay which has been shown to detect variations in the potency of anti-D serum (Urbaniak et al, 1981). It may predict the severity of haemolytic disease more accurately, even than conventional assays of liquor bilirubin by spectrophotometry. There does not seem to be any correlation between the anti-D level (IU/ml) and the ADCC activity.

Immunoglobulin subclasses of anti-D. Knowledge of the immunoglobulin class and subclasses of maternal Rh isoantibodies may be helpful in predicting the likelihood of fetal affection. Anti-D antibodies belong to the IgG class, mostly subclasses 1 and 3, and in particular are of the G1m(4) allotype. IgG_1 antibodies are present in the more severe disease forms and cord haemoglobin values are lower when the G1m(1) and G1m(4) allotypes are present. The IgG_1 antibodies may be transferred across the placenta earlier and have a longer half life than some other IgG subclasses, which could explain their association with the severe forms of HDFN.

Amniocentesis

Amniotic fluid bilirubin assays form the cornerstone of management of the isoimmunized woman and give an accurate indication of the fetal condition. It should be remembered that amniotic fluid bilirubin levels fall with advancing gestation and that the development of polyhydramnios may give a falsely low value, in which case the bilirubin trend does not then accurately reflect the fetal condition.

Spectrophotometric analysis, with a continuous recording spectrophotometer, determines the level of bilirubin by measuring the absorbance beginning at 375 μm, peaking at 450 μm and returning to normal at 525 μm. The amount of indirect bilirubin is determined by drawing an 'arbitrary line' between 375 and 525 μm and the difference between that line and the peak bilirubin at 450 μm is determined. This is called the deviation in optical density at 450 μm (ΔOD 450).

A. W. Liley, the first to formulate a systematic approach to amniotic fluid analysis (Liley, 1961), developed a graph divided into three zones (upper, middle and lower) with further subdivisions of the upper and middle zones. The initial ΔOD 450 was placed on the graph in one of the prognostic zones by week of gestation (usually 29–32 weeks). The upper zone contained the severely affected fetuses, the lower zone contained the Rh-negative or mildly affected fetuses. The middle zone contained fetuses who showed either a normal downward trend of ΔOD 450 values with increased gestation (these had milder disease) or who showed the same or higher values on subsequent examinations and had more severe disease. Values in the upper division of the upper zone predicted intrauterine or neonatal death, or infants with very low cord haemoglobin. In the lower subdivision of the upper zone, the cord haemoglobin levels were below 8 g/100 ml (8 g/dl) within 7 days of delivery. These fetuses required intrauterine transfusions if they were too premature to deliver. The prognostic value of the middle zone depended on the magnitude of deviation from normal and the trend of the deviation. Use of this method of fetal assessment reduced the perinatal mortality from 22% to 9%. Various modifications of Liley's chart now exist, but essentially the principles remain.

Amniocentesis is first done at 28–30 weeks unless the obstetric history or antibody titre indicate that it should be done earlier. Thus, it should be performed 10 weeks before the gestation of delivery of the last successful pregnancy, but not earlier than 20 weeks' gestation since intrauterine transfusion done prior to this stage is unlikely to salvage the baby. The subsequent amniocentesis will be done within 1–4 weeks, as indicated by the initial liquor bilirubin levels. The higher the level, the sooner should the test be repeated to determine the rate of progression of fetal disease. If a downward trend is observed, then the amniocentesis may be spaced every 3–4 weeks.

A good prediction of fetal outcome may be made with two or three amniotic fluid determinations, studying the trend in values and predicting the time of delivery using an 'action line'. In normal pregnancies, the trend is downwards with increasing gestation as it is in mildly affected neonates (10–14 g/100 ml [10–14 g/dl] cord haemoglobin). Severely affected fetuses (Hb < 10 g/100 ml [< 10 g/dl]) show mixed trends with some downward, unchanged or increasing. An increasing trend with advancing age, indicates impending fetal death in utero. Care should be exercised where there is polyhydramnios as a falling value will underestimate the severity of the disease. Technically, amniocentesis should be carried out under ultrasound control and the fluid placed in a brown bottle since the bilirubin reading will be falsely low if exposed to light.

Ultrasound scanning

Apart from confirming gestational age and selecting a safe amniocentesis site, ultrasound scanning is also of value in detecting the dramatic changes of hydrops fetalis and cardiac failure which precede fetal death in utero. Such scanning of the fetus can provide reassurance that continuation of the pregnancy is safe. There are limitations to its use, however, since features such as cardiomegaly, ascites, polyhydramnios, subcutaneous oedema and an enlarged placenta do not occur in a logical sequence and may develop very quickly. Furthermore, their absence does not mean that the fetus will be only mildly affected. However, in a severely affected fetus, scanning should be done twice a week. A recent report of daily ultrasound fetal scanning to detect the early signs of fetal hydrops allowed pregnancy to be continued for 8–63 days beyond the time when liquor ΔOD 450 findings indicated delivery (Benacarref and Frigoletto, 1985). The earliest signs of fetal hydrops and cardiovascular decompensation may be the visualization of both sides of the bowel wall where the presence of fluid on the outside of the bowel wall silhouettes it—thus indicating the presence of incipient ascites. This technique may allow delay of the institution of intrauterine transfusions based on history and ΔOD 450 of amniotic fluid. However, it should be noted that intrauterine fetal deaths may occur at 24–25 weeks without evidence of oedema or ascites.

Intrauterine transfusion

Since it was first introduced in 1963, this technique has undergone major advances with utilization of ultrasound and fetal immobilization techniques (Nicolaides and Rodek, 1985).

Indications and basic management. Where serial liquor ΔOD 450 values lie between the middle and high zones with rising values or when fetal hydrops develops, intrauterine transfusion is indicated. The techniques used have evolved from intraperitoneal transfusion under X-ray control to intravascular cannulation and transfusion under ultrasound or fetoscopic control.

Fetal intravascular transfusion allows the direct sampling of fetal blood with greater precision of monitoring of fetal anaemia and haematocrit so that the timing and blood volume can be better regulated to maintain the fetal haemoglobin level at 12 g/100 ml (12 g/dl). The volume to be transfused is calculated from the pre-transfusion haemoglobin and the estimated circulating blood volume of the fetoplacental unit using a haemoglobin dilution technique. Maintenance of this haemoglobin is aimed at suppressing excessive fetal red cell production in utero and in the early neonatal period, so that haemolysis is lessened and the number of exchange transfusions reduced. Hydrops may even be reversed and pregnancy thus prolonged with enhanced perinatal survival.

Once an intrauterine transfusion (IUT) has been performed it is repeated until pre-term delivery is feasible. Unfortunately, following IUT, the amniotic fluid ΔOD 450 is no longer useful in determining subsequent timing of transfusions. They are therefore repeated according to various schedules, usually at 2–3 weekly intervals, or with the assistance of ultrasound assessment of the fetal condition.

Blood for transfusion. The donor red cells selected for fetal intravascular transfusion in severe rhesus isoimmunization must be cross-matched with maternal serum with respect to the Rh-antigen and other minor systems. Enhanced antibody production to common non-rhesus antigens (e.g. Kidd [JK] and Duffy [Fy]) has been observed after intrauterine transfusion, which may themselves cause HDFN. These antibodies may then cause destruction of the transfused donor cells within the fetus. These risks appear to be greater with intravascular than with intraperitoneal transfusions. Thus, donor blood to be used for intravascular transfusion should be selected to exclude Rh, Kell, Kidd, Duffy and S antigens whenever these are absent from the maternal cells, even if the father also lacks them.

Techniques. Initially the transfusion needle was guided into the fetal abdominal cavity under X-ray fluoroscopic control for intraperitoneal transfusions. Concern over radiation to both mother and fetus led to the introduction of ultrasound techniques better to identify fetal structures and to judge the tract and depth for the transfusion needle. Real time scanning allowed simultaneous observation of the needle and the fetus. Maternal sedation has the secondary benefit of decreasing fetal movement and greatly enhanced the safety of the technique. Packed cells (5–10 ml) of type O-negative blood cross-matched with the mother are infused intraperitoneally each minute. The total volume is calculated by the formula $(n - 20) \times 10$ ml, where n is the gestational age in weeks. A further development has been to immobilize the fetus with a curarizing injection into its thigh and then to transfuse with packed red cells directly into the umbilical vein, the transfusion needle being placed under ultrasound guidance (de Crespigny et al, 1985). Fetal hydrops has been noted to resolve, allowing delivery to be delayed, thus providing an excellent chance of a successful outcome even with a hydropic fetus. The technique of paralysing the fetus would seem to be superior to placement of a transfusion line into the umbilical vein under fetoscopic guidance. Fetoscopy may be difficult in the late second trimester if the liquor is cloudy, a general anaesthetic may be required and the fetoscope has a relatively large diameter with its attendant risks.

Outcome. There are few maternal complications of intrauterine transfusion except infection, which occurs in less than 1% of cases. Premature labour, premature rupture of membranes, placental abruption and malplacement of the needle have been reported.

Fetal risks, on the other hand, are great. Fetal mortality within 48 hours may be as high as 24% with intraperitoneal transfusions, although it is usually about 4–9% in experienced hands. Using intrauterine peritoneal techniques, the major risk is puncture of a fetal vessel and exsanguination. Increased intraperitoneal pressure may compress umbilical vein blood flow if excess blood is transfused.

The number of severely affected fetuses requiring IUT is now very few. Important prognostic factors for a particular case will be influenced by the gestational age at the time of the first intrauterine transfusion, the severity of fetal involvement and the experience of the physician with the various techniques of IUT. If IUT is undertaken before 26 weeks, or in the presence of hydrops, the prognosis is poor. Initial survival rates of 24–56% were reported, with up to 68% in non-hydropic fetuses and 36% in hydropic fetuses. The use of ultrasound gives survival rates between 70–90%. The mortality of IUT also seems to be proportional to the degree of haemolysis at the time IUT is commenced. If the amniotic fluid ΔOD 450 value is < 0.3, there is a survival rate of 83%; if 0.3–0.6, it is 36%; if > 0.6, it is 0%. It is estimated that a minimum of 12–16 transfusions in 4–5 fetuses per year is required to maintain the expertise of a unit in the management of severe HDFN.

Long-term outcome studies, with control populations, suggest that there is no impairment of intellectual or behavioural abilities in surviving infants. An increase in the incidence of inguinal and umbilical hernia has been reported.

Summary of management

Since severe rhesus isoimmunization is now an infrequently occurring condition, referral centres utilizing a team approach should be established. This will enable early consultation prior to 20 weeks, to formulate a plan of management. In broad terms this includes the following:

1. The time to initiate amniocentesis for bilirubin levels based on past obstetric history and the titre of anti-D, e.g. begin amniocentesis at 25 weeks' gestation (or 20–22 weeks if previously severely affected) or a titre of $> 1:16$.
2. The frequency of amniocentesis.
3. The time of referral for intrauterine transfusion.
4. Where, when and how to accomplish delivery.

Since there is a 95% neonatal survival rate at 32 weeks' gestation in tertiary level nurseries, planned delivery of severely affected infants at this gestation will be preferred to intrauterine transfusions and prolongation of pregnancy. Thus, the decision regarding gestation for delivery will depend on the survival rate in accessible neonatal intensive care units versus the risks of intrauterine transfusion at each particular centre.

Other modes of management

An estimated minimum of 2–4 women per 10 000 confinements will continue to become isoimmunized, so the problem of Rh isoimmunization is unlikely to completely disappear. In these residual cases, the management strategies employed to treat those sensitized subjects with a severely affected fetus prior to 24–26 weeks' gestation have generally sought to alter the maternal immune response. Methods to reduce existing maternal antibody concentration or production have included repeated small volume plasmapheresis, daily administration of oral preparations of human Rh-positive erythrocyte membrane or promethazine either alone or in combination with other therapies.

Immunosuppressive drugs

Promethazine hydrochloride. Animal work suggests that promethazine hydrochloride is immunosuppressive by virtue of its ability to alter leukocyte metabolism and function, and to interfere with the phagocytosis of opsonized fetal red cells. It may also suppress humoral antibody responses. Administration of 250–500 mg/day from 14 weeks' gestation has been shown to modify the disease, and to improve the perinatal mortality, in severely Rh-sensitized patients. This has not been the case when lower doses (100–150 mg/day) have been used. The fetal effects of promethazine therapy are unknown. There is a theoretical possibility of a more global effect on the fetal immune system and an increased risk of graft-versus-host disease in treated fetuses subsequently requiring intrauterine transfusion. There does not seem to be any depression of fetal T and B cells in the infants of mothers treated with promethazine. This treatment has been recommended in those severely Rh-sensitized pregnancies where there is a significant risk of early fetal loss.

Corticosteroids. Corticosteroids decrease antibody production, impair antibody–red cell interaction and inhibit macrophage binding of antibody-coated red cells. No randomized clinical trials have been performed using these agents in the treatment of erythroblastosis. Their use has not been shown to be effective in the treatment of severe Rh-isoimmunization. Furthermore, they appear to falsely lower the amniotic fluid bilirubin values.

Plasmapheresis

Plasmapheresis involves the removal of large volumes of plasma at various intervals (daily to bi-weekly) on a chronic basis, so as to remove disease causing antibody(s). Plasma exchange was introduced in 1968, but was not shown to be beneficial until 1977, when adequate lowering of maternal anti-D concentrations was achieved, thereby reducing the degree of fetal haemolysis. A success rate of 70–75% (compared with the predicted live-birth rate of 38%) has been achieved in a small trial of 14 cases when the mean plasma volume exchanged was 3.2 litres of plasma per week over an average of 13.5 weeks (Robinson and Tovey, 1980). For plasmapheresis to be of value, the exchanges must be intensive. Between 1.6 and 2.6 litres of plasma may need to be exchanged 3–6 times a week in order to maintain the mean level of anti-D at less than 10 IU/ml. There seems to be little risk of fetal death if the maternal anti-D level remains below 15 IU/ml.

Anti-D levels will respond to plasmapheresis in one of three ways:

1. They are initially lowered and maintained at this lower level until 32 weeks' gestation, when an uncontrollable rise occurs. Since delivery can be accomplished at this gestation a 100% survival can be expected.

2. They remain high despite intensive treatment with rapid rebound to pre-exchange levels. The outlook is poor, with only a 33% survival, if anti-D levels exceed 35 IU/ml.

3. They are rapidly lowered and maintained throughout pregnancy to give a good prognosis (87%).

Such patterns may reflect the timing of, or absence of restimulation of the maternal immune system secondary to, feto–maternal antepartum bleeding. This explanation is supported by the rapid and high rise seen postnatally and sometimes after amniocentesis. Thus, if serum maternal anti-D titres are not rising, amniocentesis may be delayed until 28 weeks' gestation so as to avoid the risk of a feto–maternal leak of Rh(D)-positive cells early in pregnancy, which act as a source of maternal restimulation with resultant uncontrollably high levels of anti-D antibody.

The major maternal risk of large volume plasma exchanges is hepatitis of the non-A and non-B type, since supplementary fresh frozen plasma must be given to maintain a normal serum globulin level. A normal serum globulin level avoids stimulation of globulin synthesis which would include anti-D immunoglobulin. Furthermore, a normal serum globulin is necessary to avoid maternal predisposition to infections. Allergic reactions to random units of fresh frozen plasma have also been reported. Suxamethonium apnoea has been reported. Cholinesterase activity should therefore be measured in women requiring general anaesthesia for delivery if intensively plasmapheresed. Plasma exchange may be the only available treatment for women with severe fetal involvement before 20–25 weeks' gestation, after which time IUT becomes reasonably safe, with the recent advances in techniques described earlier in this chapter.

Oral desensitization

In animal models, oral feeding of an antigen results in failure of subsequent parenteral antigen administration to elicit an immune response. The suggested mechanisms include the following:

1. Production of local and circulating immunoglobulins (IgA) which form immune complexes that impair the secondary response.

2. Generation of specific suppressor T cells and B cells in both the intestine and the mesenteric nodes which may inhibit expression of the secondary immune response.

3. Actual diminution in the numbers of antigen-reactive B cells.

Subsequent animal work has established that the oral desensitization process involves antigen-specific IgG suppression and IgA help. Oral protein feeding induces differential, isotype-specific immunoregulation in gut-associated lymphoid tissues, which is partly mediated by an antigen-specific IgA helper T cell. Thus, in animal studies, the enteric administration of antigen will induce states of tolerance by the generation of T suppressor cells that reduce antibody responses to subsequent challenge. There is no clear evidence in animal experiments, however, that oral desensitization can be induced where prior sensitization has already occurred.

In some human studies, however, the oral administration of capsules of lyophilized Rh-positive cell membranes (erythrocyte membrane oral therapy, EMOT) has been reported to improve outcome. Severely Rh-immunized pregnant women, whose previous pregnancies had ended in an intrauterine death were treated by daily EMOT together with promethazine beginning at 12–23 weeks' gestation (Gold et al, 1983). The Rh antibody levels remained stable throughout pregnancy, as did the liquor ΔOD 450, and delivery was undertaken at 35 weeks' gestation or later in 12 of 21 women with good results. Four of 11 cases commenced EMOT at 6–15 weeks with no amelioration of the disease, and all delivered hydropic fetus at 23–37 weeks and 2 of 10 had a further fetal loss at 20–22 weeks' gestation. Such extensive administration of Rh antigen on erythrocyte membranes attempts to alter established antibody responses by changing the proportions of IgG subclasses that are produced (Barnes et al, 1987).

Prophylaxis

Before the advent of prophylaxis with anti-D, the incidence of Rh haemolytic disease was about 1:150 births (Clarke, 1982). Most women do not develop circulating titres of anti-Rh(D) antibodies without previous exposure to Rh-positive erythrocytes, so that overt haemolytic disease of the newborn rarely occurs in a first pregnancy. The possibility that Rh-negative females may be sensitized during fetal life by materno–fetal transfusion from an Rh(D)-positive mother (the 'grandmother' theory) is now considered to be unlikely.

Anti-Rh(D) antibodies usually develop from occult feto–maternal transfusion, presumably due to breaches in the chorio–decidual junction. During normal pregnancy, fetal cells can be found in the maternal circulation, as early as the 8th week of gestation; in 7% of pregnancies this occurs in the first trimester, 16% in the second trimester, and 29% in the third trimester (i.e. 20–40% near term). These small quantities of blood are usually insufficient to induce primary immunization but will stimulate a secondary response in a subject already sensitized. Of postpartum women, 20–50% will have measurable transplacental haemorrhages during or after delivery. The more sensitive fluorescence cell sorting techniques indicate that such haemorrhages are present in all pregnancies with a mean fetal volume of 1.56 ml. The initiation of the primary response depends on the frequency and quantity of Rh-positive erythrocytes transferred into the maternal circulation. The clinical significance of the ingress of small numbers of fetal red cells into the maternal circulation is uncertain, but as little as 0.1 ml of fetal blood is sufficient to sensitize Rh-negative mothers delivering Rh-positive infants.

Some naturally occurring factors may also mitigate against isoimmunization developing:

1. There may be a 'threshold effect' in pregnancy, whereby a Rh antigen concentration easily capable of invoking a response in Rh-negative males and non-pregnant females will not sensitize a pregnant woman.
2. The concomitant presence of ABO incompatibility acts to cause rapid intravascular haemolysis of the transfused red cells before the Rh(D)

antigen has time to engage the appropriate antibody-forming cells in the maternal circulation.

3. The situation in genetic non-responders who are unable to respond to any quantity of antigen.

Although larger volumes of blood may be involved in feto–maternal transfusions in the first trimester and may provoke clinically significant titres of anti-Rh(D) antibody, this phenomenon is more often caused in early pregnancy by abortion (3–4% of spontaneous abortions and 5.5% of induced abortions), or in later pregnancy by procedures which 'traumatize' the placenta, e.g. during external cephalic version or amniocentesis.

Sensitization thus usually occurs at the delivery of an ABO-compatible Rh-positive child, when separation of the placenta results in feto–maternal bleeding of variable volume in about 50% of normal deliveries. Of mothers in normal pregnancies, 25–30% will receive < 0.1 ml of fetal blood; 20–25% 0.1–5 ml, < 1% > 5 ml and 0.25% > 30 ml. Even greater volumes of feto–maternal bleeding may be associated with Caesarean section, manual manipulation of the placenta, twins, traumatic delivery, or stillbirth of unknown cause.

If the volume of transplacental bleeding is < 0.1 ml, the incidence of demonstrable immunization within 6 months of delivery is 3%; with > 0.1 ml, 14% will be immunized. Regardless of the fetal blood volume, about 1.5–2% of women will be immunized by the time they are delivered, and 7–8% of Rh-negative women will be overtly sensitized within 6 months of a first ABO-compatible Rh-positive pregnancy. A further 7–8% will show that they were Rh-immunized by mounting a secondary immune response in their next Rh-positive pregnancy, that is they were 'sensitized' by the first pregnancy but the Rh-immunization was too weak to detect. The risk of sensitization in the second pregnancy is therefore 15–16%. If the first pregnancy is with an ABO-incompatible Rh-positive fetus, then the incidence of Rh-sensitization is reduced to 1.5–3%.

Tests to detect and quantitate feto–maternal haemorrhage (FMH)

While the standard dose of anti-D will be adequate to prevent isoimmunization in most situations, there may be occasions in which it is desirable to quantitate more precisely the volume of a feto–maternal haemorrhage. Some of the available tests will be discussed.

1. Acid elution, or Kleihauer–Betke, methods rely on the greater acid resistance of fetal haemoglobin (HbF) compared with adult haemoglobin. At term, 60–80% of the infant's total haemoglobin is HbF and unlike adult haemoglobin, this is not eluted through the cell membrane in the presence of an acid buffer. Examination of a fixed blood film allows quantitation of the fetal red cell volume present in the maternal circulation. This quantitation, however, may be quite inaccurate with estimates of fetal red cells that vary from half to twice the actual volume. A modification using an enzyme-linked globulin test provides greater sensitivity and is reproducible and objective enough to identify subjects

needing more than the standard prophylactic dose of 300 µg (30 ml) which will cover a FMH of 30 ml of whole blood. Of Rh-negative mothers, 0.3% will have an FMH greater than 30 ml whole blood at delivery which is equivalent to 15 ml of red blood cells. Various other modifications of this basic method have been incorporated into commercially available test kits.

2. The microscopic fluorescent microfluorometer method for the detection of fetal erythrocytes appears to be most useful where the mother herself may normally have raised concentrations of HbF; this occurs in some Caucasians but more often in mothers of Negro origin, especially in association with sickle cell disease and trait and heterozygous β-thalassaemia. The test is relatively rapid (90 minutes), is useful where the acid elution test is doubtful, and can detect a FMH of less than 4 ml. A fluorescence-activated cell sorter may also be used for this purpose but, although it is much more sensitive than the microfluorometric method, it takes 6 hours to perform. Since the routine dose of prophylactic anti-D will cover up to 4 ml of FMH, this added sensitivity is of no practical value.

3. Serum α-fetoprotein levels have been used to monitor FMH, but unfortunately show a wide range of variability throughout normal pregnancy. Furthermore, unless routine antenatal screening is carried out, a baseline maternal blood sample may not be available prior to the FMH.

4. The D^u test is based on the ability of antiglobulin (Coombs') serum to agglutinate Rh(D) positive fetal cells in the maternal blood sample after they have been coated with the anti-Rh(D) reagent. The results are qualitative (i.e. positive or negative), but consistently detect 25 ml or more of feto–maternal haemorrhage. There is a false negative rate of 12%.

Use of anti-D prophylaxis in clinical situations

Initial studies indicated that 300 µg of Rh-immune globulin would neutralize about 30 ml of Rh-positive fetal blood; however, the currently used dosage of 100 µg appears to provide the same protection. This standard post-partum regimen fails to protect 1–2% of Rh-negative women. The most likely explanations for these apparent failures are excessive fetal bleeding into the maternal circulation at the time of delivery, for which the standard dose is inadequate, or antepartum feto–maternal haemorrhage with subsequent sensitization. Approximately 0.4% of Rh-negative women are at risk of sensitization from a large FMH. Such individuals can be detected by the acid-elution or other tests described above to quantitate the number of fetal red cells in the maternal blood. However, where it is suspected that more than 15 ml of red cells have been received from the fetus, an additional dose(s) of Rh-immune globulin should be given. There does not seem to be any value in screening the parturient woman for anti-D antibody 24–48 hours after she has received Rh-immune globulin since the low level of antibody used as a standard dose is not always detected by the usual indirect Coombs' test. Unfortunately, there is no consistent correlation between a large FMH and obstetric manipulations, complications or surgery except for manual removal of the placenta.

The majority of Rh-immune globulin failures result from antepartum transplacental FMH, usually occurring in the third trimester. The time of occurrence and the circumstances associated with a significant antepartum feto–maternal haemorrhage are virtually impossible to determine, so that susceptible women cannot be identified. Over half of those women who become sensitized in the antepartum period have no apparent predisposing cause, e.g. pre-eclampsia, antepartum haemorrhage or intrauterine growth retardation. Conversely, when patients with third trimester vaginal bleeding are tested, 60% have no detectable fetal red cells following the episode. Large feto–maternal haemorrhage can occur quite silently and may be the cause of an apparently unexplained fetal death. Other clinical situations associated with detectable FMH are non-immune fetal hydrops, antepartum haemorrhage (APH), abdominal or uterine trauma, sinusoidal fetal heart pattern, fetal death, neonatal anaemia and, of course, an Rh(D)-negative mother delivery in Rh(D)-positive baby.

Since there is a poor correlation between clinical circumstances and detection rates of FMH, the indications for administration of Rh-immune globulin include a number of antepartum events during which FMH is likely. These are induced and spontaneous abortion, ectopic pregnancy, APH, manual removal of the placenta, amniocentesis and trophoblastic tumours.

The role of D^u blood groups

The most common cause of Rh-isoimmunization is the delivery of an Rh(D)- or (D^u)-, positive child to an Rh(D)-negative woman. Rh(D^u) antigen is a weakly reacting Rh-antigen and is usually screened for in Rh-negative women. When an Rh(D)-negative (D^u-positive or D^u-negative) woman is delivered of an Rh(D) or (D^u) infant, and is not already sensitized, she should be given prophylaxis.

Routine antenatal administration of anti-D

Postpartum administration of anti-D immune globulin has reduced the incidence of maternal immunization by 90%. Some of the remaining 10% of failures are due to immunization during pregnancy. The natural incidence of antenatal sensitization varies in different populations from 1–2%. Where immunization occurs in the antenatal period, 8% of cases occur prior to 28 weeks and 16% between 29–34 weeks. Antepartum use of Rh-immune globulin aims to promote sufficient anti-D IgG in the maternal circulation to ensure rapid clearance of fetal red cells, thus preventing sensitization during pregnancy.

The early trials of antenatal Rh-prophylaxis, begun in 1968, involved the administration of anti-D IgG at 28 weeks, and sometimes at 34 weeks, to all Rh-negative women at risk. Such trials resulted in a reduction of sensitization from 1.6–2% in untreated women to 0.1–0.3% in women treated both at 28 and 34 weeks. Initial protocols recommended the use of 300 µg of

Rh-immune globulin at 28 weeks only, since passive antibody is detectable for 3 months, together with the usual postnatal dose if the child was Rh-positive. Concern for the safety of routine prophylaxis does not seem well founded.

There seems to be little risk to the mother. Only one case of anaphylaxis has been recorded. The risk of hepatitis is eliminated by the preparation method and the transplacental transfer of anti-D has not resulted in haemolysis of fetal red cells. Since Rh(D)-immune globulin is an IgG and can cross the placenta freely with a half-life of 22.5 days, it is possible that fetal red cells could be haemolysed. It has been calculated that 0.5 µg Rh-immune globulin will enter the fetal circulation following a maternally administered intramuscular dose of 150 µg which could destroy 0.1 ml of fetal blood (i.e. less than 0.6% of total fetal blood volume of 16 ml at 16 weeks). However, once attached to the fetal red cells, further antibodies would cross the placenta to establish equilibration and, therefore, theoretically could haemolyse further fetal erythrocytes. It does not appear, however, that significant fetal anaemia is produced by this mechanism. There has been no increase in fetal deaths, and no significant difference in fetal haemoglobin or bilirubin levels, following anti-D prophylaxis after genetic amniocentesis.

Other areas of concern have focused on potential adverse effects of antepartum Rh(D)-immunoglobulin on the immature fetal immune system. Studies in older children (4–12 yr) with previously normal immune function tests, given gammaglobulin therapy because of repeated respiratory infections, have shown dysfunction of T and B cell responses for up to 5 months after cessation of treatment. Theoretically, the exposed fetus' immune response to Rh-antigen in later years may be influenced if that fetus is an Rh-negative female who later bears an Rh-positive fetus.

The normal feto–maternal immune relationship with the placenta functioning as a transport and endocrine organ may be impaired if the anti-(D) interacts with the Rh(D) antigens present on the plasma membranes and cytoplasm of villous trophoblast. The greatest cause for concern is that of enhancement where potentiation, rather than suppression, of the immune response may occur later in pregnancy if the antigen (FMH) is introduced as the level of anti-D immunoglobulin falls.

These concerns appear theoretical and are not supported by clinical experience, although the possibility of enhancement raises some practical concerns. This latter fact, as well as the cost–benefit issues, seem to be the main reasons for not employing routine antenatal prophylaxis on a wide scale. It should also be remembered that the downward trend in cases of haemolytic disease of the newborn since the introduction of postpartum prophylaxis may in part be due to the changing birth order as well as to antenatal prophylactic programmes. Taking into account the trend towards low parity, it would seem rational to restrict the introduction of antepartum anti-D prophylaxis on a wide scale to primiparous patients. It may also be prudent to advise limitation of the number of pregnancies in already sensitized women, and to ensure that every eligible woman receives postpartum and selective antenatal anti-D, as the most appropriate strategies for reducing the residual small incidence of Rh-haemolytic disease.

Mechanism of antibody-mediated immune suppression (AMIS) in Rh-prophylaxis

The mechanism of antibody-mediated immunosuppression in Rh-prophylaxis is not yet established. The Rh(D) antigen may be directed away from the maternal immunological apparatus so that antibody formation is prevented. If this is the case, then cells carrying D plus other antigens must also be directed away so that anti-D should prevent the formation of antibodies to C and E as well as to D. This has proved to be so, since red cell antibodies of other specificities are almost invariably found only when anti-D is also present. The passively administered anti-D may occupy the antigenic sites, thus blocking them from the receptors in appropriate lymphoid cells. However, this simple explanation is unlikely since the quantity of antibody administered allows only a small percentage of the antigenic sites to be covered. It seems, therefore, that antigen blockade/competitive binding cannot be sustained as a complete explanation for the mechanism of anti-D prophylaxis.

The more likely mechanism involves the central anatomical sites for antigen 'recognition' and antibody synthesis. These include the white pulp of the spleen and the follicular region of the lymph node cortex. All antigens are directed to or trapped in these anatomic sites regardless of whether the immune response is normal, augmented or depressed. Within these sites cell–cell interaction is important for antigen recognition and occurs on some structural surfaces such as the macrophage surface membrane or the dendritic filamentous processes from the lining reticular cells around and within the draining lymphoid follicles. The humoral immune response relies on cooperation between T-helper lymphocytes and the epitope-specific B lymphocytes in these central sites. The HLA-DR genes are involved in this antigen presentation and there is both 'positive' and 'negative' feedback, mediated by lymphokines released by T lymphocytes and/or macrophages. All of these interactions serve to augment the immune response. On the other hand, suppressor cells (Ts) have membrane receptors for the altered Fc portion of IgG and can be stimulated by IgG containing immune complexes. Therefore, the generation of antigen-specific Ts near the time of exposure to antigen would abrogate or suppress the immune response. Thus, Rh-immunoglobulin plus Rh(D)-positive erythrocytes may generate the immune complexes needed to reduce Ts activity.

AMIS prevents a primary immune response only, and has little effect on an already existing IgG response.

Future prospects for management

High-dose intravenous immunoglobulin (IVIG)

High-dose IVIG has been used in a few cases with a history of stillbirth or a severely affected previous fetus and has resulted in live born Rh-incompatible babies requiring exchange transfusions (Berlin et al, 1985). The mode of action is unclear but possible mechanisms may be feedback inhibition of maternal antibody synthesis, partial blockade of Fc-mediated antibody transport across the placenta or Fc blockade of the reticuloendothelial system.

Chorion villous sampling (CVS)

Where the husband is heterozygous for Rh(D) antigen, CVS may be used to determine the Rh(D) group of the fetus. This will allow a decrease in the monitoring procedures if the fetus is Rh-negative or a termination of the pregnancy in a severely sensitized mother if the fetus is Rh-positive.

ISOIMMUNIZATION DUE TO THE ABO BLOOD GROUP SYSTEM

After the discovery of the ABO blood group system in 1920, and the rhesus system in 1940, jaundice occurring in the first 24 hours of life was thought to be due to ABO incompatibility between mother and fetus. This was further clarified by the development of the Coombs' test in 1946. Two-thirds of cases of HDFN involve ABO antigens, one-third rhesus antigens and about 2% of cases are due to minor blood group antigens such as Kell, E or C.

Pathophysiology

In 20–25% of pregnancies, ABO incompatibility exists between mother and fetus; that is, the maternal serum contains naturally-occurring anti-A or anti-B, while the fetal erythrocytes express the corresponding A or B antigen. Clinical disease, usually mild hyperbilirubinaemia without significant anaemia, occurs in 10–20% of such heterospecific pregnancies, with 4% having clinically significant disease which is severe in 1% of cases. The ABO incompatibility may be so mild as to make the distinction between physiological jaundice and pathological neonatal jaundice obscure. In some cases, however, it may be severe enough to require exchange transfusion.

The heterospecific combinations (mother A–infant B; mother B–infant A; mother O–infant A or B) are important determinants of the disease severity. Group O mothers with group B or group A (particularly A_1) infants, are affected almost exclusively. Maternal A with infant B, or maternal B with infant A, combinations are rarely associated with haemolytic disease. The density of the A and B receptors on fetal erythrocytes is much less than in the adult and they are not as sensitive to maternal antibodies (iso-agglutinins) which cross the placenta in small amounts. Haemolysis is therefore less dramatic than with high density antigens and high affinity antibodies, such as in the rhesus D system. Placental cells also contain A and B antigens, so that maternal antibodies may be 'trapped' in the placenta thereby limiting access to the fetal antigens.

Isoantibodies are produced early in life by those who lack the corresponding antigen after encountering it in food, plants and bacteria. Group A or B individuals produce anti-A or anti-B that is predominantly 19S IgM anti-

body. These 'naturally' occurring antibodies are not involved in the haemolytic process of ABO incompatibility. Group O individuals, on the other
hand, produce anti-A or anti-B which is predominantly 7S IgG antibody and
able to cross the placenta. This so-called 'incomplete or immune antibody' is
involved in non-complement dependent haemolysis in ABO haemolytic
disease. The erythrocyte destruction occurs extravascularly, usually in the
spleen.

Clinical features

ABO haemolytic disease affects first-born children in 50% of cases
(Lockyer, 1982). Multiple siblings may be affected with comparable severity. Some studies suggest that the severity may increase with successive
pregnancies at risk, particularly in group A mothers, although there is no
linear correlation between antibody titre and disease severity. Prenatal
prediction is not reliable. Characteristically jaundice occurs within the first
24 hours of life and is of variable severity. Hepatosplenomegaly is minimal
or absent. Stillbirth and hydrops are rarely seen. A variable elevation of
indirect bilirubin occurs. Significant disease is present with values of 10–
12 mg/100 ml (10–12 mg/dl) at 24 hours of age, and levels may approach
20 mg/100 ml (20 mg/dl) in severe disease. Very high serum bilirubin levels
may cause kernicterus.

Severe anaemia is uncommon and haemoglobin values are usually normal
(13.5–20 g/100 ml [13.5–20 g/dl]) at birth. However, haemolysis is reflected
by an elevated reticulocyte count. The peripheral blood film shows sphero-
cytes which indicate antigen–antibody interaction and steric alteration by
the splenic macrophages. The diagnosis is largely based on excluding other
causes of early onset haemolytic disease in the presence of a heterospecific
pregnancy, usually involving group O mothers and group A or B infants.
The direct Coombs' test on cord blood is weakly positive in 30–50% cases,
and is most likely to be so in the first 24 hours of life. A positive indirect
Coombs' test establishes the diagnosis (anti-A present in group A, or anti-B
in a group B infant), but does not quantitate the haemolytic process.

Management of the newborn depends upon bilirubin surveillance, phototherapy and exchange transfusion. Phototherapy is required in about 10% of
cases and exchange transfusion only rarely. Adjustments need to be made
where other conditions, such as asphyxia, respiratory distress or infection,
are present which enhance the clinical significance of bilirubin values, thus
requiring the use of the various treatment modalities at lower bilirubin
levels. Where an exchange transfusion is necessary, group O blood should
be selected to avoid severe haemolytic reactions, which the use of antigen-
rich adult type-specific A or B cells in the presence of circulating antibody
would cause.

ISOIMMUNIZATION DUE TO OTHER BLOOD GROUP ANTIGENS

As HDFN caused by antibodies to the Rh(D) antigen has decreased, there has been a relative increase in HDFN due to other irregular antibodies (Beal, 1985). This may be secondary to the liberal use of blood transfusions. From 2–5% of all cases of HDFN, and up to 50% of antibodies to clinically significant antigens found during pregnancy, are to antigens other than D. Of the Rh antigens, antibodies to E, C and C_w are the most commonly occurring in Rh(D)-positive women. Antibodies in the Kell (K) and Duffy (FY^a) systems are second in importance to those of the P$_s$ system in frequency and severity. Haemolytic disease due to irregular antibodies may be very severe and the clinical management more difficult in rhesus anti-D situations.

An adequate antibody screen must be performed on all antenatal patients, whether Rh-positive or negative, to detect the presence of irregular antibodies. It is important to emphasize that at least 40% of new cases of isoimmunization within the Rh, Kell and Duffy systems are found in Rh-*positive* women. This figure may be a conservative estimate since few Rh-positive women are re-tested later in pregnancy. The clinical importance of these irregular antibodies rests in the potential cross-matching difficulties and the need for amniotic fluid spectrophotometric analysis to predict the severity of disease in the fetus, and to assist in selecting the time of delivery for optimum neonatal outcome.

The gestational age at which irregular antigens have been identified on fetal red cells varies with the antigen: Duffy antigen at 6 weeks; Kell and Kidd antigens at 12 weeks; Xg^a and Lutheran antigens at 14 weeks. The last two are poorly developed in frequency and antigenic strength, even at term, compared with the adult, so that the disease is usually mild.

Kell blood group system

Although Kell sensitization is an uncommon cause of haemolytic disease of the newborn, the disease may be severe. The genotypes and their frequencies are KK < 1%; Kk 8.7%; kk 91%. There are two subgroups of Kell, Kp^a and Kp^b, which are rarely involved in haemolytic disease, and the Sutter system, Js^a and Js^b, which occurs almost exclusively in black races.

Severe haemolytic disease with hydropic neonates occurs secondary to anti-K, with the appearance of antibody and progression of the haemolytic process being much more rapid than that with anti-D, thus contributing to the high morbidity and mortality associated with anti-K. Amniotic fluid bilirubin levels may rise suddenly over a short time, so that more frequent amniocentesis should be carried out to detect any sudden rise into the severely affected zone, in which case premature delivery or intrauterine transfusion may be needed. Greater reliance must be placed on ultrasound to detect early changes of hydrops, ascites or placental thickening, with weekly or even daily assessment in the Kell-sensitized pregnant woman.

Apart from the K antigen, isoimmunization to the other antigens of the Kell system is associated with mild disease only, requiring no active intervention.

Duffy blood group system

In most cases of maternal sensitization to the Duffy antigens, the disease is mild to moderate but all grades of severity of HDFN occur. The sensitizing event in 50–65% of cases is blood transfusions prior to the affected pregnancy. The relevant antigen is Fy^a since there are no reported cases of haemolytic disease due to anti-Fy^b. Pregnancy management is largely dependent on serial liquor bilirubin analysis in all women with anti-Fy^a since there is poor correlation with maternal antibody titres. A neonatal mortality rate of 15% has been reported, and an exchange transfusion rate of 35% may be anticipated in affected infants.

Lewis blood group system

Antibodies to the antigens of this system (Le^a and Le^b) do not cause haemolytic disease since they are mostly IgM and do not therefore cross the placenta. Recently, sensitive ELISA assays have shown IgG Lewis antibodies to be present in cord sera. However, since the Lewis antigen only develops in early childhood, fetal red cells have a low level of Lewis antigens so that they do not bind the IgG anti-Le^a to cause significant HDFN.

Kidd blood group system

Pregnancy, rather than blood transfusions, seems to be the triggering sensitizing event in the Kidd system. All grades of severity of HDFN including stillbirth have been reported with anti-Jk^a, while anti-Jk^b causes mild haemolytic disease generally requiring no treatment. A third antibody, anti-Jk^3, has been reported in one case of mild disease.

MNSs blood group system

Antibodies to these antigens are predominantly naturally-occurring complete cold agglutinins of the IgM class, and therefore not able to cause haemolytic disease. However, anti-M and anti-N have been reported in the IgG fraction and can be pathological. Similarly, antibodies to S and s have also been associated with haemolytic disease. The other major antigen of this system is U. All whites are U^+; the U^- phenotype is only encountered in African negroes. As all grades of severity of disease can occur with all of these antigens, sensitized patients should be followed with serial amniotic fluid studies.

Lutheran blood group system

The antigens, Lu^a and Lu^b, are both associated with mild disease requiring no treatment, with Lu^a being most common. The Lutheran antigen on the fetal red cell is not fully developed, so that maternal sensitization is not marked, nor is the relevant fetal antigen expressed sufficiently to be involved in a significant antibody response.

Xg blood group system

The antigen for this system is carried on the X chromosome and only one case of haemolytic disease is reported following the development of maternal autoimmune anti-Xg^a antibodies.

Diego blood group system

This antigen system (Di^a and Di^b) is considered to be Mongolian in origin and is rare in whites or blacks. It is present in 5–15% of Orientals and 36% of South American Indians. A few cases of all grades of severity of haemolytic disease have been reported, so that serial amniotic fluid studies should be performed in the management of sensitized pregnant women.

P blood group system

Only anti-PP_1P_k has been associated with haemolytic disease of the newborn of all grades of severity. Amniotic fluid studies are therefore necessary.

Private and public antigens

Public antigens are those which occur in 99% of the population, so that only the remaining 1% are at risk of becoming sensitized. Eight public antigens have been associated with haemolytic disease of varying severity, but only three are of clincal significance. A private antigen occurs in only 0.25% of the population, and 6 have been associated with isolated cases of HDFN. Management of these rare cases should include serial amniotic fluid analysis.

The known clinically significant antigens associated with HDFN are summarized in Table 4. The clinically most significant 'immune antibodies', other than anti-D, are anti-Kell and anti-Fy^a (Duffy). The majority of antibodies are naturally occurring. Optimum management includes antenatal screening on several occasions throughout pregnancy, with amniotic fluid analysis if indicated, and appropriate neonatal support for the prematurely delivered infant.

Table 4. Clinically significant irregular antigens.

Kell	K
Duffy	Fy^a
Kidd	Jk^a/JK^b
MNSs	M, S, s, U
I	Mi^a, Mt^b
Diego	Di^a Di^b
P	PP_1pk
Public	Yt^a, En^a, Co^a
Private	Biles, Good, Heibel, Radin, Wright, Zd

LEUKOCYTE ISOIMMUNIZATION

Pregnant and parous women frequently possess leukocyte isoantibodies (Shulman et al, 1964). The incidence and titre of antibodies increases with parity and may also be influenced by prior blood transfusions which deliver human leukocyte antigens (HLA) determined by haplotypes that are common to those of the paternal contribution(s) to the fetal genetic constitution. Leukocyte antibodies may appear for the first time in the maternal circulation by mid-pregnancy in primiparous women and as early as 8 weeks' gestation in multiparous pregnancies. Implicit in the occurrence of these isoantibodies is the passage of sensitizing leukocytes into the mother across the placenta during pregnancy or at the time of placental separation. This accords with similar mechanisms relating to the traffic of fetal erythrocytes; however, direct evidence for maternal exposure to fetal leukocytes is scanty. It was demonstrated in the 1960s that both leukocytes and platelets derived from fluoresceinated donor blood used in intrauterine fetal transfusions could be detected subsequently in maternal blood within hours of the procedure.

Other studies carried out during pregnancy using chromosome markers for fetal cells have suggested that between 0.1% and 2.0% of leukocytes in maternal blood are of fetal origin and that their transfer may commence as early as 15 weeks' gestation. The results of these studies have been questioned both on methodological grounds and by reference to the calculated extent of feto–maternal 'leakage' of blood, as extrapolated from accurate estimates of the concentration of fetal erythrocytes in maternal blood in late pregnancy. Given that the volume of fetal blood gaining excess to the mother during pregnancy may on occasions reach 2.0 ml, but may be as low as 0.1 ml, the maximum ratio of fetal to maternal leukocytes to be expected in the mother would be of the order of 1:1500, at which level fetal cells would be virtually impossible to detect by any known means (see Chapter 11). The ability to identify fetal leukocytes in maternal blood would also depend on the presence of pre-existing leukocytotoxic antibodies in the mother since these would rapidly clear any 'foreign' cells containing their target antigen(s). Conversely, relative histocompatibility of the mother with her fetus would theoretically allow the longer survival and easier detection of fetal cells in her circulation. Greater numbers of fetal leukocytes might be expected to gain entry to the maternal circulation at the time of placental separation but comprehensive data on postpartum blood samples are unavailable.

The high incidence of leukocyte isoimmunization in the face of such a low level of exposure to fetal cells can be construed as a testimony to the immunogenicity of leukocyte antigens. There are other mechanisms, however, whereby the mother may be sensitized to such antigens. HLA antigens in soluble form may cross the placenta and contribute to maternal isoimmunization. In addition, there is evidence for the existence of antigens that are common to both leukocytes, trophoblast and spermatozoal cells, and these could be a source of cross-reactive sensitization.

Clinical significance

Maternal isoimmunization against fetal leukocytes is common, more so than similar reactions involving the less immunogenic erythrocyte antigens.

Leukocytes carry erythrocyte antigens, including those of the ABO, MN and P systems, but not of the Rh system. In addition, they have antigens (particularly the HLA system) not present on erythrocytes; these antigens have been detected and characterized using sera from individuals who have received multiple blood transfusions or from multiparous women. The sera of parous women contain monospecific antibodies (i.e. directed against paternal genotype) more often than do the sera of transfusion recipients in whom antibodies of different specificities are found. Pregnancy sera have therefore proved useful as a convenient source of HLA typing antibodies. The incidence of multispecific antibodies in maternal sera appears to increase with parity.

Leukocyte antibodies have been detected and characterized using techniques of agglutination, cytotoxicity and complement-fixation. The incidence and pattern of appearance of antibodies varies with the method used for their detection, and may be influenced by the source of the test cells. The greater the range of antigen specificities present in the test cell panel, the more antibodies are likely to be revealed.

Overall about 30% of maternal sera contain HLA antibodies. Their incidence increases with parity and, somewhat curiously, they may disappear in some instances within several months postpartum. One intriguing aspect of isoimmunization against leukocyte antigens is the fact that this phenomenon reflects a possible mechanism whereby the allogenic conceptus, and ultimately the placenta, escapes recognition and attack by the maternal immune system. There is evidence that an appropriate 'protective' maternal immune response to fetal (paternal) antigens is necessary to circumvent reproductive failure manifest in conditions such as recurrent abortion (Chapter 4) and pregnancy-induced hypertension (Chapter 5). Thus, women with these disorders may demonstrate a high degree of histocompatibility with their male partner and may fail to develop antibodies directed against paternal antigens coded for by the MHC or related gene loci in their first pregnancy. The 'markers' that have been most studied in this regard are cytotoxic and non-cytotoxic antibodies directed against both T and B lymphocytes.

In contrast to the potential protective effect of maternal recognition of fetal antigens, it is reasonable to assume that leukocyte isoimmunization might have direct deleterious effects on pregnancy, particularly since HLA antibodies can be demonstrated in up to 20% of the newborn of isoimmunized women. This does not appear to be the case, however, apart from the evidence from infrequent reports of cases of neonatal leukopaenia, admittedly some of which have been severe, even fatal. There has been one unconfirmed study describing a high incidence of prematurity, increasing with parity, in women with leukocyte agglutinins in their sera but there appears to be no association between leukocyte isoantibodies and the rates of abortion, perinatal mortality, neonatal infection or congenital abnormalities.

The reasons why leukocyte isoimmunization appears to be a benign phenomenon are conjectural, but the following explanations have been advanced:

1. Leukocyte numbers vary widely in neonates and it may be difficult to distinguish a pathological count from one at the lower limit of the physiological range.
2. The leukocyte pool in the bone marrow is large by contrast with the erythrocyte pool, so that mild cell destruction is easily compensated.
3. Variations in the specificity, titre and IgG subclass of the maternal antibodies.
4. The role of the placenta as an immunoabsorbent filtering out at least some of the cytotoxic HLA antibodies which might otherwise attack fetal leukocytes. This presupposes a mechanism whereby the binding of HLA antibodies within the placenta is at sites (probably in the villous stroma) which circumvent a potentially equally harmful effect on the syncytiotrophoblast.
5. Fetal tissues themselves may also be capable of absorbing low titres of leukocyte antibodies, thereby protecting the white cells.

PLATELET ISOIMMUNIZATION

There is no direct evidence for the presence of fetal platelets in maternal blood under physiological conditions. However, in view of the clear evidence for the existence of platelet isoimmunization, and by analogy with the mechanisms described above for leukocytes, there can be no doubt that the pregnant woman is exposed to platelet antigens.

Platelets carry antigens which are common to erythrocytes or leukocytes but, in addition, at least six which are platelet-specific. Isoimmune neonatal thrombocytopaenia is rare and is due to the transplacental passage of antibodies to the platelet antigen systems, PLA1 (most commonly), PLB1 and PLE (Kelton et al, 1980; Chandler and Daniel, 1985). These antibodies are designated as platelet-bindable IgG (PBIgG), in contrast to those present in individuals with autoimmune thrombocytopaenic purpura (ATP) which are called platelet-associated IgG (PAIgG).

Clinical significance

The detection of PBIgG antibodies in maternal and neonatal serum has proved vexatious using methods such as agglutination, cytotoxicity and complement fixation but has become more accurate with the advent of solid phase antigen–antibody binding techniques. The incidence of platelet isoimmunization is unclear but its clinical importance is confined to the situation where a newborn baby develops purpura in the absence of serological or clinical evidence of ATP in the mother. In the latter situation, the placental transfer of platelet autoantibodies (PA IgG) is a common cause of passive ATP in the infants of mothers so affected.

Isoimmune neonatal thrombocytopaenia may be severe and fatal due to intracranial haemorrhage, but if treated adequately is benign and self-limiting in keeping with the half-life of the offending antibodies. Its serological distinction from neonatal ATP is vital since the management is different in each instance. In contrast to neonatal ATP, where corticosteroids and random donor platelet infusions are effective, the baby affected by platelet isoantibodies of maternal origin requires treatment with maternal platelets, which, lacking the relevant iso- (allo-) antigen, will escape immune destruction.

REFERENCES

Barnes RMR, Duguid JKM, Roberts FM et al (1987) Oral administration of erythrocyte membrane antigen does not suppress anti-Rh(D) antibody responses in humans. *Clinical and Experimental Immunology* **67:** 220.

Beal RW (1985) Non-Rhesus (D) blood group isoimmunization in obstetrics. *Clinical Obstetrics and Gynaecology* **6:** 493.

Benacarref BR & Frigoletto FD (1985) Sonographic sign for the detection of early fetal ascites in the management of severe isoimmune disease without transfusion. *American Journal of Obstetrics and Gynaecology* **152:** 1039.

Berlin G, Selbing A & Ryden G (1985) Rhesus haemolytic disease treated with high-dose intravenous immunoglobulin. *Lancet* **i:** 1153.

Chandler D & Daniel SJ (1985) Isoimmune neonatal thrombocytopaenia: A case report and review. *American Journal of Clinical Pathology* **83:** 766.

Clarke C (1982) Historical annotation: Rhesus haemolytic disease of the newborn and its prevention. *British Journal of Haematology* **52:** 525.

Coombs RRA, Mourant AE & Race RR (1945) Detection of weak and incomplete Rh agglutinations: a new test. *Lancet* **ii:** 15.

de Crespigny L Ch, Robinson HP, Quinn M et al (1985) Ultrasound-guided fetal blood transfusion for severe Rhesus isoimmunization. *Obstetrics and Gynecology* **66:** 529.

Davey M (1979) The prevention of Rhesus-isoimmunisation. *Clinical Obstetrics and Gynaecology* **6:** 493.

Gold WR, Queenan JT, Woody J & Sacher RA (1983) Oral desensitisation in Rh disease. *American Journal of Obstetrics and Gynecology* **146:** 980.

Hughes-Jones NC (1975) Red-cell antigens, antibodies, and their interaction. *Clinical Haematology* **4:** 29.

Johnson PM & Brown PJ (1981) Fc_γ receptors in the human placenta. *Placenta* **2:** 355.

Kelton JG, Blanchette VS, Wilson WE et al (1980) Neonatal thrombocytopaenia due to passive immunisation. *New England Journal of Medicine* **302:** 1401.

Kochenour NK & Scott JR (1985) Rh isoimmunization in pregnancy. In Scott JR & Rote NS (eds) *Immunology in Obstetrics and Gynaecology*, p 141. Norwalk: Appleton-Century-Crofts.

Liley AW (1961) Liquor amnii analysis in management of pregnancy complicated by rhesus sensitization. *American Journal of Obstetrics and Gynecology* **82:** 285.

Lockyer WJ (1982) ABO haemolytic disease of the newborn: Laboratory prediction and postnatal diagnosis. *Medical Laboratory Science* **39:** 287.

Nicolaides KH & Rodek CH (1985) Rhesus disease: The model for fetal therapy. *British Journal of Hospital Medicine* **34:** 141.

Race RR & Sanger R (1975) *Blood Groups in Man.* Oxford: Blackwell.

Robinson A & Tovey LAD (1980) Intensive plasma exchange in the management of severe Rh disease. *British Journal of Haematology* **45:** 621.

Shulman NR, Marder JV, Hiller MC & Collier EM (1964) Platelet and leucocyte isoantigens and their antibodies: Serology, physiology and clinical studies. *Progress in Haematology* **4:** 222.

Urbaniak SJ, Ayoub GM, Crawford, RJ & Fergusson MCJ (1981) Prediction of the severity of Rhesus haemolytic disease of the newborn by an ADCC assay. *Lancet* **ii:** 142.

Wiener AS (1944) The Rh series of allelic genes. *Science* **100:** 595.

4

Recurrent miscarriage

P. M. JOHNSON
G. H. RAMSDEN

CLINICAL BACKGROUND

The terms miscarriage and spontaneous abortion are synonymous and are the commonest complication of pregnancy. It is generally accepted that the frequency of clinically recognized miscarriage is approximately 15%, mostly in the first trimester; with sensitive and specific β-human chorionic gonadotrophin (hCG) estimation, detection of unsuspected pregnancy loss can increase the incidence to 30–60%. Recurrent miscarriage (RM) is defined by the occurrence of three or more consecutive spontaneous abortions and the population incidence has been put at up to 1% of the gravida 3 or more female population (Alberman, 1988). Chromosomal, anatomical and endocrinological causes have traditionally been implicated (Stirrat, 1983), but RM remains a distressing and frustrating condition since as many as 50% of all RM patients have no recognized cause (Tho et al, 1979; Stray-Pedersen and Stray-Pedersen, 1984; see also Figure 1).

Treatment is often empirical, although most evidence suggests the chance of success in the next pregnancy after three previous consecutive miscarriages is in the range 40–70% (Warburton and Fraser, 1964; Poland et al,

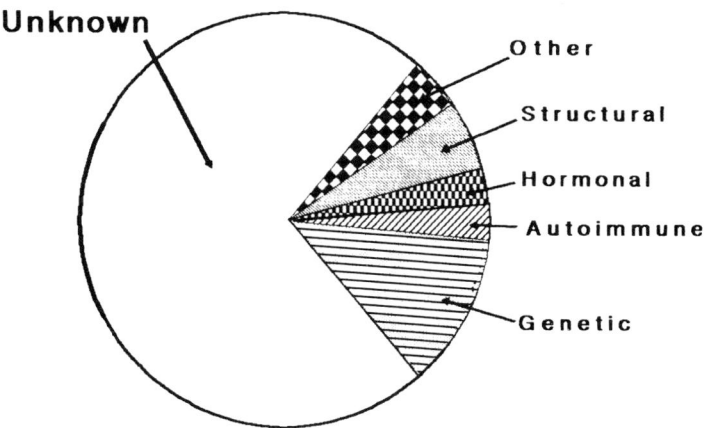

Figure 1. A notional distribution of identified causes of *recurrent* miscarriage.

1977; Alberman, 1988). Investigations in RM have been beset by inconsistencies related to variations in local patient selection or referral policies from a large and often disillusioned potential pool of RM patients. Similar considerations apply in the assessment of therapeutic modalities, including the absence of double-blind controlled trials. There has been growing interest, however, in the last decade regarding possible immunological causes of previously unexplained RM (Beer, 1986; Johnson et al, 1986; McIntyre et al, 1986; Scott et al, 1987). This chapter reviews this work.

It is necessary first to mention briefly other aetiologies of RM since it is only after detailed exclusion that an immunological basis can be proposed. These include genetic causes and, with newer banding techniques, the number of detected abnormalities of parental karyotypes is rising. Tharapel et al (1985) showed an overall prevalence of chromosomal abnormalities in couples with two or more pregnancy losses to be 2.9%, five to six times higher than the general population. It has been reported that 50–60% of *culturable* spontaneous abortions have chromosomal abnormalities (Simpson, 1980; Tharapel et al, 1985), although most arise spontaneously from non-inheritable random errors in meiosis and mitosis or from polyspermy. The risk of recurrence is low and, indeed, the chromosomal abnormality rate in abortuses of RM couples may be only 6% (Simpson, 1980). Other aetiologies may include malformations of the uterus or cervix, corpus luteum deficiencies, persistent infection, thyroid disease, diabetes and other possible contributory maternal medical disorders (Glass and Golbus, 1978; Beer, 1986; Ramsden and Johnson, 1988).

We have investigated at a miscarriage clinic 300 RM couples with a mean of 4.42 ± 2.15 prior consecutive spontaneous abortions (range 3–17). Surprisingly, two women demonstrated marked thrombocythaemia with platelet counts in excess of 700×10^9/litre, one of whom subsequently had an uncomplicated term pregnancy following chemotherapy to reduce the platelet count to within the normal range. A similar prevalence of overt thrombocythaemia in unexplained RM patients has also been noted by Dr Cowchock at Thomas Jefferson University, Philadelphia; the overall prevalence of 0.7% at the two centres is significantly increased compared with the general antenatal population ($< 0.05\%$) (Cowchock and Johnson, unpublished data).

LUPUS ANTICOAGULANT AND RECURRENT INTRAUTERINE FETAL DEATH

Between 2–4% of RM women attending the miscarriage clinic have clearly detectable lupus anticoagulant autoantibody (anti-phospholipid autoantibody, APA; see Chapter 7 for a full description including that for APA immunoassay and phospholipid-dependent coagulation tests). Of these RM women, a majority had a significant clinical history involving thrombosis, pulmonary disease or vasculitis. Two patients had strong APA activity which had not been identified in pre-pregnancy screening and became detectable only during early pregnancy. Both pregnancies resulted in subsequent intrauterine fetal death.

Although only 15% of APA-positive individuals may present as clearcut cases of systemic lupus erythematosus (SLE), there is undoubtedly a strong association between the occurrence of these antibodies and recurrent fetal death (Lockshin et al, 1985; Branch, 1987). The mechanism of adverse action of APA in pregnancy has been attributed to several mechanisms (Scott et al, 1987). It is thought that APA acts on vascular tissues to inhibit release of EDRF (endothelial-derived relaxin factor) and prostacyclin, a potent vasodilator, as well as inhibiting endothelial cell-mediated activation of protein C to promote a net effect of vasoconstriction and local vascular thrombosis (Lubbe and Liggins, 1985; Scott et al, 1987). Purified antibody fractions with APA activity have not been isolated for experimental purposes and no suitable animal model has yet been derived for testing either therapeutic models or hypothetical mechanisms of action by passive antibody transfer. Lupus anticoagulant has classically been associated with fetal loss in the second trimester; however, with improved laboratory detection of APA, it is now becoming clear that the incidence of fetal loss may be highest (>50%) in the first trimester, compared with 25% in the second and 15% in the third. In these later cases, pregnancy failure may be more clearly identified with an increased degree of placental infarction and utero-placental thrombosis.

Treatment for lupus anticoagulant RM patients in pregnancy has largely been carried out on an empirical basis although, without treatment, fetal prognosis is very poor. The risk of utero-placental thrombosis can be reduced by low-dose aspirin (75 mg daily), which may often be effective in uncomplicated patients with mildly elevated APA antibodies but not necessarily those with markedly prolonged activated partial thromboplastin time (APTT) or kaolin-cephalin clotting time (KCCT) or pronounced previous clinical history. Otherwise, combined aspirin and high-dose steroid therapy may be the combination of choice, particularly during early pregnancy, to suppress coagulation times and APA levels to within the normal range (Lubbe and Liggins, 1985). Maternal complications can arise with continuing successful pregnancy associated with high-dose steroid therapy, including osteoporosis or increased hypertension during pregnancy (Branch, 1987). In general, the risk to the fetus from use of prednisone is minimal. Azathioprine has not proven a useful alternative to prednisone. Plasmapheresis can be used to attain rapid reduction in circulating APA levels in high-risk situations or if there is concern about continuing use of high-dose prednisone; intravenous gammaglobulin, although expensive, may also prove effective in similar situations. Subcutaneous heparin has been administered to lupus anticoagulant patients with apparent success (Scott et al, 1987), but will alter plasma coagulation times and may complicate interpretation of regular laboratory monitoring of patient progress. Initial indications have also suggested that heparin may be useful in some patients with repeated second-trimester fetal loss, with or without detectable APA or lupus anticoagulant, although the mode of action of heparin remains obscure in such cases. All treatments of lupus anticoagulant in pregnancy need regular laboratory monitoring of coagulation times and APA antibody for predicting the course of the condition and possible adverse effects to the fetus or mother. Because fetal prognosis is so poor without treatment, it is difficult to justify placebo-controlled randomized trials; however, comparative randomized therapeutic studies would be of considerable benefit.

IMMUNOGENETIC STUDIES IN UNEXPLAINED RECURRENT MISCARRIAGE

Polymorphisms within the major histocompatibility gene complex (MHC) substantially contribute to materno-fetal genetic disparity which is of considerable potential biological relevance in human pregnancy. Since cell surface HLA antigens encoded within the MHC region are the focus of mechanisms of T cell restriction, rejection of allografts and control of the immune response, they are presumed to be of crucial importance in the immunogenetic enigma of successful reproduction (Beer and Billingham, 1977; Johnson and Stern, 1986).

Extensive data has now accumulated to show that chorionic villous trophoblast normally lacks expression of any class I or II MHC antigen, and this must be of fundamental significance in passive protection of trophoblastic tissue from maternal immune attack (Bulmer and Johnson, 1985; Lessin et al, 1988). However, there is now current interest in a 40 kD class I-like MHC antigen detected on most extravillous cytotrophoblast in the placental bed and extraembryonic tissues, as well as on certain choriocarcinoma cells, and also in possible factors that might regulate class I MHC antigen expression by trophoblast (Ellis et al, 1986; Johnson and Stern, 1986; Head et al, 1987; Bulmer et al, 1988; Hsi et al, 1988). This antigen may represent either the translated product of a novel human class I MHC gene or an unusual product, perhaps closely related to HLA-C, resultant from atypical post-transcriptional processing of a class I MHC gene in invasive cytotrophoblast.

In addition, antibodies in placental eluates and some multiparous sera may identify HLA-related determinants of limited polymorphism which are separate from classical HLA alloantigens (Johnson and Stern, 1986; Konoeda et al, 1986). Current speculation suggests that fetal trophoblastic expression of a class I MHC antigen may contribute to induction of specialized pregnancy-associated maternal immunological mechanisms involving both antibody and suppressor-type cellular activities which protect the fetus from adverse allograft rejection responses. Such host responses would be expected to be more elusive to identify than, for example, classical cytotoxic responses to HLA antigens.

Evolutionary mechanisms which have generated polymorphisms within MHC gene loci, and the selective pressures to maintain them within a species, are little understood. There is evidence ranging from primitive tunicates to inbred mammalian species indicating a superior reproductive proficiency of MHC heterozygotes (Beer and Billingham, 1977; Gill and Repetti, 1979). This has often been interpreted as showing materno-fetal histoincompatibility to be advantageous for reproductive performance, with selection in favour of the heterozygote in offspring of inbred animals taking place in utero, although syngeneic matings do not prominently involve recurrent fetal wastage. There is HLA data from closed communities supporting a similar effect in humans (Ober et al, 1983). It is uncertain whether this may result from either essential maternal immunoregulatory recognition of paternally-inherited fetal alloantigens or MHC hetero-zygosity favouring a broader capacity for antigen presentation (e.g. in the spectrum of immune responses to intrauterine pathogens). Although appearing to represent natural selection contributing to maintenance of genetic polymorphism within MHC, this effect is not absolute and must involve many complex genetic factors. Thus, for example, HLA-identical feto-maternal combinations can be found among normal term pregnancies (Kilpatrick, 1984; Jazwinska et al, 1987). Conversely, completely HLA-non-identical feto-maternal combinations are found in examples of donor oocyte pregnancies.

Significant HLA segregation distortion does not seem to occur in humans, as determined by inheritance patterns (Klitz et al, 1987), apart from some diabetic families where there may be prenatal intrauterine selection to the advantage of HLA-DR3 and HLA-DR4 bearing haplotypes (Vadheim et al, 1986). It is, nonetheless, attractive to propose a relationship between parental HLA haplotypes and risk of miscarriage (Diamond, 1987; Gill, 1987). A genetic variation within the MHC complex (i.e. deletion, dupli-cation, mutation or recombination), or linkage disequilibrium with a disease-associated gene, could pronouncedly influence intrauterine prenatal selection. This could act either through a direct biological consequence or through defective immunogenetic signalling which may be necessary for the normal protective response of the mother to the fetal allograft. Other considerations have centred on the concepts that feto-maternal histocom-patibility may be associated either with a greater likelihood of entry of maternal lymphocytes to cause fetal engraftment leading to graft-versus-host disease or with decreased activation of decidual leukocytes and local production of cytokines that could normally benefit placental growth and development (Clark et al, 1987).

It is against this background that there has been much recent enthusiasm for parental HLA studies in unexplained recurrent miscarriage, although the initial promise of this approach has failed yet to reach fruition. Parental HLA sharing in RM compared with controls has been reported both as significantly increased (Komlos et al, 1977; Unander and Olding, 1983; Beer et al, 1985; McIntyre et al, 1986; Coulam et al, 1987; Ober et al, 1987) and as not significantly increased (Oksenberg et al, 1984; Cauchi et al, 1987; Johnson et al, 1985, 1988a). The data is mostly fragmentary and inconsistent between centres, although Reznikoff-Etievant et al (1988) have analysed pooled data from 21 centres and shown statistically significant increased sharing for HLA-DR and, less so, for HLA-B. Nevertheless, on closer analysis, results from individual centres have tended to fall just on either side of a line of significance at the 1% level. This variation could be expected because of inconsistent definition of RM, the choice of control couples, low numbers in the study groups and different tissue typing methodology (particularly the number of HLA-DR antigens assessed with the typing antiserum panel). General population studies have shown that parental HLA compatibility is not a significant selective factor in determining which paternal haplotype is expressed in live-born offspring (MacQueen and Sanfilippo, 1984).

Similar conclusions have been reached when HLA data has been analysed for HLA homozygosity: thus, significantly increased apparent HLA-DQ and HLA-DR locus homozygosity (Coulam et al, 1987), as well as apparent HLA-B and C4 locus homozygosity (Johnson et al, 1985, 1988a), has been reported in unexplained RM women. These observations do not involve the majority of RM women and may not necessarily be repeated in results from all other centres. Indeed, it is likely that HLA tissue typing will prove to be of little clinical usefulness in the identification or determination of prognosis in RM patients. Because these serological HLA studies may reflect weak phenomena resultant from adjacent genetic effects within the MHC region, it is possible that a detailed study of DNA restriction fragment length polymorphisms (RFLPs) could identify more precisely any MHC gene-linked event associated with RM. However, our preliminary work to date has noted no unusual RFLP patterns in RM women compared with controls using cDNA or genomic probes for tumour necrosis factor (TNF_α), C4, $HLA-DQ_\alpha$ or various 'locus-specific' class I MHC probes (Risk and Johnson, unpublished observations).

IMMUNOLOGICAL STUDIES

Cell-mediated immunity

Initial observations suggested decreased maternal cellular responsiveness to paternal stimulator cells in a mixed lymphocyte reaction (MLR) for RM couples compared with controls (Lauritsen et al, 1976; Beer et al, 1981; McIntyre et al, 1986). However, this has not proven to be a consistent or clinically exploitable phenomenon of intrinsic cellular hyporesponsiveness (Chia and Johnson, unpublished data). Reported data may result from the marginally increased maternal–paternal HLA sharing and, notably when the assay is performed in autologous serum, the presence of serum blocking factors (see below). There are no significant differences in mean absolute numbers or relative percentages of the major T lymphocyte subpopulations in peripheral blood of RM women compared with controls (Fiddes et al, 1986; Chia and Johnson, 1987).

There have been no consistent reports of histopathological evidence of immune-mediated attack in the placenta of an abortus (see Chapter 8). Indeed, local cellular events at the feto-maternal interface in spontaneously aborted material have been little studied because of difficulties in obtaining such fresh tissues and confusion with post-abortion inflammatory cellular changes. It has been proposed from murine studies that soluble factors in decidual tissues which suppress interleukin-2 (IL-2) dependent cellular responses may be absent in certain situations of intrauterine fetal demise

(Daya et al, 1987). The mechanism of induction of soluble suppressor activity from human decidual mononuclear cells is unclear, but could involve a contribution from direct molecular signals provided by pre-implantation embryos and trophoblast cell surface components (Daya and Clark, 1988; Daya et al, 1988).

Humoral immunity

Production of serum antibodies which inhibit a wide variety of in vitro lymphocyte proliferation or function assays is a common feature in normal pregnancy, notably arising after the first-trimester. This phenomenon is not observed in RM women, either during or after unsuccessful pregnancies (Rocklin et al, 1976; Stimson et al, 1979; Unander et al, 1983; Beer et al, 1985; Power et al, 1986). Such activity may require a concentration of up to 29% serum for optimal assay in MLR inhibition studies (Takakuwa et al, 1986). However, it is not an entirely consistent phenomenon, and hence could be a consequence rather than cause of repeated early pregnancy failure.

The origin of so-called 'blocking antibodies' normally found in pregnancy cannot be fully explained by discrete anti-HLA specificities. It could also involve variable contributions from antibodies reactive with other leukocyte differentiation antigens (some of which may be common also to tropho-blast), or auto-anti-idiotypic specificities (Editorial, 1983; Johnson and Stern, 1986), or even soluble fetal HLA in maternal blood. Indeed, blocking effects that are not mediated by antibody may be of central importance in these assay systems, such as the inhibition of IL-2 activity given by retro-placental sera (Nicholas and Panayi, 1986). The role of any immunoglobulin effector specificity in immunobiological events central to establishment of pregnancy or survival of the intrauterine fetal allograft has been cogently challenged by Rodger (1985), based on normal pregnancies in B cell deficient agammaglobulinaemic mice, as indeed is also the case in agamma-globulinaemic women. Thus, the basis for this blocking phenomenon remains obscure, but perhaps this functional assay, rather than direct sero-logical binding assays, may still be the most fruitful area for further research in normal pregnancy and in RM women before and after immunotherapy (see next section).

Other approaches have identified two separate groups of women suffering repeated fetal loss: (i) no live birth or pregnancy exceeding 28 weeks gestation (primary RM), and (ii) a single live birth or pregnancy of at least 28 weeks gestation preceding the unbroken series of pregnancy losses (secondary RM). In contrast to the reports above, which generally favour absence of blocking antibody effects in unexplained RM women without immunotherapy, one group has identified maternal serum inhibition of materno-paternal MLR that occurs only in the secondary RM grouping (McIntyre et al, 1986). This appears also to be associated with strong serum lymphocytotoxic antibody (LCA) activity with wide panel reactivity (McIntyre et al, 1986). However, other centres have not noted a significantly increased prevalence of LCA in secondary RM compared with primary RM women (Cauchi et al, 1987;

Johnson et al, 1988a). Approximately 15–20% of women develop LCA detectable by microlymphocytotoxicity assay after their first term pregnancy, often with a wider specificity than solely for discrete paternal HLA allo-antigens. Conversely, LCA have been detected in only 10–20% of all unexplained RM women (Mowbray and Underwood, 1985; Cauchi et al, 1987; Johnson et al, 1988a). This was interpreted initially as being in line with immunological hyporesponsiveness to fetal antigens in RM. However, a more pertinent comparison with women who have had three or more elective abortions has shown that only 4% of this latter multigravid group had detectable LCA compared with 13% RM patients (Biddle et al, 1987).

Other parameters of specific immune responsiveness have also been studied which could be particularly relevant. One interesting example is evidence that both humoral and cellular immunity to cytomegalovirus (CMV) is significantly impaired in RM women, unlike for their male partners or age-matched female controls, whereas humoral immunity to other herpes viruses (*Herpes simplex* virus and Epstein–Barr virus) is not reduced in RM women (Radcliffe et al, 1986). These observations highlight the point that investigation of the interrelationship of immunity and infection in RM women has largely been ignored. Studies of tissue-reactive autoantibodies or total serum IgE levels have failed to identify parameters characteristic of any clinical subset of RM women (Johnson et al, 1988a). Several groups have attempted to develop laboratory assays for detection of any serum antibodies reactive with human placental trophoblast membrane antigens. There is some controversy regarding the performance and interpretation of these binding assays, which are usually based on ELISA. We have been unable to detect significant serum immunoglobulin binding activity to isolated tropho-blast membrane antigen preparations for multiparous pregnant women or primary RM women compared with controls, although a small number of LCA-positive secondary RM women did demonstrate significantly elevated binding activity (Hole et al, 1987).

IMMUNOTHERAPY

The earlier investigational studies formed the original basis for immunization with paternal or third-party unmatched leukocytes as immunotherapy in unexplained RSA (Beer et al, 1981; Taylor and Faulk, 1981). The general concept was that occasional RM women had abnormalities in the immuno-logical recognition response to early pregnancy (Rocklin et al, 1976; Unander et al, 1985; Johnson et al, 1986; McIntyre et al, 1986; Clark et al, 1987). This could involve either intrinsic maternal hyporesponsiveness (which would be partner-nonspecific) or incomplete maternal recognition due to materno-fetal allelic identity of a relevant genetically polymorphic antigen (which would be partner-specific). The rationale for immunization involves priming for immunoregulatory alloresponses other than by pregnancy.

Selection of RM women is principally by exclusion of all other known causes as determined by taking a thorough clinical history, examination and investigations to include karyotypic analyses, hysterosalpingogram, endo-

Table 1. Examples of immunotherapy in RM patients.

Immunogen	Route	Patients with subsequent pregnancies	Live births (%)	Reference
Paternal leukocytes	Intradermal Intravenous Subcutaneous	22	77	Mowbray et al, 1985
Paternal leukocytes	Intradermal	7	71	Takakuwa et al, 1986
Paternal leukocytes	Intradermal	37	70	Beer et al, 1985
Paternal leukocytes	Intradermal Intravenous Subcutaneous	28	93	Reznikoff-Etievant et al, 1988
Third-party leukocytes	Intravenous	21	82	Taylor et al, 1985
Third-party leukocytes	Intravenous	12	92	Unander & Lindholm, 1986
Trophoblast membrane vesicles	Intravenous	21	76	Johnson et al, 1988c

cervical swab cultures and thyroid function tests. Most immunotherapeutic studies would also exclude women with a history of aneuploidic pregnancy loss, detectable serum anti-nuclear or anti-phospholipid autoantibody, clinical evidence of autoimmune disease or an abnormal full blood count (Beer, 1986; Johnson et al, 1988b; Ramsden and Johnson, 1988). These women fall into an, as yet, unexplained group of RM patients and it would be unjustified to assume a single common mechanism for all such cases of RM.

Reports of successful pregnancy outcome after leukocyte immunization are accumulating steadily (Table 1). Although the cell source (paternal or third-party), dose (from 10^8 cells to large multiple transfusions) and route of administration (intravenous, intradermal, subcutaneous, with or without repeated immunization) has varied significantly between centres, initial studies have described successful pregnancies in 70–93% of cases. Patient referral and selection has varied significantly between centres; for example, some exclude LCA-positive women, partly because of risk of anaphylactic reaction and partly because the presence of LCA would indicate that maternal immune responses to fetal alloantigens had indeed occurred in a previous pregnancy. The strength of the 'placebo' effect in these studies remains obscure, although undoubtedly psychological support plays an important role in the clinical approach to women with unexplained RM (Grimm, 1962). Thus, for example, there have also been strikingly success-ful claims for the success of supportive psychotherapy (Stray-Pedersen and Stray-Pedersen, 1984; Vlaanderen and Treffers, 1987). Only one controlled trial of immunotherapy has been reported, showing 78% success in RM women immunized with paternal leukocytes compared with 37% in RM women receiving their own leukocytes (Mowbray et al, 1985). Most epi-demiological studies have indicated the likelihood of successful pregnancy after three previous miscarriages to be of the order or 60% (Alberman, 1988). Whether RM women who fulfil selection criteria for immunotherapy represent a particularly poor prognosis without active therapy is still to be fully evaluated (Reginald et al, 1987).

Although convenient, immunization of healthy women with viable leukocytes should be approached with caution, and only carried out at research centres with appropriate multidisciplinary interests. Thus, for example, concomitant sensitization to platelet or blood group antigens may compromise a subsequent pregnancy, although leukocyte immunization can be given with anti-Rh(D) immunoglobulin cover when necessary. Sensitization to fetal HLA or other leukocyte antigens may occur, and the full significance of such events for any possible clinical sequelae in mother or fetus remain unclear. Severe intrauterine growth retardation has been reported following immunization (Beer et al, 1985; Cauchi et al, 1987), but no increased risk has been noted at other centres (Taylor et al, 1985; Mowbray et al, 1987). Preterm labour may also be common in RM patients following immunotherapy. Transfusion-related risks have to be considered, including possible viral (e.g. CMV or HIV) transmission by viable leukocytes (Radcliffe et al, 1986). Following leukocyte immunization, Hofmeyr et al (1987) found systemic side-effects to be common. Finally, some genetic developmental abnormalities have occurred in pregnancies following immunization but, since RM patients tend to be in the higher age-groups, it is difficult to ascertain whether there is any increased risk apart from possibly in those couples with pronounced parental HLA sharing (Beer et al, 1985). It should still be remembered that it is quicker to identify successful outcome than risk factors in these therapeutic approaches to RM, an area with substantial emotive pressure. Long-term follow-up of RM patients and their infants is required before these controversial issues are finally settled.

Alternative approaches may also require exploration. Intravenous infusion with isolated sterile syncytiotrophoblast microvillous plasma membrane vesicle preparations, although less convenient than leukocyte immunization, has the advantage of being HLA-negative and mimics one example of fetal cellular contact with the maternal immune system in normal pregnancy (Johnson et al, 1988b,c). Initial results have shown a similar success for trophoblast membrane infusion (TMI) as that reported following leukocyte immunization (Table 1), without any significant adverse reactions (Johnson et al, 1988b). Secondary RM patients appear to respond as well as primary RM patients from this approach (Johnson et al, 1988c). Another novel approach under current investigation is the repeated use of intravaginal seminal plasma suppositories (Coulam et al, personal communication). Thus, central questions remain focussed on the most rational approach and further placebo-controlled or comparative studies need to be completed to assess the efficacy of active immunotherapy.

The immunobiological mechanism whereby immunization might confer a beneficial effect is not clearly understood, but presupposes the development of an appropriate immunological recognition response which would involve complex interactions between direct cellular, regulatory antibody and cytokine stimulation effects. A candidate antigen system to be involved is the trophoblast–leukocyte common (TLX) antigen. This antigen is expressed on all populations of peripheral blood lymphocytes and fetal trophoblast (Bulmer and Johnson, 1985). It was originally described using polyclonal antisera and has been claimed also to be present in seminal plasma (McIntyre et al, 1986). A murine monoclonal antibody (H316) has been used to characterize a cell-surface glycoprotein antigen of similar tissue distribution, except that it is expressed on spermatozoa rather than in seminal plasma (Stern et al, 1986; Anderson et al, 1988). There is no evidence that the TLX antigen system is linked to the MHC, but instead may be encoded from chromosome 1 (Stern et al, 1986).

Laboratory monitoring of RM patients is clearly difficult, although perhaps the most successful monitoring following leukocyte immunization has been based on determination of blocking antibody activity (Unander and Lindholm, 1986; Takakuwa et al, 1986). This could not be detected in RM patients following TMI (Chia and Johnson, unpublished data). Development of LCA following leukocyte immunization does not appear necessarily to indicate a favourable prognosis and may not be of particular clinical usefulness (Regan and Braude, 1987); indeed, there is even one report that the LCA-positive women following leukocyte immunization fare worse than the persistently LCA-negative RM women (Beer, 1988). Comprehensive studies of specific non-cytotoxic lymphocyte-reactive antibodies induced by pregnancy or immunization of RM patients have yet to be described. Women with anti-sperm antibodies may also be less successful following leukocyte immunization (Haas et al, 1986), perhaps because the early embryo expresses similar antigens to some of the surface antigens of spermatozoa and hence there can be an interrelationship between embryotoxic and anti-sperm antibodies in certain cases of recurring occult or early fetal loss.

ANIMAL MODELS

Animal models of immunologically-mediated recurrent early fetal loss could greatly facilitate our understanding of basic mechanisms. Two mating combinations of inbred mouse strains have been identified in which, with increasing maternal age, there can be a marked incidence of spontaneous fetal resorption: these are CBA/J female × DBA/2 male (most studied) and B10 female × B10.A male. The resorption in the former appears to involve a specific genetic contribution independent of major histocompatibility loci since both CBA/J(H-2k) females mated to other H-2d male strains (e.g. Balb/c) and other H-2k female strains (e.g. C3H) mated to DBA/2 (H-2d) males have normal low resorption rates. The fetal resorption model of B10(H-2b) females mated with B10.A(H-2a) males behaves similarly, but may not give such marked resorption rates (Melnick et al, 1981; Chaouat et al, 1988).

Much interest has been generated by the discovery that prior immunization of CBA/J females with Balb/c or C57BL male spleen cells (but not DBA/2 spleen cells) significantly reduces the subsequent fetal resorption rate following mating with DBA/2 males (Chaouat et al, 1985). This phenomenon has now been studied in detail using a variety of congenic or F1 splenocytes for immunization. It has been concluded to centre on an anti-MHC response that itself is dependent on the correct allogeneic environment furnished by minor histocompatibility antigens (Kiger et al, 1985; Chaouat et al, 1988). Others have shown that maternal–fetal disparity at multiple minor histocompatibility antigens can have significant effects on the weight of the feto-placental unit (Hamilton and Hamilton, 1987a).

It is also of note that the protective effect of systemic immunization with splenocytes in the CBA/J × DBA/2 model can be reproduced by maternal pre-immunization with placental cell preparations of the correct strain type or with the B6 trophoblast cell line, as well as by intrauterine immunization (Clark et al, 1986; Chaouat et al, 1988). Similarly, the high resorption rate is abrogated by a prior pregnancy (Chaouat et al, 1985; Chavez et al, 1987). Strong evidence for direct immunological effects in this murine model of recurrent early fetal loss is provided by the display of memory effects from previous mating combinations (Chavez et al, 1987; Chaouat et al, 1988). Most, if not all, 'protection' following appropriate immunization can be transferred passively to non-mated recipients with either serum or immune cells, most notably LyT2+ cells (Chaouat et al, 1988). The protective effect of maternal immunization correlates with induction of anti-H-2d antibodies and also with detection of strong suppressor activities in cultures of mononuclear cells derived from the decidualized endometrial tissue (Clark et al, 1987).

It has been noted by various investigators that the fetal resorption rates for CBA/J × DBA/2 and control matings may vary considerably between centres. Hamilton and Hamilton (1987b) have reported, intriguingly, that the precise figures may be influenced by the environment in which the animals are maintained, notably that the resorption rate was lower for mice maintained in a specific pathogen-free room than for those maintained in a conventional animal housing facility. This effect could involve a specific microbial pathogen or other environmental differences between the two rooms. It is of further interest to note, however, that maternal pre-immunization with heat-aggregated serum or gammaglobulin can also abrogate the CBA/J × DBA/2 resorption effect (Chaouat et al, 1988).

One interpretation has been along the lines of the 'placental immunotrophism hypothesis' that growth and function of placental cells may be favourably enhanced by cytokines derived from maternal leukocytes in decidual tissues (Wegmann, 1987). Thus, preliminary data has indicated that maternal treatment with GM-CSF may lower the resorption rate in the CBA/J × DBA/2 model whereas treatment with IL-2 may increase the rate (Chaouat et al, 1988). However, administration of recombinant cytokines to experimental animals may have to be interpreted with caution since contaminating bacterial products could also influence cellular events and placental function. It would be preferable to control each cytokine with a separate biologically inactive gene product derived using the same expression vector. Similar considerations apply also to recombinant protein production from mammalian cell vectors. Nevertheless, the importance of these emerging concepts may be illustrated by the fact that epidermal growth factor (EGF) deficiency in mice produced by pregestational removal of the submandibular glands significantly reduced the subsequent number of viable pregnancies (Tsutsumi and Oka, 1987).

A separate murine model of fetal resorption has been described by Tartakovsky and Gorelik (1988) where, conversely, prior immunization causes rather than abrogates the effect. This involves immunization of C57BL/6J female mice with the syngeneic repressor BL6 melanoma tumour which had been reacted with N-methyl-N'-nitronitrosoguanidine to obtain an immunogenic variant (BL6-T2). Mice subsequently mated with DBA/2 or B6D2F1 males, but not those with CBA/J or C57BL/6J mice, undergo a high proportion of fetal resorption in a subsequent pregnancy. This effect may be due to an immune response to tumour-associated antigens cross-reacting with fetal antigens in allopregnant mice.

Two animal models of fetal death following adoptive embryo transfer also deserve mention. Preimplantation embryos from the wild mouse species *Mus caroli* transferred to the laboratory mouse *Mus musculus* implant and develop normally to mid-term when they fail and resorb. Detailed investigation of this model has used preimplantation chimaeras, constructed such that the trophoblast component may be of varying genotype, as well as embryo transfer experiments into either mice carrying the *scid* mutation or immunologically compromised *Mus musculus* animals (e.g. by prior infusion with antibodies to L3T4 or to the IL-2 receptor). These studies have led to the conclusion that the failure of *Mus caroli* embryos is not due to conventional allograft rejection responses but rather a primary non-immunological failure of *Mus caroli* trophoblast giant cells (Croy et al, 1987; Crépeau et al, 1988).

A separate model is that of donkey-in-horse xenogeneic pregnancy, where some 75% of pregnancies end in abortion between days 80 and 95 of gestation. This appears to be a non-genetic defect of trophoblast function unresponsive to exogenous hormone therapy. Initial indications have shown a beneficial effect on pregnancy outcome following transfer of large volumes of serum from mares carrying normal intraspecies horse pregnancies or by immunization with lymphocytes from the genetic parents of the transferred donkey embryo (Allen et al, 1987). Further development of this model, however, is hindered by the obvious constraints on numbers of pregnancies that can be studied.

CONCLUDING REMARKS

There is much attractiveness in the concept that certain cases of unexplained RM may represent natural models of failure in the normal maternal immunological adaptation to the early embryo. This mechanism of fetal loss may be more common than examples of recurrent miscarriage due to the action of anti-phospholipid autoantibodies. However, extensive laboratory investigations have provided many leads but no consistent results applicable to clinical use in the identification of an immunoregulatory background for unexplained RM patients. Several immunotherapeutic trials based on immunization with leukocytes, trophoblast membrane or seminal plasma antigens are currently in progress and their results are awaited with interest. In the meantime, animal models may provide important clues as to how alterations in the immune system might be involved in recurrent fetal loss and its treatment.

Acknowledgements

The authors wish to thank Birthright and the Mersey Regional Health Authority for their support to this work.

REFERENCES

Alberman E (1988) The epidemiology of repeated abortion. In Sharp F & Beard RW (eds) *Early Pregnancy Loss: Mechanisms and Treatment*, pp 9–17. London: Royal College of Obstetricians and Gynaecologists.

Allen WR, Kydd JH & Antczak DF (1987) Maternal immunological response to the trophoblast in xenogeneic equine pregnancy. In Gill TJ III & Wegmann TG (eds) *Immunoregulation and Fetal Survival*, pp 263–285. New York: Oxford University Press.

Anderson DJ, Michaelson JA & Johnson PM (1988) Trophoblast–leukocyte common antigen is also expressed on human testicular germ cells and capacitated sperm. *Biology of Reproduction* (in press).

Beer AE (1986) New horizons in the diagnosis, evaluation and therapy of recurrent spontaneous abortion. *Clinics in Obstetrics and Gynaecology* 13: 115–124.

Beer AE (1988) Pregnancy outcome in couples with recurrent abortions following immunological evaluation and therapy. In Sharp F & Beard RW (eds) *Early Pregnancy Loss: Mechanisms and Treatment*, pp 337–349. London: Royal College of Obstetricians & Gynaecologists.

Beer AE & Billingham RE (1977) Histocompatibility gene polymorphisms and materno-fetal interaction. *Transplantation Proceedings* 9: 1393–1401.

Beer AE, Quebbeman JF, Ayers JWT & Haines RF (1981) Major histocompatibility complex antigens, maternal and paternal immune responses, and chronic habitual abortions in humans. *American Journal of Obstetrics and Gynecology* 141: 987–999.

Beer AE, Semprini AE, Xiaoyn Z & Quebbeman JF (1985) Pregnancy outcome in human couples with recurrent spontaneous abortion: HLA antigen profiles, HLA antigen sharing, female serum MLR blocking factors and paternal leukocyte immunization. *Experimental and Clinical Immunogenetics* 2: 137–153.

Biddle PK, Friedman CI & Johnson PM (1987) Lymphocyte-reactive antibodies and recurrent early pregnancy failure. *American Journal of Obstetrics & Gynecology* 157: 785–786.

Branch DW (1987) Immunologic disease and fetal death. *Clinical Obstetrics and Gynecology* 30: 295–311.

Bulmer JN & Johnson PM (1985) Antigen expression by trophoblast populations in the human placenta and their possible immunobiological relevance. *Placenta* 6: 127–140.

Bulmer JN, Johnson PM, Sasagawa M & Takeuchi S (1988) Immunohistochemical studies of fetal trophoblast and maternal decidua in hydatiform mole and choriocarcinoma. *Placenta* 9: 183–200.

Cauchi MN, Koh SH, Tait B, Mraz G, Kloss M & Pepperell RJ (1987) Immunogenetic studies in habitual abortion. *Australian and New Zealand Journal of Obstetrics and Gynaecology* 27: 52–54.

Chaouat G, Kolb JP, Kiger N, Stanislawski M & Wegmann TG (1985) Immunological consequences of vaccination against abortion in mice. *Journal of Immunology* 134: 1594–1598.

Chaouat G, Clark DA & Wegmann TG (1988) Genetic aspects of the CBA × DBA/2 and B10 × B10.A models of murine pregnancy failure and its prevention by lymphocyte immunisation. In Sharp F & Beard RW (eds) *Early Pregnancy Loss: Mechanisms and Treatment*, pp 89–102. London: Royal College of Obstetricians & Gynaecologists.

Chavez DJ, McIntyre JA, Colliver JA & Faulk WP (1987) Allogeneic matings and immunization have different effects on nulliparous and multiparous mice. *Journal of Immunology* **139:** 85–88.

Chia KV & Johnson PM (1987) T-lymphocyte subsets in unexplained recurrent spontaneous abortion. *Fertility and Sterility* **48:** 685–687.

Clark DA, Chaput A & Tutton D (1986) Active suppression of host-versus-graft reaction in pregnant mice. VII. Spontaneous abortion of allogeneic CBA/J × DBA/2 fetuses in the uterus of CBA/J mice correlates with deficient non-T suppressor cell activity. *Journal of Immunology* **135:** 1668–1675.

Clark DA, Chaouat G, Guennet JL & Kiger N (1987) Local active suppression and successful vaccination against spontaneous abortion in CBA/J mice. *Journal of Reproductive Immunology* **10:** 79–85.

Coulam CB, Moore SB & O'Fallon WM (1987) Association between major histocompatibility antigen and reproductive performance. *American Journal of Reproductive Immunology and Microbiology* **14:** 54–58.

Crépeau MA, Yamashiro S & Croy BA (1988) Anatomical and immunological aspects of fetal death in the *Mus musculus/Mus caroli* model of pregnancy failure. In Sharp F & Beard RW (eds) *Early Pregnancy Loss: Mechanisms and Treatment*, pp 69–83. London: Royal College of Obstetricians & Gynaecologists.

Croy BA, Crépeau M, Yamashiro S & Clark DA (1987) Further studies on the transfer of *Mus caroli* embryos to immunodeficient *Mus musculus*. *Colloque INSERM* **154:** 101–112.

Daya S & Clark DA (1988) Identification of two species of suppressive factor of differing molecular weight released by in vitro fertilised human oocytes. *Fertility and Sterility* **49:** 360–363.

Daya S, Rosenthal KL & Clark DA (1987) Immunosuppressor factor(s) produced by decidua-associated suppressor cells: a proposed mechanism for fetal allograft survival. *American Journal of Obstetrics and Gynecology* **156:** 344–350.

Daya S, Johnson PM & Clark DA (1988) Trophoblast induction of suppressor-type cell activity in human endometrial tissue. *American Journal of Reproductive Immunology and Microbiology* (in press).

Diamond JM (1987) Causes of death before birth. *Nature* **329:** 487–488.

Editorial (1983) Maternal blocking antibodies, the fetal allograft and recurrent abortion. *Lancet* **ii:** 1175–1776.

Ellis SA, Sargent IL, Redman CWG & McMichael AJ (1986) Evidence for a novel HLA antigen found on human extravillous trophoblast of a choriocarcinoma cell line. *Immunology* **59:** 595–601.

Fiddes TM, O'Reilly DB, Cetrulo CL et al (1986) Phenotypic and functional evaluation of suppressor cells in normal pregnancy and in chronic aborters. *Cellular Immunology* **97:** 407–418.

Gill TJ III (1987) Genetic factors in fetal loss. *American Journal of Reproductive Immunology and Microbiology* **15:** 133–137.

Gill TJ III & Repetti CF (1979) Immunologic and genetic factors influencing reproduction. *American Journal of Pathology* **95:** 465–470.

Glass RH & Golbus MH (1978) Habitual abortion. *Fertility and Sterility* **29:** 257–265.

Grimm EB (1962) Psychological investigation of habitual abortion. *Psychosomatic Medicine* **23:** 369–378.

Haas GG, Kubota K, Quebbeman JF, Jijon A, Menge AC & Beer AE (1986) Circulating antisperm antibodies in recurrently aborting women. *Fertility and Sterility* **45:** 209–215.

Hamilton BL & Hamilton MS (1987a) Effect of maternal–fetal histoincompatibility on the weight of the feto-placental unit in mice: the role of minor histocompatibility antigens. *American Journal of Reproductive Immunology and Microbiology* **15:** 153–155.

Hamilton MS & Hamilton BL (1987b) Environmental influences on immunologically associated spontaneous abortion in CBA/J mice. *Journal of Reproductive Immunology* **11:** 237–241.

Head JR, Drake BL & Zuckermann FA (1987) Major histocompatibility antigens on trophoblast and their regulation: implications in the maternal–fetal relationship. *American Journal of Reproductive Immunology and Microbiology* **15:** 12–18.

Hofmeyr GJ, Joffe MI, Bezwoda WR & van Iddekinge B (1987) Immunologic investigation of recurrent pregnancy loss and consequences of immunization with husbands' leukocytes. *Fertility and Sterility* **48:** 681–684.

Hole N, Cheng HM & Johnson PM (1987) Antibody reactivity against human trophoblast membrane antigens in the context of normal pregnancy and unexplained recurrent miscarriage. *Colloque INSERM* **154:** 213–224.

Hsi B-L, Samson M, Grivaux C, Fénichel P, Hunt JS & Yeh C-JG (1988) Topographical expression of class I major histocompatibility complex antigens on human amniotic epithelium. *Journal of Reproductive Immunology* **13:** 183–191.

Jazwinska EC, Kilpatrick DC, Smart GE & Liston WA (1987) Feto-maternal HLA compatibility does not have a major influence on human pregnancy except for lymphocytotoxin production. *Clinical and Experimental Immunology* **68:** 116–122.

Johnson PM & Stern PL (1986) Antigen expression at human materno-fetal interfaces. In Cinader B & Miller RG (eds) *Progress in Immunology VI*, pp 1056–1069. Orlando: Academic Press.

Johnson PM, Barnes RMR, Risk JM, Molloy CM & Woodrow JC (1985) Immunogenetic studies of recurrent spontaneous abortion in humans. *Experimental and Clinical Immunogenetics* **2:** 77–83.

Johnson PM, Chia KV & Risk JM (1986) Immunological question marks in recurrent spontaneous abortion. In Clark DA & Croy BA (eds) *Reproductive Immunology 1986*, pp 239–245. Amsterdam: Elsevier Biomedical Press.

Johnson PM, Chia KV, Risk JM, Barnes RMR & Woodrow JC (1988a) Immunological and immunogenetic investigation of recurrent spontaneous abortion. *Disease Markers* **6:** 163–171.

Johnson PM, Ramsden GH & Chia KV (1988b) Trophoblast membrane infusion (TMI) in the treatment of recurrent spontaneous abortion. In Sharp F & Beard RW (eds) *Early Pregnancy Loss: Mechanisms and Treatment*, pp 389–396. London: Royal College of Obstetricians & Gynaecologists.

Johnson PM, Chia KV, Hart CA, Griffith HB & Francis WJA (1988c) Trophoblast membrane infusion for unexplained recurrent miscarriage. *British Journal of Obstetrics and Gynaecology* **95:** 342–347.

Kiger N, Chaouat G, Kolb JP, Wegmann TG & Guennet JL (1985) Immunogenetic studies of spontaneous abortion in mice. Preimmunization of females with allogeneic male cells. *Journal of Immunology* **134:** 2966–2970.

Kilpatrick DC (1984) A case of materno-foetal histocompatibility—implications for leucocyte transfusion for recurrent aborters. *Scottish Medical Journal* **29:** 110–112.

Klitz W, Lo SK, Neugebauer M, Baur MP, Albert ED & Thomson G (1987) A comprehensive search for segregation distortion in HLA. *Human Immunology* **18:** 163–180.

Komlos L, Zamir R, Joshua H & Halbrecht I (1977) Common HLA antigens in couples with repeated abortions. *Clinical Immunology and Immunopathology* **7:** 330–335.

Konoeda Y, Terasaki PI, Wakisaka A, Park MS & Mickey MR (1986) Public determinants of HLA indicated by pregnancy antibodies. *Transplantation* **41:** 253–259.

Lauritsen JG, Kristensen T & Grunnet N (1976) Depressed mixed lymphocyte culture reaction in mothers with recurrent spontaneous abortion. *American Journal of Obstetrics and Gynecology* **125:** 35–39.

Lessin DL, Hunt JS, King CR & Wood GW (1988) Antigen expression by cells near the maternal–fetal interface. *American Journal of Reproductive Immunology and Microbiology* **16:** 1–7.

Lockshin MD, Druzin ML, Goei S et al (1985) Antibody to cardiolipin as a predictor of fetal distress or death in pregnant patients with systemic lupus erythematosus. *New England Journal of Medicine* **313:** 152–156.

Lubbe WF & Liggins CG (1985) Lupus anticoagulant and pregnancy. *American Journal of Obstetrics and Gynecology* **153:** 322–327.

McIntyre JA, Faulk WP, Nichols-Johnson VR & Taylor CG (1986) Immunologic testing and immunotherapy in recurrent spontaneous abortions. *Obstetrics and Gynecology* **67:** 169–175.

MacQueen JM & Sanfilippo FP (1984) The effect of parental HLA compatibility on the expression of paternal haplotypes in offspring. *Human Immunology* **11:** 155–161.

Melnick M, Jaskoll T & Slavkin HE (1981) The association of H-2 haplotype with implantation, survival and growth of murine embryos. *Immunogenetics* **14:** 303–308.

Mowbray JF & Underwood JL (1985) Immunology of abortion. *Clinical and Experimental Immunology* **60:** 1–7.

Mowbray JF, Gibbings C, Liddell H, Reginald PW, Underwood JL & Beard RW (1985) Controlled trial of treatment of recurrent spontaneous abortion by immunisation with paternal cells. *Lancet* **i**: 941–943.

Mowbray JF, Underwood JL, Michel M, Forbes PB & Beard RW (1987) Immunisation with paternal lymphocytes in women with recurrent miscarriage. *Lancet* **ii**: 679–680.

Nicholas NS & Panayi GS (1986) Inhibition of interleukin-2 production by retroplacental sera: a possible mechanism for human fetal allograft survival. *American Journal of Reproductive Immunology and Microbiology* **9**: 6–11.

Ober CL, Martin AO, Simpson JL et al (1983) Shared HLA antigens and reproductive performance among Hutterites. *American Journal of Human Genetics* **35**: 994–1004.

Ober C, Simpson JL, Ward M et al (1987) Prenatal effects of maternal–fetal HLA compatibility. *American Journal of Reproductive Immunology and Microbiology* **15**: 141–149.

Oksenberg JR, Persitz E, Amar A & Brautbar C (1984) Maternal–paternal histocompatibility: lack of association with habitual abortions. *Fertility and Sterility* **42**: 389–395.

Poland BJ, Miller JR, Jones DC et al (1977) Reproductive counselling in patients who have had a spontaneous abortion. *American Journal of Obstetrics and Gynecology* **127**: 685–691.

Power DA, Mather AJ, Macleod AM, Lind T & Catto DRG (1986) Maternal antibodies to paternal B lymphocytes in normal and abnormal pregnancy. *American Journal of Reproductive Immunology and Microbiology* **10**: 10–13.

Radcliffe JJ, Hart CA, Francis WJA & Johnson PM (1986) Immunity to cytomegalovirus in women with unexplained recurrent spontaneous abortion. *American Journal of Reproductive Immunology and Microbiology* **12**: 103–105.

Ramsden GH & Johnson PM (1988) Tests for pregnancy failure. In Liu DTY (ed.) *Clinical Tests for Obstetrics and Gynaecology*, London: Chapman & Hall (in press).

Regan L & Braude PR (1987) Is antipaternal cytotoxic antibody a valid marker in the management of recurrent abortion? *Lancet* **ii**: 1280.

Reginald PW, Beard RW, Chapple J et al (1987) Outcome of pregnancies progressing beyond 28 weeks gestation in women with a history of recurrent miscarriage. *British Journal of Obstetrics and Gynaecology* **94**: 643–648.

Reznikoff-Etievant MF, Durieux I, Huchet J, Salmon C & Netter A (1988) Human MHC antigens and paternal leucocyte injections in recurrent spontaneous abortions. In Sharp F & Beard RW (eds) *Early Pregnancy Loss: Mechanisms and Treatment*, pp 375–384. London: Royal College of Obstetricians & Gynaecologists.

Rocklin RE, Kitzmiller JL, Carpenter CB, Garovoy MR & David JR (1976) Maternal–fetal relation: absence of an immunological blocking factor from the serum of women with chronic abortions. *New England Journal of Medicine* **295**: 1209–1213.

Rodger JC (1985) Lack of a requirement for a maternal humoral immune response to establish or maintain successful allogeneic pregnancy. *Transplantation* **40**: 372–375.

Scott JR, Rote NS & Branch DW (1987) Immunologic aspects of recurrent abortion and fetal death. *Obstetrics and Gynecology* **70**: 645–656.

Simpson JL (1980) Genes, chromosomes and reproductive failure. *Fertility and Sterility* **33**: 107–113.

Stern PL, Beresford N, Thompson S, Johnson PM, Webb PD & Hole N (1986) Characterisation of the human trophoblast–leucocyte antigenic molecules defined by a monoclonal antibody. *Journal of Immunology* **137**: 1064–1069.

Stimson WH, Strachan AF & Shepherd A (1979) Studies on the maternal immune response to placental antigens: absence of a blocking factor from the blood of abortion-prone women. *British Journal of Obstetrics and Gynaecology* **86**: 41–45.

Stirrat GM (1983) Recurrent abortion—a review. *British Journal of Obstetrics and Gynaecology* **90**: 881–883.

Stray-Pedersen B & Stray-Pedersen S (1984) Etiological factors and subsequent reproductive performance in 195 couples with a prior history of habitual abortion. *American Journal of Obstetrics and Gynecology* **148**: 140–146.

Takakuwa K, Kanazawa K & Takeuchi S (1986) Production of blocking antibodies by vaccination with husband's lymphocytes in unexplained recurrent aborters: the role in successful pregnancy. *American Journal of Reproductive Immunology and Microbiology* **10**: 1–9.

Tartakovsky B & Gorelik E (1988) Immunization with a syngeneic regressor tumour causes resorption in allo-pregnant mice. *Journal of Reproductive Immunology* **13**: 113–122.

Taylor CG & Faulk WP (1981) Prevention of recurrent abortion with leucocyte transfusions. *Lancet* **ii:** 68–70.

Taylor CG, Faulk WP & McIntyre JA (1985) Prevention of recurrent spontaneous abortions by leukocyte transfusions. *Journal of the Royal Society of Medicine* **78:** 623–627.

Tharapel AT, Tharapel SA & Bannerman RM (1985) Recurrent pregnancy losses and parental chromosome abnormalities: a review. *British Journal of Obstetrics and Gynaecology* **92:** 899–914.

Tho PT, Byrd JR & McDonagh PG (1979) Etiologies and subsequent reproductive performance of 100 couples with recurrent abortion. *Fertility and Sterility* **32:** 389–395.

Tsutsumi O & Oka T (1987) Epidermal growth factor deficiency during pregnancy causes abortion in mice. *American Journal of Obstetrics and Gynecology* **156:** 241–244.

Unander AM & Lindholm A (1986) Transfusions of leukocyte-rich erythrocyte concentrates: a successful treatment in selected cases of habitual abortion. *American Journal of Obstetrics and Gynecology* **154:** 516–520.

Unander AM & Olding LB (1983) Habitual abortion: parental sharing of HLA antigens, absence of maternal blocking antibody and suppression of maternal lymphocytes. *American Journal of Reproductive Immunology* **4:** 171–178.

Unander AM, Lindholm A & Olding LB (1985) Blood transfusions generate/increase previously absent/weak blocking antibody in women with habitual abortion. *Fertility and Sterility* **44:** 766–771.

Vadheim CM, Rotter JI, Maclaren NK, Riley WJ & Anderson CE (1986) Preferential transmission of diabetic alleles within the HLA gene complex. *New England Journal of Medicine* **315:** 1314–1318.

Vlaanderen W & Treffers PE (1987) Prognosis of subsequent pregnancies after recurrent spontaneous abortion in first trimester. *British Medical Journal* **295:** 92–93.

Warburton D & Fraser FC (1964) Spontaneous abortion risks in man: data from reproductive histories collected in a medical genetics unit. *Human Genetics* **16:** 1–13.

Wegmann TG (1987) Placental immunotrophism: maternal T cells enhance placental growth and function. *American Journal of Reproductive Immunology and Microbiology* **15:** 67–70.

5

Pre-eclamptic toxaemia

D. M. JENKINS

It has been tempting to seek an immunological cause for pre-eclampsia in the context of the fetal allograft. The clinical picture is heterogeneous and, not surprisingly, the aetiology would appear to be multifactorial.

HISTORICAL NOTES

Eclampsia was referred to by Hippocrates and other ancient writers. Convulsions, stupor and fetal death featured in the clinical picture. Mauriceau (1668) drew attention to the particular association of the disease with primigravidity and, realizing that the convulsions ceased after delivery, logically advocated prompt delivery as treatment.

Eclampsia and epilepsy were only distinguished by the cessation of convulsions after delivery in eclampsia. This distinction was not absolute and some confusion still occurs for patients with single post-natal fits. Lever (1843) noted that the proteinuria he had found in eclamptics disappeared after delivery, whilst that in women with the clinically similar condition of glomerulonephritis did not. It was not until the beginning of the twentieth century, when measurement of the blood pressure was introduced, that the 'strong swollen pulse' of the ancient writers was recognized as hypertension.

The incidence of eclampsia today in the third world is higher than it was in the British Isles twenty five years ago. I append two actual case histories so that the non-clinician has some idea of the disease. Both occurred more than twenty five years ago and neither represent good or modern management.

1. In the 34th week of her first pregnancy, 27 year old Mrs X called her General Practitioner. Until that time she had felt extremely well and regular antenatal examinations had been unremarkable. But now she felt ill with a pounding headache, a sharp abdominal pain and nausea. Occasionally curious flashing lights danced across her field of vision. Her doctor examined her at home and noted that her blood pressure, previously normal, was now 180/120; he tested her urine and found 300 mg% of protein. He diagnosed pre-eclampsia, prescribed a sedative and left.

    That evening she called again to say she felt no better. The doctor asked his midwife to visit Mrs X, at which time the hypertension and proteinuria were confirmed. A further sedative was prescribed and Mrs X had a restless and uncomfortable night at home. In the morning, feeling considerably worse, she asked her doctor to come again but, before he arrived, she collapsed and died shortly afterwards from a cerebral haemorrhage.

2.   The patient, a 28 year old primigravida, was admitted to hospital at 38 weeks' gestation with a blood pressure of 150/110 and moderate proteinuria. She was given sodium gardinal (3 g intramuscularly every four hours for the next twelve hours) and then transferred to the Labour Ward for surgical induction of labour. The patient had her first fit whilst in the lithotomy position with her legs supported in stirrups. The patient's apnoea and deep cyanosis were memorable. One marvelled that the fetal heart was still present at the end of the fit. Over the next 30 hours Avertin (Bromethal) was administered rectally every six hours. The patient had a further fit 24 hours after the first. A live baby was delivered six hours later, its appearance far from lively, raising the question as to how much brain damage it had suffered during the hypoxia of the previous 30 hours. The mother looked little better than the baby, having been virtually anaesthetized for the duration of labour. The condition of the attending obstetrician was not strikingly different from that of his two patients.

CLINICAL SUMMARY

The disease is bedevilled by different names and controversy concerning definitions and classifications. Ignorance of the cause of disease, variable manifestations in terms of clinical signs, and extremely variable progression with and without therapy explain the classification difficulties. The disease is asymptomatic until far advanced and eclampsia, the convulsive phase, imminent. Oedema remains the only sign the patient can perceive and, in parts of the third world where little antenatal care exists, remains the only recognized abnormality that might lead to self-referral for medical help. The clinical symptoms of imminent eclampsia, abdominal pain, vomiting and visual disturbances are rarely seen in the developed world.

    The clinical signs of pre-eclampsia are those of hypertension, proteinuria and oedema. Disagreement exists about the absolute value of blood pressure that is diagnostic of the disease and its severity. Similar problems exist concerning the significance of oedema which may also occur to a degree in normal pregnancies. An erratic relationship exists between the rise in blood pressure, proteinuria and oedema.

    A rise in blood pressure to 140 mmHg systolic and 90 mmHg diastolic which persists having been normal before 20 weeks' gestation, serves well enough as the upper limit of normal pressure. In the presence of proteinuria of more than 0.3 g in 24 hours, this is diagnostic of the disease state or syndrome. The clinician who has no time for terminological wrangles usually settles for pre-eclamptic toxaemia (PET) in the British Isles when there is pregnancy-induced hypertension even if there is no proteinuria and only physiological oedema. The older European term, gestosis, is favoured by some. Severity of disease is best and most easily based on the amount of protein in 24-hour urine collections, with mild to moderate disease being below 2 g/litre and severe disease over 5 g/litre. Treatment of the hypertension makes its subsequent use limited for classifying the severity of the disease.

Prevalence

Problems of definition and classification make estimates of prevalence of the disease problematical; there appears also to be wide geographic variations. Confounding variables, for example, the high proportion of primigravidae in Chinese maternity statistics, again hamper comparison. The incidence in Burma is reported to be lower in primigravidae than among all births. This is quite contrary to all other geographic and historical data, and indicates the likelihood of some hidden bias. The prevalence of the disease, especially the severe variety, is falling in the developed world but eclampsia remains common in developing countries where antenatal care is deficient (Ghose and Das, 1985).

Parity

The disease occurs in about 12% of primigravidae in the UK with an incidence of 4% in second pregnancies rising to double figures again by the fifth pregnancy. Whether the disease of the multiparous patient is the same as that of the primigravida is contentious, and renal biopsy of high parity patients has shown much chronic renal disease.

Age

MacGillivray (1958) has described a 'J-shaped' curve of incidence of the disease with increasing maternal age. The incidence of severe PET for a small group of pregnant girls under the age of 15 was three times the mean in an American collaborative study (Vollman, 1970). The increased incidence in women over 35 years of age may be related to underlying essential hypertension. Elderly primigravidas have a particularly high incidence, especially of severe disease.

Diet

Dietary factors seem to play little part in the incidence of PET. Dietary intervention, in the form of low calorie or high protein low calorie diets, has not been shown to alter the incidence (Campbell and MacGillivray, 1975; Grieve et al, 1979).

Pathophysiology

There is general agreement that the plasma volume expansion normally seen in pregnancy is reduced in PET. There is no agreement on changes in cardiac output in PET compared with normal pregnancy. Although cerebral and hepatic blood flow is not abnormal in pre-eclamptic pregnancy, there is marked individual variation with respect to renal blood flow and function with a general decreased filtration fraction in PET. There is general agreement that in established PET the utero-placental blood flow is decreased. Gant et al (1976) have reported a 50–65% decrease in utero-placental blood flow 3–4 weeks before onset of overt hypertension. There are contradictory reports of plasma viscosity in PET but the haematocrit tends to increase in PET and eclampsia in association with increasing severity of disease.

Blood constituents

No differences in plasma electrolyte concentrations are found in PET, whereas there is a well-recognized fall in plasma protein concentrations. An expected fall in serum osmolarity occurs in the first eight weeks of pregnancy and a further fall in osmotic pressure was found by Campbell (1981) in pre-eclampsia compared with normal pregnancy. This is presumably consequent upon the leakage of protein through vessels in PET (Campbell, 1981).

Although not different in number, erythrocytes in PET show an increased proportion of deformed cells (Thorburn et al, 1982). The platelet count falls in pregnancy, occasionally more so in PET.

PET is considered to be associated with disseminated intravascular coagulation, although MacGillivray (1983) states with typical caution that 'in PET there is a disturbance in the coagulation/fibrinolytic system. . . .'

Excess weight gain in pregnancy may be associated with PET. However, those with low weight gain who develop PET have higher perinatal mortality rates. Put simply, the babies of women with 'wet' PET are bigger and do better than the babies of women with 'dry' PET. Some 40% of women with normal blood pressure in pregnancy have oedema. Sodium and potassium are retained in proportion to the increase in body water (MacGillivray, 1967); there is no change, therefore, in sodium concentration in body fluids.

Endocrinology

There are endocrine changes in PET not seen in normal pregnancy. These are generally resultant from the disease process. Thus, oestriol excretion in urine and plasma oestrogen concentration fall in PET and have been used to monitor the feto-placental unit. Gant et al (1977) have suggested increased oestrogen activity before the development of PET. Jenkins and Perry (1978) and Jenkins and Soltan (1980) showed, and then failed to confirm, an association between high plasma prolactin levels in pregnancy and incidence of PET. Circulating adrenaline, but not noradrenaline, is increased in PET (Sammour et al, 1980). Symonds and Broughton-Pipkin (1978) have reported changes in the renin angiotension system in PET. Sensitivity to angiotension decreases in normal pregnancy but to a reduced extent in PET—a situation that can be predicted with angiotension II stress testing early in pregnancy (Gant et al, 1971).

The role of prostaglandins in maintaining vascular tone is still being defined but the interaction of different prostaglandins with other agents, such as prolactin, progesterone and adrenaline, would seem to be central to understanding the mechanism of pregnancy-associated hypertension.

CLINICAL MANAGEMENT

Initial diagnosis of PET is straightforward using the criteria of raised blood pressure and proteinuria, detected by simple albustix. Prediction of the course of the condition is less easy. There are two patients to observe. The fetus is observed for growth both clinically and with ultrasound, and for its well-being with biophysical tests (such as fetal movement counts, fetal heart response to its own movement) and biochemical tests of fetal or feto-placental function. Arduini et al (1987) recently reported accurate prediction of pregnancy-induced hypertension using a pulsed duplex Doppler system at the level of the uterine vessels to measure utero-placental blood flow velocity wave forms. This report is preliminary but, if confirmed, is important. Blood tests may not be used much by clinicians although some find guidance from changes in particular parameters. Recent research has indicated the clinical value of sophisticated measurement of blood flow in fetal and uterine vessels but clinical observation from day to day (even from hour to hour) may be more valuable than most biochemical data, the results of which can take days or weeks to arrive.

The identification of women likely to develop PET would be of enormous help in management. Eclampsia is rare where antenatal care allows diagnosis of PET and delivery before eclampsia may develop. The number of cases of PET that would, untreated, progress to eclampsia is unknown but, in parts of the developing world in the absence of antenatal care, eclampsia remains common. Death rates associated with eclampsia have fallen from 22.5% in the UK in 1922 to a current incidence of eclampsia of about 1 per 1000 deliveries with a mortality of 1%. The confidential report on maternal deaths in the UK (1972) in the three years 1970–1972 reported 29 deaths from eclampsia. Mortality is higher in older and parous women than younger primigravidas. Ghose and Das (1985) reported a maternal mortality rate of 5.92% in a series of 152 consecutive cases of eclampsia in Calcutta between 1976 and 1983, with a perinatal mortality rate of 36.6%.

The major cause of death in eclampsia is cerebral haemorrhage which accounts for 70% of deaths. The highest blood pressure in women with cerebral haemorrhage associated with PET was reported by Sheehan and Lynch (1973) to be not more than 140 mm Hg systolic and 100 mm Hg diastolic. As many women have higher rises in blood pressure without haemorrhage it seems likely that those who do bleed are in some way susceptible and their vessels do not make the 'pregnancy accommodative changes' which prevent many more women showing a similar pathology with pregnancy hypertension. Other fatal complications of eclampsia include respiratory, hepatic, renal and cardiac failure, disseminated intravascular coagulation, postpartum haemorrhage, placental abruption and septic shock. Death can often be associated with more than one of these complications.

Perinatal mortality rate (PMR) is approximately three times more common in association with hypertensive disease of pregnancy other than eclampsia. Perinatal mortality rates in association with eclampsia are approximately 30% when figures from both the developing and developed world are included. When proteinuria occurs with hypertension, PMR increases threefold. Perinatal mortality follows antepartum and intrapartum fetal anoxia due to reduced placental blood flow; this is consequent upon changes in placental bed maternal arterial vessels which remain narrow due to the failure of physiological expansion of these vessels in early pregnancy, and the constricting effect of the atherosis in these vessels (see Chapter 8). Brosens et al (1972) reported that the mean diameter of myometrial spiral arterioles of 50 normal pregnant women was 500 µm, compared with 200 µm in 36 women with PET.

PET is usually a disease of the third trimester and the disease is cured by terminating the pregnancy. With recent advances in neonatology, death from prematurity is much less common than a decade ago. It follows that the disease can be effectively and successfully treated for mother and baby as soon as the last eight weeks of pregnancy have been reached, or even earlier. This can be further aided by the use of corticosteroids to mature the fetal lung, so reducing the risk of respiratory distress for the newborn. Methods of induction of labour have also improved, making early intervention the treatment of choice in most cases. Clearly, very early intervention is only employed for severe disease whilst mild uncomplicated hypertension without proteinuria needs no intervention until term has been reached.

Treating the signs of PET with anti-hypertensives and diuretics is of debatable value and may be positively harmful. Although therapy and even bed-rest alone may be associated with disappearance of signs of the disease, the underlying vascular pathology in the placental bed persists and the risk to the fetus remains. Masking the signs of the disease with diuretics and anti-hypertensives can obscure the severity and progress of the disease. Apart from mild or moderate disease, where bed-rest may be all that is needed until delivery in the last two weeks of pregnancy, the optimal course of action is delivery with therapy aimed at controlling blood pressure and avoiding eclampsia before and immediately after delivery.

IMMUNOLOGICAL CONSIDERATIONS

The fetus, having inherited half of its transplantation antigen content from its father, may be considered a semi-allograft on its mother. Absence of evidence of fetal rejection has been considered an apparent paradox. Considerable research to identify evidence of immune rejection in cases of pregnancy failure, e.g. spontaneous abortion and pre-eclampsia, have been unrewarding. Yet, feto-maternal immune interaction, as for example in the case of rhesus isoimmunization, undoubtedly influences pregnancy outcome (see Chapter 3).

Because pre-eclampsia is not seen outside pregnancy, and is cured by removing the placenta, it has been concluded that the placenta in some way 'causes' the syndrome. The association of increased placental mass (hyper-placentosis), e.g. twins, with increased incidence of pre-eclampsia has been cited as proof of the causal relationship between placental tissue and pre-eclampsia. However, the majority of cases of hyperplacentosis may not be associated with pre-eclampsia. These tenuous associations between placental mass, incidence of pre-eclampsia and feto-maternal immune interaction has proved irresistible to the research workers who then searched for evidence to support the guilt of the suspect placenta. Much of that evidence has been circumstantial and no specific causal antigen has been identified.

One current working hypothesis proposes that women with severe pre-eclampsia are hypoimmune with respect to non-specific responses as well as specific responses to paternal antigens (Scott et al, 1978). This may or may not be associated with increased histocompatibility between the patient and her partner. It is further argued that this hypoimmune state is consistent with the first pregnancy preponderance of the syndrome, representing a primary immune response to pregnancy and/or paternal antigens and therefore of lower magnitude than to be expected with secondary responses after repeated exposure.

Feto-maternal interaction

Penrose (1946) and Kalmus (1946) both considered that an 'offending' fetal antigen might be responsible for PET, whilst Platt et al (1958) considered the opposite with fetal reactions to an offending maternal antigen leading to the condition. If such antigens are genetically determined, then a woman suffering from PET would not be expected to have a mother or daughter also suffering the disease since she could not differ from her own mother and her own daughter in exactly the same way. Yet there is evidence of a strong familial factor in PET (Chesley, 1962, 1978; Adams and Finlayson, 1961). This reveals an increased incidence of severe pre-eclampsia and eclampsia in daughters and grand-daughters of eclampsia sufferers and in sisters rather than sisters-in-law of patients with severe pre-eclampsia. Thus, a single gene disparity between mother and fetus causing the disease is not supported by the family studies. Again, feto-maternal immune interaction as a cause of PET would be expected to have an association with parity similar to rhesus isoimmunization, which is clearly not the case. Chesley et al (1986) have suggested maternal homozygosity is associated with PET; testing of his unique data being 'in good agreement with the predictions made by the hypothesis that a single recessive gene acting in the mother determines pre-eclampsia.'

Placental studies

Jones and Fox (1980) concluded that the changes in the placenta in PET were secondary to changes in the maternal vessels in the placental bed (see also Chapter 8). There is disagreement about which changes are characteristic of

PET but no single lesion is pathognomonic. Readers are recommended to read *Pathology of the Placenta* (Fox, 1978). Evidence for immune rejection of the placental graft is absent, although Sinha and Faulk (1982) have reported quantitatively increased deposition of complement components in pre-eclamptic placentae as compared with placentae from normal pregnancies.

Jaameri et al (1965) reported a twentyfold increase in numbers of trophoblast cells in uterine vein blood in PET, although this observation has not yet been confirmed. The massive embolization of fetal tissue in the form of trophoblastic cellular elements into the maternal circulation from early pregnancy (Chapter 11) would seem likely to affect the accommodation of the maternal immune system to pregnancy. The effect of hyperplacentosis on trophoblast embolization has not been studied.

Molar pregnancy is associated with increased incidence and early presentation of PET. Placental mass is increased. All fetal tissue antigens are derived from paternal genes in complete mole and hence this represents an entire rather than semi-allograft on the maternal host (Chapter 6) which could be associated with an increased magnitude of antigenic challenge to the maternal host. Multiple pregnancy is also associated with increased incidence of PET and increased placental mass. Stevenson et al (1971) found pre-eclampsia to be more common in unlike rather than like twins, whereas studies by McFarlane and Scott (1976) and McGillivray (1975) found no such difference. Unlike twins would increase the possibilities of feto-maternal incompatibility but not the volume of pregnancy or trophoblast-associated antigenic challenge.

Triploidy is another condition associated with early and severe PET and hyperplacentosis. In triploidy associated with dispermy the degree of materno-fetal disparity may be greater for a given amount of placental tissue.

Hydrops fetalis may be due to both immune and non-immune pathology and is also associated with early and severe PET and increased placental mass. These situations of hyperplacentosis associated with early and severe PET suggest that there is a placental mass effect. This may not be immunological but rather an endocrine effect acting either directly or via suppression of immune response by pregnancy-associated proteins produced by the placenta (Jenkins et al, 1972). If the effect of hyperplacentosis is directly immunological then increased or excessive antigenic challenge to the maternal host by fetal or pregnancy-associated antigens may be causally related to PET. Immune responses are influenced by dose of antigen, mode of administration, primary or repeated exposure, recipient genetic competence to respond to that particular antigen, as well as other endocrine, nutritional and drug-related factors. It follows that the effect on a pregnant woman of increased size of pregnancy-associated antigenic challenge may range from an increased response to a failure to respond at all. Failure of an adequate immune response may occur in a patient with normal or defective immune capacity with respect to the specific antigen involved, especially if the occasion represents a primary immune challenge as in first pregnancies. Indeed, a high incidence of severe PET has been reported in oocyte-donated embryo transfer patients (Serhal and Craft, 1987). This involves antigens from two genetic sources, both 'foreign' to the maternal recipient, and in this situation it is not the mass of the antigenic challenge but its 'density' in the placental graft that may be significant.

The influences of placental mass and antigenicity may add to the effect of whether an immune response may be primary, as in first pregnancy, or secondary, as in subsequent pregnancies. Twins in a first pregnancy are associated with higher risk of PET than twins in a subsequent pregnancy. However, these considerations are speculative in the absence of any defined causal antigen.

MacGillivray (1958) reported a protective effect of previous miscarriage on PET incidence in first full-term pregnancies. This may be understood in terms of the miscarriage priming the maternal immune response which would be adequate in a subsequent full-term pregnancy associated with second exposure to a causal antigen.

The risk of PET is reduced in those women with prolonged prior exposure to seminal antigens, e.g. women avoiding pregnancy using the contraceptive pill (Marti and Herrmann, 1977). If pregnancy tissues and semen share antigens then prolonged exposure to seminal fluid may again be seen as priming the maternal immune response prior to challenge in first pregnancy. The high incidence of PET in very young women with presumed limited exposure to seminal antigens prior to first pregnancy (MacGillivray, 1958), may be understood along similar lines. Similar considerations relating to changed paternity and previous blood transfusion will be discussed later (Feeney, 1980; Feeney et al, 1977).

Need et al (1983) studied 584 AID pregnancies and found evidence supporting the 'fresh mating' aetiological concept of PET. No role for HLA was evident rather than for a seminal component sensitizing the female partner in a chronic manner in oligospermic males. Prior full-term pregnancy was 'protective' with respect to PET but not 'partial' pregnancy, i.e. associated with abortion. These results provided clear support for immunological enhancement induced by prior coital antigen exposure in the genesis of PET.

Placental bed

The second invasive wave of trophoblast into the decidua and myometrium is not seen in PET (Robertson et al, 1976; Figure 1). This cellular migration normally occurring at 12 and 16 weeks results in 'physiological' dilatation of the spiral arteries, so accommodating the increased blood flow to the fetus and perhaps also the increased maternal blood volume (Figure 2). Whether these waves of trophoblast invasion are controlled by immune mechanisms is not known (see Chapter 8). Sheppard and Bonnar (1976) have noted a similar failure of physiological response in the maternal vessels in placental bed tissues in cases of intrauterine growth retardation in the absence of pre-eclampsia.

The relationship between feto-maternal interaction and placentation has been studied. Evidence in the mouse has indicated that feto-maternal histocompatibility or maternal tolerance of paternal antigens is associated with placental failure, whilst maternal disparity or hypersensitivity to paternal

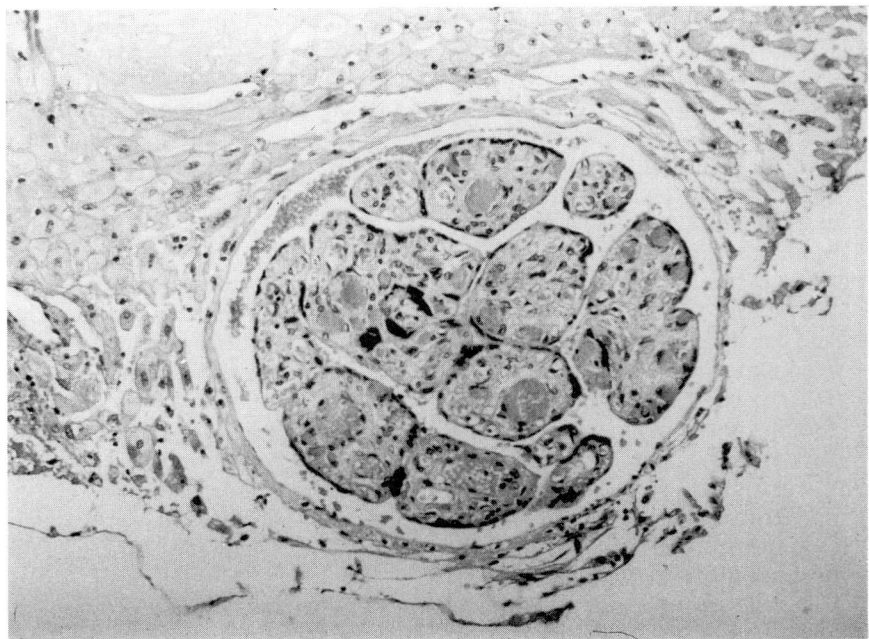

Figure 1. Chorionic villus in uterine vein. Evidence of fetal invasion of maternal host. Kindly donated by Dr Hans Kohler.

Table 1. Lymphocyte response to PHA in the presence of patient's own serum.

| Time of observation | Lymphocyte response to PHA (cpm $\times 10^3$) Mean $\pm$ SD | | | |
	Pre-eclampsia (a)	Normal pregnancy (b)	Never been pregnant (c)	p value
Pregnant	55.4 ± 58.0 (41)	93.2 ± 73.3 (39)		a:b<0.01 a:c<0.005 b:c<0.025
			248.3 ± 249.9 (14)	
Postnatal	81.6 ± 72.8 (29)	132.0 ± 65.1 (21)		a:b<0.01 a:c<0.0125 b:c<0.05

The number of observations is shown in brackets.

antigens favoured pregnancy outcome (James, 1965). Using materno-fetal mixed lymphocyte culture reactions as a measure of materno-fetal disparity, Jenkins and Good (1976) showed an association of larger placentas with increasing disparity. The presence of fetal tissue as cytotrophoblast in maternal spiral arteries suggests a possible immune challenge to the maternal host, but whether this influences the degree of uterine invasion by trophoblast is not clear. The association of increased placental mass with histoincompatibility (Jenkins and Good, 1976) and increased incidence of PET is not in accord with later evidence of increased histocompatibility in severe PET (Jenkins et al, 1978).

Cooper and Liston (1979) have concluded that data from Aberdeen and America was consistent with severe PET being inherited as a Mendelian recessive but they were unable to determine whether it was the genotype of the mother or the offspring which led to the condition. Chesley's data in North America (Chesley et al, 1962; Chesley et al, 1968) favoured the maternal genotype. Recurrent severe PET seems to have the same genetic basis as the more common primigravid type. Mild non-proteinuria PET seems usually to be inherited independently of the severe form. The apparent recessive inheritance of severe PET could be due to common environmental factors within families. Recent evidence (Boyd et al, 1987) related to increased PET prevalence in trisomy 13 has implicated a gene or genes on fetal chromosome 13 in the aetiology of PET.

Cell-mediated immune response

Need et al (1976) reported a greater degree of immunosuppression during pre-eclamptic pregnancies than in normal pregnancies. This was apparent both in the presence and absence of maternal serum when maternal lymphocytes were treated with phytohaemagglutinin (PHA). The patients were women with carefully defined severe pre-eclampsia and controls were age- and parity-matched (Table 1).

Table 2. Mean ($\pm$ SD) values for one-way mixed lymphocyte reactions (MLR) performed at delivery in 25 pre-eclamptic women and 33 normal controls and their husbands and babies.*

MLR study	Pre-eclamptic patients	Controls	p value†
Mother–father	1.35 ± 1.19 ($n = 25$)	2.62 ± 1.76 ($n = 33$)	<0.01
Mother–child	0.59 ± 1.26 ($n = 11$)	1.38 ± 1.50 ($n = 30$)	NS

* Studies on fresh cord blood were sometimes not possible due to perinatal deaths.
† Two-sample rank sum test. NS = Not significant.

These same patients were studied by Jenkins et al (1978) with respect to human leukocyte antigens (HLA) and mixed lymphocyte reactions. Thirty eight women and their husbands formed the study group, and 39 women with normal pregnancies as well as their husbands served as controls. Parental HLA compatibility was increased in the pre-eclamptic group compared with matched controls and with theoretical estimates for possible matings (Figure 3). The one-way mixed lymphocyte reaction at delivery showed a diminished response of maternal to paternal and cord blood cells in pre-eclamptic women (Table 2). It is postulated that this reduced maternal reactivity may have a role in PET and that paternal–maternal histocompatibility may be a feature of the severe form. HLA antigen distribution in patients with severe pre-eclampsia and their husbands was not different from controls, an observation consistent

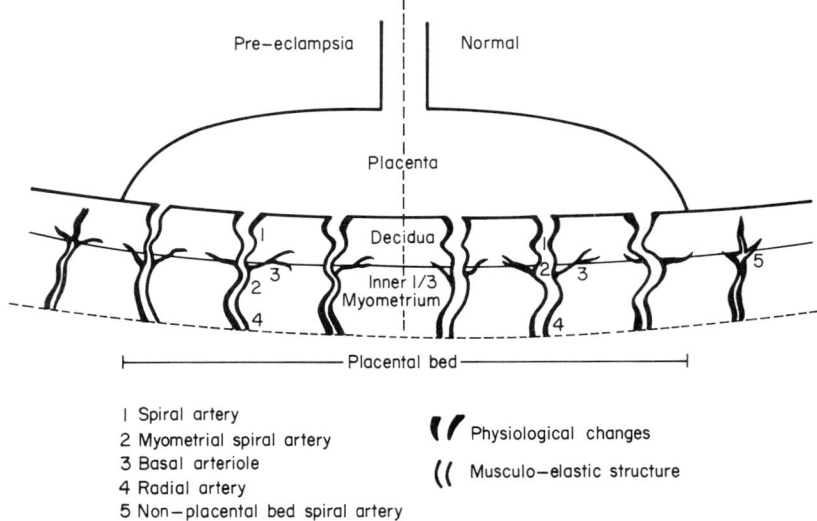

I Spiral artery
2 Myometrial spiral artery
3 Basal arteriole
4 Radial artery
5 Non-placental bed spiral artery

𝟔𝟔 Physiological changes

((Musculo-elastic structure

Figure 2. Diagrammatic demonstration of failure of physiological 'dilation' of spiral arteries in PET in comparison with similar vessels in normal pregnancy.

with that of Scott and Beer (1976). Redman et al (1978) reported similar results with increased homozygosity in both patient and her male partner. Gille et al (1977) also reported evidence of reduced lymphocyte reactivity in pre-eclamptic pregnancies.

Sargent et al (1982) reported an increase in spontaneous lymphocyte transformation in all pregnant women but no evidence of hyperactivity in pre-eclampsia. Their MLR time-course studies in pre-eclampsia showed a consistent and significant difference between maternal and paternal responses due to a diminished primary, rather than an enhanced or secondary, maternal reaction. No explanation for their diminished primary response was established.

Alanen and Lassila (1982), unlike Need et al (1976), showed no difference in lymphocyte reactivity between women with pre-eclampsia or uncomplicated pregnancy using phytohaemagglutinin, concanavalin A and purified protein derivative of tuberculin. Both groups of women exhibited normal numbers of circulating T and B lymphocytes. The number of active E

Table 3. Anti-HLA antibodies in severe pre-eclampsia/eclampsia and matched controls.

Time of sample	Toxaemic	Control
Antenatal	−(8)	5 (22)
Delivery	−(35)	6 (29)
Postnatal	−(27)	7 (21)
Totals	−(70)	7 (72)

The figures in parentheses are the number of samples.

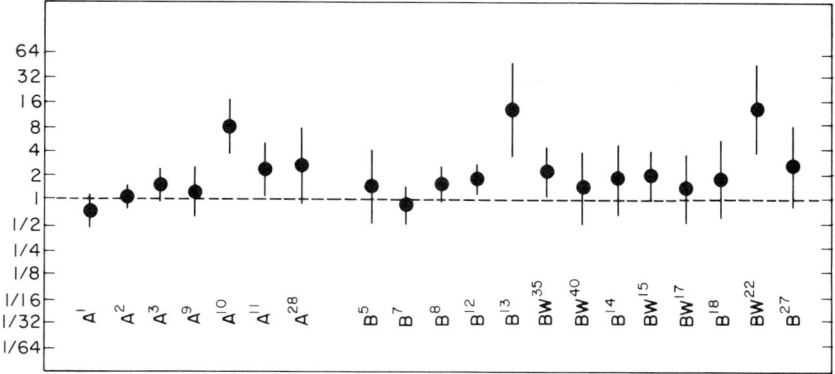

Figure 3. Matching of HLA antigens in pre-eclamptic pairs compared with estimates from general population data. Bold dots on display relate to frequency of matchings (± SD). Marks on vertical axis represent doubling or halving in incidence of matching from that expected. Eighteen of the twenty antigens were more commonly matched in pre-eclamptic pairs than controls.

rosette-forming cells was significantly higher in peripheral blood of pre-eclamptic patients.

Studies of sub-populations of T cells have not shown altered numbers of suppressor or helper T cells in pre-eclampsia compared with controls. Jenkins and Cumberbatch (1980), in a prospective study of peripheral lymphocyte response to PHA in pregnancy-induced hypertension (as distinct from pre-eclampsia), showed no difference from controls at any stage in pregnancy. The difference between these findings and those of Need et al (1976) may be seen as suggesting that pregnancy-induced hypertension and severe pre-eclampsia could have different pathologies. Kilpatrick (1987) studied full HLA-A,B and DR types in 22 families associated with severe PET, 21 with mild PET and 132 control families. There was an increased frequency of HLA-DR4 in both neonates and mothers of the severe PET families compared with controls. There was no difference between the PET groups and controls in HLA antigen homozygosity, HLA antigen sharing or in lymphocytotoxin production. They speculated that the maternal susceptibility for PET is located on chromosome 6 and is in positive linkage disequilibrium with HLA-DR4. A 'substantial proportion' of their PET patients had the maximum number of HLA mismatches between mother and fetus, showing that a high degree of HLA compatibility (Jenkins et al, 1978) is not a prerequisite for the development of the disease.

Humoral immune response

Data on changes in plasma immunoglobulin levels, particularly IgG, in pre-eclampsia and normal pregnancy are conflicting. Kelly and McEwan (1973) reported that urinary excretion of IgA is related to fetal mortality in pre-eclampsia and this IgA may have been produced in the renal tubule in response to an antigen associated with the condition.

Table 4. Numbers of patients in different 'changed paternity' groups associated with PET in a pregnancy subsequent to the first which was normal (Feeney, 1980).

	Patients	Controls	
Definite record of changed paternity	9	1	$(p<0.05$
Strong suggestive evidence of changed paternity	4	2	$\}$ $(p<0.01)$
Recorded evidence gives rise to doubt	5	2	
No evidence of changed paternity	29	42	
Total	47	47	

Jenkins et al (1977), in a prospective study of cases of severe pre-eclampsia, found a significantly reduced incidence of serum antibody to paternal histocompatibility antigens (Table 3). These results suggested a maternal hypo-response to fetal antigens in severe pre-eclampsia which differed from previous reports indicating the opposite in less severe or ill-defined pre-eclampsia (Tiilikainen, 1971). Caretti et al (1974) also reported a significant association between pre-eclampsia and the presence of anti-HLA antibodies. Differences in severity of the disease in different studies may explain conflicting results.

Immune complexes

Kirkwood (1975) has suggested that PET is an immune complex disease based on the observation of mild arthritic features in some PET patients. She proposed PET as a possible type III hypersensitivity state involving a maternal antibody response to a fetal antigen; poor maternal antibody response in primigravidas experiencing fetal antigens for the first time would result in antigen excess and no immune complex formation, whilst an intermediate immune response may yield complexes with slight antigen or antibody excess which persist in the circulation, activate complement and cause the disease. Multiparous patients with a good immune response resulting in antibody excess would be free of immune complex disease. However, the study of immune complexes in normal pregnancy and PET has yielded contradictory results, probably the consequence of methodological problems (McLaughlin et al, 1979). Stirrat et al (1978) reported increased levels of circulating immune complexes in PET compared with normal pregnancy. Petrucco et al (1979) reported the presence of IgM deposits in renal glomeruli in seven of eleven patients with severe disease, with arteriolar and glomerular complement deposition in nine of these eleven cases. Antibody and/or complement deposition has also been reported in the liver and in decidual blood vessels in PET (Arias and Mancilla-Jimenez, 1978; Kitzmiller and Benirschke, 1973).

It is attractive to speculate that an as yet undefined antigen might immunize in certain pregnancies resulting in immune complex disease at tissue sites with appropriate ratios of antigen to antibody, notably the kidney, liver and placental bed vasculature. There are similarities between pre-eclampsia and acute immune complex glomerulonephritis and its resemblance to the generalized Schwartzmann reaction is of note.

CONCLUDING REMARKS

There is some circumstantial evidence to support the hypothesis that the pre-eclamptic woman has failed to make adequate immune adaptation to the pregnant state. This is more evident in first pregnancies and in the presence of increased placental mass. It may be inherited as a recessive trait together with a defective immune response to histocompatibility or pregnancy-associated antigens. This might be further exacerbated in histo-compatible matings. The evidence of Feeney (1980) showing an increased incidence of changed paternity in multiparous women with pre-eclampsia (Table 4), having had normal first pregnancies, as well as the protective effect of previous blood transfusions on the first pregnancy incidence of pre-eclampsia, is consistent with this hypothesis.

However, the relationship of these immune changes to the low grade intra-vascular coagulation or decreased fibrinolysis observed in pre-eclampsia, as well as changes in the renin angiotensin system, remain largely undefined. The falling incidence of the disease in the developed world, whilst it still persists in the Third World, seems unlikely to be completely explained by better antenatal care.

Immune factors may act as trigger mechanisms if other variables are 'permissive' in a 'domino effect'. The remarkable variability in presentation and progress of the disease may reflect the presence of a variable number of these permissive factors or the absence of others.

The disease remains the main killer of pregnant women and their unborn children in the Third World but is fast disappearing as a cause of such in the developed world. This 'disease of theories' may eventually disappear without its complex aetiology having been unravelled. Those thousands of researchers who have tackled its mysteries in vain would then have to acknowledge defeat as the disease disappeared from the stage. Alternatively, the disease may return with a vengeance as new reproductive technologies alter feto-maternal relationships.

REFERENCES

Alanen A & Lassila O (1982) Cell mediated immunity in normal pregnancy and pre-eclampsia. *Journal of Reproductive Immunology* 4: 349–354.
Arduini D, Rizzo G, Romanini C & Mancuso S (1987) Utero-placental blood flow velocity wave forms as predictors of pregnancy induced hypertension. *European Journal of Obstetrics and Gynaecology and Reproductive Biology* 26: 335–341.
Arias F & Mancilla-Jimenez R (1978) Hepatic fibrinogen deposits in pre-eclampsia. Immuno-fluorescent evidence. *New England Journal of Medicine* 295: 578–582.
Brosens K, Robertson WB & Dixon HG (1972) The role of the spiral arteries in the pathogenesis of pre-eclampsia. In Wynn RM (ed.) *Obstetrics and Gynecology Annual*, p 177. New York: Appleton Century Crofts.
Campbell DM (1981) Further studies on Evans blue disappearance rate in normal and pre-eclamptic pregnancies. *British Meeting of the International Society of the Study of Hypertension in Pregnancy*. Leeds.
Campbell DM & MacGillivray I (1975) The effect of a low calorie diet or a thiazide diuretic on the incidence of pre-eclampsia and on birthweight. *British Journal of Obstetrics and Gynaecology* 82: 572.

Caretti N, Fagiola V, Zanetti M & Chairamonte P (1974) Association of anti-HLA antibodies with toxaemia of pregnancy. In Centara A & Caretti N (eds) *Immunology in Obstetrics and Gynaecology*, pp 221–225. New York: Excerpta Medica.

Chesley LC, Cosgrove RA & Annitto JE (1962) Pregnancies in the Sisters and Daughters of Eclamptic Women. *Obstetrics and Gynaecology* **20:** 39–46.

Chesley LC (1978) *Hypertensive disorders in pregnancy*. New York: Appleton-Century-Crofts.

Chesley LC, Annitto JD & Cosgrove RA (1968) The Familial Factor in Toxaemia of Pregnancy. *Obstetrics and Gynaecology* **32:** 303–311.

Chesley LC & Cooper DW (1986) Genetics of Hypertension in Pregnancy: Possible single gene control of pre-eclampsia and eclampsia in the descendants of eclamptic women. *British Journal of Obstetrics and Gynaecology* **93:** 898–908.

Confidential Enquiries into Maternal Deaths in England and Wales 1967–1969 (1972). London: Her Majesty's Stationery Office.

Cooper D & Liston WA (1979) Genetic control of severe pre-eclampsia. *Journal of Medical Genetics* **16:** 409–416.

Feeney JG (1980) Pre-eclampsia and changed paternity. In Bonnar J, Symmonds E & MacGillivray I (eds) *Proceedings of the First Congress of the International Society for the Study of Hypertension in Pregnancy*, pp 41–44. MTP Press.

Feeney JG, Tovey LAD & Scott JS (1977) Influence of previous blood transfusion on incidence of pre-eclampsia. *Lancet* **i:** 874–875.

Fox H (1978) *Pathology of the Placenta*. London: WB Saunders.

Gant NF, Daley GL, Chand S, Whalley PJ & McDonald PC (1971) A study of angiotensin II, pressor response throughout primigravid pregnancy. *Journal of Clinical Investigation* **52:** 2682.

Gant NF, Chand S, Cunningham SG & McDonald PC (1976) Control of vascular reactivity to angiotensin II in human pregnancy. In Lindheimer MD, Katz AI & Zuspan FP (eds) *Hypertension in Pregnancy*. New York: J Wiley, p 148.

Gant NF, Porter JC & McDonald PC (1977) Relationship of maternal placental blood flow to the placental clearance of maternal plasma dehydroisoandrosterone sulphate through oestradiol. In Symonds EH (ed.) *Clinics in Obstetrics and Gynaecology*, Vol. 4, p 632. Hypertensive States in Pregnancy. London: WB Saunders.

Ghose N & Das B (1985) Treatment of Eclampsia. *Journal of the Indian Medical Association* **83:** 299–302.

Gille J, Williams JH & Hoffman CP (1977) *European Journal of Obstetrics, Gynaecology and Reproductive Biology* **7:** 227.

Grieve IFK, Campbell-Brown BM & Johnstone FD (1979) Dieting in pregnancy: A study of the effect of a high protein, low carbohydrate diet on birthweight in an obstetric population. In Sutherland HS & Stowers JM (eds) *Carbohydrate Metabolism in Pregnancy and the Newborn*. p 518. Berlin: Springer.

Jaameri KEV, Koivuniemi AP & Carpen ED (1965) Occurrence of trophoblasts in the blood of toxaemic patients. *Gynaecologia* **160:** 315.

James DA (1965) *Nature* (London) **205:** 613.

Jenkins DM & Cumberbatch KM (1980) *Journal of Reproductive Immunology* **2:** 93–97.

Jenkins DM & Good S (1976) Mixed lymphocyte reaction and placentation. *Nature, New Biology* **240:** 211.

Jenkins DM & Perry LA (1978) Plasma prolactin in pregnancy induced hypertension. *British Journal of Obstetrics and Gynaecology* **85:** 754–757.

Jenkins DM & Soltan HM (1980) Plasma prolactin and puerperal blood pressure. *British Journal of Obstetrics and Gynaecology* **87:** 597–599.

Jenkins DM, Acres MD, Peters J & Riley J (1972) Human chorionic gonadotrophins and the fetal allograft. *American Journal of Obstetrics and Gynecology* **114:** 13–16.

Jenkins DM, Need JA & Rajah SM (1977) Deficiency of specific HLA antibodies in severe pregnancy pre-eclampsia/eclampsia. *Clinical and Experimental Immunology* **27:** 485–486.

Jenkins DM, Need JA, Scott JS, Morris H & Pepper M (1978) Human leucocyte antigens and mixed lymphocyte reaction in severe pre-eclampsia. *British Medical Journal* **1:** 542–544.

Jones CJP & Fox H (1980) An ultrastructural and ultrahistochemical study of the human placenta in maternal pre-eclampsia. *Placenta* **1:** 61.

Kalmus H (1946) On the familial appearances of maternal and fetal incompatibility. *Annals of Eugenics* **13:** 141–145.

Kelly AM & McEwan HP (1973) Proteinuria in pre-eclamptic toxaemia of pregnancy. *Journal of Obstetrics and Gynaecology of the British Commonwealth* **80:** 520–524.

Kilpatrick DC (1987) Immune mechanisms and pre-eclampsia. *Lancet* **ii:** 1460.

Kirkwood E (1975) Is pre-eclampsia an immune complex disease? *Lancet* **ii:** 1100.

Kitzmiller JL & Benirschke K (1973) Immunofluorescent study of placental bed vessels in pre-eclampsia of pregnancy. *American Journal of Obstetrics and Gynecology* **115:** 248–251.

Lever ICW (1843) Cases of puerperal convulsions with remarks. In Barlow GH (ed.) *Guy's Hospital Reports, 2nd Series*, p 495. London: Samuel Highley.

McFarlane A & Scott JS (1976) Pre-eclampsia/eclampsia in twin pregnancies. *Journal of Medical Genetics* **13:** 208–211.

MacGillivray I (1958) Some observations on the incidence of pre-eclampsia. *Journal of Obstetrics and Gynaecology of the British Commonwealth* **65:** 536.

MacGillivray I (1967) The significance of blood pressure and body water changes in pregnancy. *Scottish Medical Journal* **12:** 237.

MacGillivray I (1975) Complications of twin pregnancies. In MacGillivray I, Nylander PPS & Cornay G (eds) *Human Multiple Reproduction*, p 116. Toronto: WB Saunders.

MacGillivray I (1983) Pre-eclampsia, the Hypertensive Disease of Pregnancy, London: WB Saunders.

McLaughlin PJ, Stirrat GM, Redman CWG & Levinsky RJ (1979) Immune complexes in normal and pre-eclamptic pregnancy. *Lancet* **i:** 934.

Marti JJ & Herrmann U (1977) Immunogestosis: A new aetiological concept of 'essential' EPH gestosis with special consideration of the primigravid patient. *American Journal of Obstetrics and Gynecology* **128:** 489–493.

Mauriceau F(1668) Des maladies et fennes grosses. *Accuoches avec la Bonne et Veritable Methode*, Paris: Circle du Linne Precieux.

Need JA, Jenkins DM, Scott JS (1976) The response of lymphocytes to phytohaemagglutinin in women with pre-eclampsia. *British Journal of Obstetrics and Gynaecology* **83:** 438–440.

Need JA, Bell P, Meffin E, Iowes WR (1983) Pre-eclampsia in pregnancies from donor inseminations. *Journal of Reproductive Immunology* **5:** 329–338.

Penrose LS (1946) On the familial appearances of maternal and fetal incompatibility. *Annals of Eugenics* **13:** 141–145.

Petrucco PM, Woodroffe AJ, McKenzie PE & Clarkson AR (1979) A study of immune complexes in normal pregnancy and pre-eclampsia. In Studd J (ed.) *Progress in Obstetrics and Gynaecology*, Vol. 1, p 68. Edinburgh: Churchill Livingstone.

Platt R, Stewart AE & Emery EW (1958) The aetiology incidence and heredity of pre-eclamptic toxaemia of pregnancy. *Lancet* **i:** 552–556.

Redman CWG, Bodmer WF, Bodmer JF, Beilin LJ & Bonnar J (1978) HLA antigens in severe pre-eclampsia. *Lancet* **ii:** 397–399.

Robertson WB, Brosens I & Dixon HG (1976) Maternal uterine vascular lesions in the hypertensive complications of pregnancy. In Lindheimer MD, Katz AI & Zuspan FP (eds) *Hypertension in Pregnancy*, p 15. New York: John Wiley and Sons.

Sammour MD, Ammar AR, Tash F & Dawood S (1980) Catecholamines during labour in normal and pre-eclamptic pregnancy. In Bonnar J, MacGillivray I & Symonds EM (eds) *Pregnancy Hypertension*, p 167. Lancaster: MTP Press.

Sargent IL, Redman CWG & Stirrat GM (1982) Maternal cell mediated immunity in normal and pre-eclamptic pregnancy. *Clinical and Experimental Immunology* **50:** 601–609.

Scott JR & Beer AE (1976) *Journal of the American Medical Association* **235:** 402.

Scott JS, Jenkins DM & Need JA (1978) Immunology of Pre-eclampsia. *Lancet* **i:** 704–706.

Serhal JJ & Craft I (1987) *Lancet* **ii:** 744.

Sheehan H & Lynch JB (1973) *Pathology of Toxaemia of Pregnancy*. London: Churchill Livingstone.

Sheppard BL & Bonnar J (1976) The ultrastructure of the arterial supply of the human placenta in pregnancy complicated by fetal growth retardation. *British Journal of Obstetrics and Gynaecology* **83:** 948.

Sinha DP & Faulk WP (1982) Clotting and immunological factors in pre-eclampsia. In Sammour MD, Symonds EM, Zuspan FP & El-Tomi N (eds) *Proceedings of the 2nd Congress of the International Society for the Study of Hypertension in Pregnancy*. p 527. Cairo: Aim-Shams University Press.

Stevenson AC, Davison BCC, Say B et al (1971) Contribution of feto-maternal incompatibility to aetiology of pre-eclamptic toxaemia *Lancet* **ii:** 1286–1289.

Stirrat GM, Redman CWG & Levinsky RJ (1978) Circulating immune complexes in pre-eclampsia. *British Medical Journal* **1:** 1450.

Symonds EM & Broughton-Pipkin F (1978) Pregnancy hypertension parity and the renin angiotension system. *American Journal of Obstetrics and Gynecology* **132:** 473.

Thorburn J, Drummond MM, Wigham KA et al (1982) Blood viscosity and haemostatic factors in late pregnancy, pre-eclampsia and fetal growth retardation. *British Journal of Obstetrics and Gynaecology* **89:** 117.

Vollman RF (1970) Rates of toxaemia by age and parity. In Rippman ET (ed.) *Die Spatgestose (EHO Gestose)*, p 338. Basel-Schwalie: EPH Gestosis Press.

6

Gestational trophoblastic disease

ROSS S. BERKOWITZ
DONALD P. GOLDSTEIN

Gestational trophoblastic tumours (GTT) are one of the rare human malignancies that are highly curable even with disseminated disease (Bagshawe, 1976; Goldstein and Berkowitz, 1982). GTT comprise a spectrum of interrelated neoplasms including invasive mole and choriocarcinoma that have varying tendencies for local invasion and spread. While GTT most commonly follow a molar pregnancy, they may ensue after any gestation including ectopic and term pregnancy or spontaneous and therapeutic abortion. Exciting advances have occurred in the detection, management and follow-up of patients with gestational trophoblastic disease during recent years. Furthermore, our understanding of the cytogenetic origin and immunobiology of gestational trophoblastic diseases has also substantially advanced. This chapter will review current knowledge of the clinical management and immunobiology of GTT.

MOLAR PREGNANCY

Complete vs partial molar pregnancy: pathologic and chromosomal features

Molar pregnancy may be categorized as either a complete or partial mole on the basis of gross morphology, histopathology and karyotype (Table 1).

Complete moles have no identifiable embryonic or fetal tissues. The chorionic villi are diffusely hydropic and are enveloped by hyperplastic trophoblast. Complete hydatidiform moles usually have a 46XX karyotype

Table 1. Complete vs partial molar pregnancy.

	Complete mole	Partial mole
Fetal or embryonic tissue	Absent	Present
Hydatidiform swelling of chorionic villi	Diffuse	Focal
Trophoblastic hyperplasia	Diffuse	Focal
Scalloping of chorionic villi	Absent	Present
Trophoblastic stromal inclusions	Absent	Present
Karyotype	46XX; 46XY	Triploid

and the molar chromosomes are entirely of paternal origin (Kajii and Ohama, 1977). Complete moles generally arise from an ovum which has been fertilized by a haploid sperm which then duplicates its own chromosomes; maternal chromosomes may be either absent or inactivated (Yamashita et al, 1979). While most complete moles have a 46XX chromosomal pattern, about 10% of complete moles have a 46XY karyotype (Pattillo et al, 1981). The molar chromosomes in the 46XY complete mole are also entirely of paternal origin and result from a dispermic fertilization (Surti et al, 1979).

Partial hydatidiform moles are characterized by the following features: (i) varying-sized chorionic villi with focal hydropic swelling and cavitation, (ii) marked villous scalloping with stromal trophoblastic inclusions, (iii) focal trophoblastic hyperplasia, and (iv) identifiable fetal or embryonic tissues (Szulman and Surti, 1978a). Partial moles usually have a triploid karyotype which results from fertilization of an ovum by two sperm (Szulman and Surti, 1978b). When fetuses are identified with partial moles, they generally have stigmata of triploidy including growth retardation, syndactyly, pulmonary hypoplasia, and cleft palate.

Complete molar pregnancy

Presenting signs and symptoms

Vaginal bleeding. Vaginal bleeding is the most common presenting sign of complete mole occurring in 97% of our patients (Berkowitz and Goldstein, 1981). Molar villi may separate from the decidua and disrupt maternal vessels causing vaginal bleeding. The uterine cavity may be expanded by large volumes of retained clot.

Excessive uterine size. The uterus is excessively enlarged for gestational age in 51% of our patients with complete mole. The endometrial cavity may be expanded by both chorionic tissue and clot. Excessive uterine size is associated with markedly elevated human chorionic gonadotrophin (hCG) levels because the uterus is partially expanded by chorionic tissues with hyperplastic trophoblast.

Pre-eclampsia. Pre-eclamptic toxaemia is diagnosed in 27% of our patients with complete mole. Although pre-eclampsia is often associated with hypertension, proteinuria and hyperreflexia, convulsions rarely occur. Pre-eclampsia develops almost exclusively in patients with markedly elevated hCG values and excessive uterine size (Curry et al, 1975). The diagnosis of molar pregnancy should be considered in any patient who develops pre-eclampsia early in pregnancy.

Hyperemesis gravidarum. Of our patients with complete mole, 26% experience hyperemesis requiring anti-emetic therapy. Hyperemesis occurs primarily in patients with excessive uterine size and markedly elevated hCG values. Depue et al (1987) reported that hyperemesis is associated with elevated serum levels of free oestradiol in pregnant women. Furthermore, patients with molar pregnancy and markedly elevated hCG values tend to have particularly elevated serum oestradiol levels (Osathanondh et al, 1986).

Hyperthyroidism. Hyperthyroidism is observed in 7% of our patients with complete mole and is clinically manifested by tachycardia and tremor. The diagnosis of hyperthyroidism is confirmed by measuring elevated serum levels of free thyroxine (T_4) and tri-iodothyronine (T_3). If hyperthyroidism is suspected, it is important to administer β-adrenergic blockers prior to molar evacuation since anaesthesia or surgery may precipitate thyroid storm. Thyroid storm may cause hyperthermia, convulsion, atrial fibrillation or cardiovascular collapse.

Human chorionic gonadotrophin has been implicated as the thyroid stimulator in patients with molar pregnancy (Nisula and Taliadouros, 1980). Correlations between serum hCG and total T_4 or total T_3 concentrations have been observed in some but not all studies. We found no significant correlation, however, between serum hCG levels and free T_4 or T_3 index levels in 47 patients with complete mole (Amir et al, 1984). The identity of the thyrotropic factor in molar pregnancy is, therefore, still in question.

Trophoblastic embolization. Of our patients with complete mole, 2% develop acute respiratory distress presumably due to pulmonary trophoblastic embolization (Kohorn et al, 1978). Patients may develop tachypnoea and tachycardia in the recovery room after molar evacuation. Auscultation of the chest may demonstrate diffuse rales and chest roentgenogram may show bilateral pulmonary infiltrates. The signs and symptoms of respiratory insufficiency generally resolve within 72 hours with cardiovascular and respiratory support.

Interestingly, Hankins et al (1987) detected only scanty amounts of trophoblast in pulmonary arterial blood of six women undergoing evacuation of large molar pregnancies. None of these women developed significant pulmonary compromise. Hankins et al postulated that respiratory compromise in molar pregnancy may be due at least in part to the cardiopulmonary changes induced by pre-eclampsia, hyperthyroidism and vigorous transfusion therapy.

Theca lutein ovarian cysts. Prominent theca lutein ovarian cysts (>6 cm in diameter) develop in about half of our patients with complete mole (Berkowitz and Goldstein, 1981). The cysts are usually multilocular and bilateral and contain serosanguineous or amber-coloured fluid. Markedly elevated hCG levels hyperstimulate the ovaries and induce theca lutein cysts. The formation of theca lutein cysts may also be related to increased serum levels of prolactin (Osathanondh et al, 1986). While theca lutein cysts are usually noted at presentation, they may also develop shortly after uterine evacuation. Montz et al (1987) studied the natural history of theca lutein cysts in 99 patients and the mean time for spontaneous disappearance was 8 weeks. Only three patients developed acute surgical complications of cystic haemorrhage or adnexal torsion.

Partial molar pregnancy

Presenting signs and symptoms

Between January 1979 and August 1984, 81 patients were followed with partial hydatidiform mole at the New England Trophoblastic Disease Center (NETDC) (Berkowitz et al, 1986b). The uterine size was small for dates in 54 (66.7%) patients, appropriate for dates in 24 (29.6%) patients and large for dates in only three (3.7%) patients. The presenting clinical diagnosis was either incomplete or missed abortion in 74 (91.3%) patients and hydatidiform mole in only 5 (6.2%) patients. Pre-evacuation hCG levels exceeded 100 000 mIU/ml in only two (6.6%) of 30 patients and no patient had prominent theca lutein ovarian cysts. Patients with partial mole usually do not present with the clinical features that are characteristic of complete mole. These patients generally present with the signs and symptoms of incomplete or missed abortion, and the diagnosis of partial mole may be considered only after histological review of the curettage specimens (Szulman and Surti, 1982).

Diagnosis of hydatidiform mole: ultrasonography

Ultrasonography is a sensitive technique for differentiating between a normal intrauterine gestation and a complete molar pregnancy. Because of the diffuse hydropic swelling of the chorionic villi, complete mole produces a characteristic vesicular pattern on the ultrasound. However, molar villi may be too small to be resolved by ultrasound in the first trimester. It may, therefore, be difficult to distinguish by ultrasound an early mole from degenerating products of conception. However, the accuracy of sonographic interpretation may be enhanced by consideration of the hCG level (Romero et al, 1985).

Ultrasonography may also contribute to the diagnosis of partial molar pregnancy (Berkowitz et al, 1986b). Sixty-one of our patients with partial mole, who were clinically thought to have an incomplete or missed abortion, underwent a pre-evacuation pelvic ultrasound. Pelvic ultrasound suggested a diagnosis of mole in 16 (26.2%) patients due to the presence of multiple cystic spaces in the placenta.

Natural history of molar pregnancy

Complete hydatidiform moles are well recognized to have a potential for developing uterine invasion or distant spread. Following evacuation, uterine invasion occurs in 15% of patients and metastasis develops in 4% (Berkowitz and Goldstein, 1986).

We have reviewed 858 patients with complete mole at the NETDC to identify factors that predispose to persistent GTT (Table 2). At the time of presentation, 41% of the patients had the following signs of marked tropho-blastic proliferation: hCG level of > 100 000 mIU/ml, large uterine size for

Table 2. Sequelae of low- and high-risk complete hydatidiform mole.

Outcome	Number of patients (%)	
	Low-risk	High-risk
Normal involution	486/506 (96)	212/352 (60.2)
Persistent GTT		
Non-metastatic	17/506 (3.4)	109/352 (31.0)
Metastatic	3/506 (0.6)	31/352 (8.8)
Totals	506/858 (59)	352/858 (41)

GTT: gestational trophoblastic tumour.
All patients managed by evacuation with no prophylactic chemotherapy.

gestational age, and theca lutein cysts greater than 6 cm in diameter. After evacuation, 31% of these patients developed uterine invasion and 8.8% developed metastases. The risk for persistent GTT is considerably less for patients who do not present with signs of marked trophoblastic growth. Following molar evacuation, only 3.4% of these patients developed local invasion and 0.6% developed metastases. Therefore, patients with complete moles with markedly elevated hCG levels and excessive uterine size are at increased risk of developing persistent GTT.

Eight (9.9%) of our 81 patients with partial mole developed non-metastatic persistent GTT (Berkowitz et al, 1986b). These eight patients were all thought to have missed abortion before evacuation. None of the patients had theca lutein cysts, markedly elevated hCG levels or excessive uterine size before molar evacuation. The patients with partial mole who developed persistent tumour did not have clinical characteristics that distinguished them from other patients with partial mole.

Treatment

Suction curettage is the preferred method of evacuation regardless of uterine size in patients who desire to preserve fertility (Berkowitz et al, 1987b). An oxytocin infusion may be begun prior to the induction of anaesthesia. When suction evacuation is thought to be complete, a sharp curettage should be performed to remove any residual chorionic tissue. The tissue from suction and sharp curettage are separately submitted for pathological review.

If the patient no longer wishes to preserve fertility, hysterectomy may be performed. The ovaries may be conserved even though prominent theca lutein cysts are present.

Prophylactic chemotherapy

The use of prophylactic chemotherapy at the time of molar evacuation remains controversial. However, several studies have indicated that chemoprophylaxis reduces the risk of post-molar GTT.

Between July 1965 and June 1979 at the NETDC, 247 patients with complete mole received actinomycin-D prophylactically at the time of evacuation (Berkowitz et al, 1987b). Local uterine invasion subsequently developed in only 10 (4%) patients and no one developed metastases. Furthermore, all ten patients who developed local invasion later achieved remission after only one additional course of chemotherapy.

Kim et al (1986) performed a prospective randomized trial of chemoprophylaxis in patients with complete mole. Chemoprophylaxis reduced the incidence of persistent GTT from 47 to 14% in patients with high-risk mole.

We reviewed recently our experience with prophylactic chemotherapy in patients with high-risk mole (Berkowitz et al, 1987b). Following chemoprophylaxis, only 10 (11%) of 93 patients with high-risk mole developed persistent GTT. The risk for chemoprophylaxis failure was significantly related to the pre-evacuation hCG level. Prophylactic chemotherapy may be helpful in the management of patients with high-risk mole, particularly when hormonal follow-up is either unavailable or unreliable.

Human chorionic gonadotrophin

Human chorionic gonadotrophin is a constant and predictable secretory product of the trophoblast cell. Like the other glycoprotein hormones, hCG is composed of two polypeptide chains α and β attached to a carbohydrate moiety. The β-chain is biochemically unique and confers both biological and immunological specificity. The β-subunit radioimmunoassay is the most reliable commercial assay currently available and allows measurement of low concentrations of hCG without interference from physiological values of luteinizing hormone.

Highly sensitive and specific monoclonal immunoradiometric assays have recently been developed for measuring minute amounts of intact hCG and its free α- and β-subunits (Ozturk et al, 1988). During normal gestation, the β-hCG/intact hCG ratio is under stringent control and remains remarkably constant at about 0.5% after 5 weeks of pregnancy. In contrast, the β-hCG/intact hCG ratio in gestational choriocarcinoma ranges from 5 to 15%. This ratio in complete mole is intermediate between normal pregnancy and choriocarcinoma. The measurement of absolute serum concentrations of intact hCG and its subunits, and calculation of the ratios, may distinguish complete mole and choriocarcinoma from normal pregnancy with high probability. The free β-hCG/intact hCG ratio appears to reflect differentiation of the trophoblast.

The composition of sugar molecules that are linked to hCG has also been studied in both normal pregnancy and gestational choriocarcinoma. Choriocarcinoma hCG molecules are characterized by an eightfold increase in hexasaccharides as compared with normal pregnancy (Cole, 1986). hCG molecules that are secreted by malignant trophoblast are, therefore, structurally different from hCG molecules produced by normal trophoblast.

Hormonal follow-up

After molar evacuation, all patients must be followed with hCG measurements to detect persistent GTT promptly. Patients are monitored with weekly β-hCG levels until normal for three weeks, and then monthly levels until normal for six months.

Patients are encouraged to use reliable contraception during the entire interval of hormonal follow-up. Intrauterine devices should not be inserted until the patient attains normal hCG values because of the risk of perforation with invasive tumour. If the patient does not desire sterilization, she is then confronted with the choice of either oral contraceptives or barrier methods.

The incidence of post-molar GTT has been reported to be increased in patients who used oral contraceptives before gonadotrophin remission (Stone et al, 1976). Data from the University of Southern California and the NETDC indicate, however, that oral contraceptives do not increase the risk of post-molar trophoblastic disease or influence the hCG regression time (Morrow et al, 1985; Berkowitz et al, 1981b). We believe, therefore, that oral contraceptives may be safely prescribed after molar evacuation during the entire interval of hormonal follow-up.

GESTATIONAL TROPHOBLASTIC TUMOURS

Following a molar pregnancy, persistent GTT may have the histological pattern of either molar tissue or choriocarcinoma. Choriocarcinoma does not contain chorionic villous structures, but is composed of sheets of both anaplastic cyto- and syncytiotrophoblast. After a non-molar gestation, persistent GTT may only have the histological features of choriocarcinoma.

Placental site trophoblastic tumour (PSTT) represents an uncommon variant of choriocarcinoma. PSTT does not contain chorionic villi, but is composed almost entirely of cytotrophoblast with very minimal syncytiotrophoblast. PSTT secrete very limited amounts of hCG and are generally resistant to chemotherapy. There are few, if any, long-term survivors with metastatic PSTT despite intensive multimodal therapy. Because of their poor response to chemotherapy, a diagnosis of non-metastatic PSTT should be followed by prompt hysterectomy.

Natural history

Non-metastatic disease

Locally invasive GTT develops in 15% of patients following molar evacuation and infrequently after other gestations (Berkowitz and Goldstein, 1981). These patients may present with irregular vaginal bleeding, uterine sub-involution and/or elevated hCG values. The trophoblastic tumour may perforate through the myometrium producing intraperitoneal bleeding or erode into uterine vessels causing vaginal haemorrhage.

Metastatic disease

Metastatic GTT occurs in 4% of patients after molar evacuation and infrequently following other pregnancies. Metastatic GTT is usually associated with the presence of choriocarcinoma. Choriocarcinoma has a propensity for early vascular invasion with widespread dissemination. The most common metastatic sites in patients with GTT are as follows: lung 80%, vagina 30%, liver 10% and brain 10%. Because trophoblastic tumours are supplied by many fragile vessels, metastatic lesions are often haemorrhagic and patients commonly present with signs and symptoms of bleeding from metastases.

Staging system

The International Federation of Gynecology and Obstetrics has begun reporting data on GTT using an anatomical staging system (Table 3). Stage I includes all patients with persistently elevated hCG values and tumour confined to the uterine corpus. Stage II comprises all patients with tumour outside of the uterus but localized to the vagina and/or pelvis. Stage III includes all patients with pulmonary metastases with or without uterine, vaginal or pelvic involvement. Stage IV patients have far-advanced disease with involvement of the brain, liver, kidneys or gastrointestinal tract.

Table 3. Staging of gestational trophoblastic tumours.

Stage	Characteristics
I	Confined to uterine corpus
II	Metastases to pelvis and vagina
III	Metastases to lung
IV	Distant metastases

Patients with Stage IV disease are at highest risk to be resistant to chemotherapy. Stage IV tumours generally have the histological pattern of choriocarcinoma and commonly follow a non-molar pregnancy.

In addition to anatomical staging, it is helpful to employ other prognostic variables to predict the likelihood of drug resistance and to aid the clinician in selecting appropriate chemotherapy. The World Health Organization has proposed a prognostic scoring system, based on one developed by Bagshawe, which reliably predicts the potential for chemotherapy resistance (Table 4). When the prognostic score is 8 or greater, the patient is placed in a high-risk category and requires intensive combination chemotherapy to achieve remission. Patients with Stage I disease generally have a low-risk score and patients with Stage IV disease have a high-risk score.

Diagnostic evaluation

The optimal management of GTT requires a thorough assessment of the extent of the disease prior to the initiation of treatment. The metastatic work-up should include a chest roentgenogram, liver isotope scan, ultrasonography of the abdomen and pelvis, head computed tomography scan

Table 4. Scoring system based on prognostic factors.

Prognostic factors	Score†			
	0	1	2	4
Age (years)	≤39	>39		
Antecedent pregnancy	HM	Abortion	Term	
Interval*	4	4–6	7–12	12
hCG (IU/litre)	10^3	10^3–10^4	10^4–10^5	10^6
ABO groups (female × male)		O × A	B	
		A × O	AB	
Largest tumour, including uterine tumour		3–5 cm	5 cm	
Site of metastases		Spleen	GI tract	Brain
		Kidney	Liver	
No. of metastases identified		1–4	4–8	8
Prior chemotherapy			Single drug	2 or more drugs

* Interval: time (months) between end of antecedent pregnancy and start of chemotherapy.
† The total score for a patient is obtained by adding the individual scores for each prognostic factor. Total score:
  ≤4: low-risk.
  5–7: middle-risk.
  ≥8: high-risk.

and, in some cases, selective angiography of abdominal and pelvic organs. In the absence of pulmonary or vaginal metastases, involvement of other distant sites is uncommon. While the liver isotope scan may be useful, small scattered lesions may be missed by this technique. Selective angiography may be more sensitive in detecting hepatic metastases, but is associated with the risks of an invasive procedure. Ultrasound and computed tomography scan of the liver will, it is hoped, contribute to detection of hepatic lesions. The introduction of the head computed tomography scan has greatly facilitated the early detection of asymptomatic cerebral lesions (Athanassiou et al, 1983).

Human chorionic gonadotrophin levels may be measured in the cerebrospinal fluid (CSF) in patients with choriocarcinoma and/or metastatic disease to detect cerebral metastases. Bagshawe and Harland (1976) have reported that a plasma:CSF hCG ratio less than 60 strongly suggests central nervous system involvement by GTT. However, hCG levels in the CSF take time to equilibrate with the levels in the plasma. When plasma levels of hCG are rapidly changing, a single plasma:CSF hCG ratio may be misleading.

Radioimmunolocalization using ^{131}I-labelled antibodies to hCG has proved helpful in identifying occult sites of drug-resistant disease (Begent et al, 1980). Uptake by a lesion does not, however, absolutely exclude necrotic tumour tissue because necrotic trophoblast may still bind antibodies to hCG.

Management of Stage I GTT

Table 5 reviews the NETDC protocol for the management of Stage I disease. The selection of treatment is based primarily on the patient's desire to retain fertility.

If the patient no longer wishes to preserve fertility, hysterectomy with adjuvant single-agent chemotherapy may be performed. Adjuvant chemotherapy is administered for three reasons: (i) to reduce the likelihood of disseminating viable tumour at surgery, (ii) to maintain a cytotoxic level of chemotherapy in the bloodstream and tissues in case viable tumour cells are disseminated, and (iii) to treat any occult metastases that may be already present. Occult pulmonary metastases may be detected by computed tomography scan in about 40% of patients with presumed non-metastatic disease (Mutch et al, 1986). Twenty-three patients were treated by primary hysterectomy and adjuvant chemotherapy at the NETDC, and all achieved complete remission.

Single-agent chemotherapy is the preferred treatment in patients with

Table 5. Treatment protocol for Stage I GTT (NETDC).

Initial
Sequential MTX/Act-D *or*
Hysterectomy with adjunctive chemotherapy
Resistant
Combination chemotherapy
Hysterectomy with adjunctive chemotherapy
Local resection
Pelvic infusion
Follow-up
hCG
Weekly until normal × 3
Monthly until normal × 12
Contraception
12 consecutive months of normal hCG levels

MTX, Methotrexate.
Act-D, Actinomycin-D.

Stage I disease who desire to retain fertility. Primary single-agent chemotherapy was administered to 299 patients with Stage I GTT and 283 (94.6%) patients achieved complete remission. The remaining 16 resistant patients later attained remission with either further chemotherapy or surgical intervention. When the patient desires to preserve fertility but is resistant to single agent therapy, we favour administering combination chemotherapy. If the patient is resistant to both single-agent and combination chemotherapy, local uterine resection may be considered.

All patients with Stages I, II and III GTT are followed with weekly hCG levels until normal for three weeks and then monthly levels until normal for 12 months. Patients are encouraged to use effective contraception during the entire interval of hormonal follow-up.

Management of Stage II and III GTT

The NETDC protocol for the management of Stage II and III disease is outlined in Table 6. While low-risk patients are treated with primary single-agent chemotherapy, high-risk patients are managed with primary combination chemotherapy. Between July 1965 and December 1986, 25 patients with Stage II disease were managed at the NETDC and all achieved remission. Single-agent chemotherapy induced complete remission in 15 (88.2%) of 17 low-risk patients. In contrast, only two of eight high-risk patients attained remission with single-agent treatment.

Vaginal metastases may bleed profusely because they are highly vascular and friable. When blood loss is considerable, bleeding may be controlled by packing the lesion or performing wide local excision. Bilateral hypogastric artery ligation or angiographic procedures may also be required to control haemorrhage from vaginal tumour.

Between July 1965 and December 1986, 103 patients with Stage III disease were treated at the NETDC and 102 achieved complete remission.

Table 6. Treatment protocol for Stage II and III GTT (NETDC).

Low risk*	
Initial	Sequential MTX/Act-D
Resistant	Combination chemotherapy
High risk*	
Initial	Combination chemotherapy
Resistant	Second-line combination chemotherapy
Follow-up	
hCG	Weekly until normal × 3
	Monthly until normal × 12
Contraception	12 consecutive months of normal hCG levels

* Local resection optional.
MTX, Methotrexate.
Act-D, Actinomycin D.

Gonadotrophin remission was induced with single-agent chemotherapy in 63 (87%) of 72 patients with low-risk disease and in 13 (42%) of 31 patients with high-risk disease. All patients, who were resistant to single-agent treatment, later achieved remission with combination chemotherapy.

Thoracotomy has a limited role in the management of Stage III GTT. It should be undertaken if the diagnosis is seriously in doubt; furthermore, if a patient has a persistent viable pulmonary nodule despite intensive chemotherapy, thoracotomy may be performed to resect the resistant focus. Fibrotic nodules may, however, persist for months on chest roentgenogram after complete gonadotrophin remission is achieved.

Hysterectomy may be necessary in patients with metastatic disease to control uterine haemorrhage or sepsis. Furthermore, in patients with bulky uterine tumour, hysterectomy may reduce the tumour burden and limit the need for chemotherapy (Hammond et al, 1980).

Management of Stage IV GTT

Table 7 outlines the NETDC protocol for the management of Stage IV disease. These patients are at greatest risk of developing rapidly progressive and resistant tumours despite intensive therapy.

All patients with Stage IV disease should be treated with primary intensive combination chemotherapy and the selective use of radiation therapy and surgery (Surwit and Hammond, 1980). Before 1975, only six (30%) of 20 patients with Stage IV GTT achieved complete remission at the NETDC. After 1975, however, 12 (75%) of 16 patients with Stage IV tumours achieved gonadotrophin remission. This dramatic improvement in survival resulted from the use of primary combination chemotherapy in conjunction with radiation and surgical treatment.

If cerebral metastases are detected, whole brain irradiation is promptly instituted at our Center. The risk of spontaneous intracranial bleeding may be limited by the concurrent use of combination chemotherapy and irradiation

Table 7. Treatment protocol for Stage IV GTT (NETDC).

Initial
  Combination chemotherapy
  Brain
    Whole head irradiation (3000 rad)
    Craniotomy to manage complications
  Liver
    Resection to manage complications

Resistant*
  Second-line combination chemotherapy

Follow-up
  hCG
    Weekly until normal × 3
    Monthly until normal × 24

Contraception
  24 consecutive months of normal hCG levels

* Local resection optional.

(Weed and Hammond, 1980). Yordan et al (1987) reported that deaths due to cerebral involvement occurred in 11 (44%) of 25 patients treated with chemotherapy alone, but in none of 18 patients treated with irradiation and chemotherapy.

In contrast, Athanassiou et al (1983) have reported excellent remission rates in patients with brain metastases who were treated with chemotherapy alone. Of their patients with cerebral lesions, 80% achieved sustained remission when they were treated with intensive combination chemotherapy including high-dose intravenous and intrathecal methotrexate.

Craniotomy should be performed to manage life-threatening complications with the hope that the patient will ultimately be cured with chemotherapy. Craniotomy may be required to provide acute decompression or to control bleeding. Fortunately, patients with cerebral metastases who achieve remission generally have no residual neurological deficits.

Patients with Stage IV GTT are monitored with weekly hCG values until normal for three weeks and then monthly values until normal for 24 months.

These patients require prolonged follow-up because they have an increased risk of late recurrence.

Chemotherapy

Single-agent chemotherapy

Single-agent chemotherapy with either actinomycin D (ActD) or methotrexate (Mtx) has induced comparable and excellent remission rates in both non-metastatic and low-risk metastatic GTT (Osathanondh et al, 1975; Berkowitz et al, 1982a). An optimal regimen should maximize the cure rate while limiting toxicity.

Methotrexate–folinic acid (Mtx–FA) has been the preferred single-agent regimen in the treatment of GTT at the NETDC since 1974 (Berkowitz et al, 1981a, 1986a). Between September 1974 and September 1984, 185 patients with GTT were treated with primary Mtx–FA at the NETDC. Complete remission was induced with Mtx–FA in 162 (87.6%) patients and 132 (81.5%) of these patients required only one course of Mtx–FA to achieve remission. Mtx–FA induced remission in 147 (90.2%) of 163 patients with Stage I GTT and in 15 (68.2%) of 22 patients with low-risk Stages II and III disease. Following Mtx–FA, granulocytopaenia, thrombocytopaenia, and hepatotoxicity occurred in only 11 (5.9%), 3 (1.6%) and 26 (14.1%) patients, respectively. Mtx–FA not only induces an excellent remission rate with minimal toxicity but also effectively limits chemotherapy exposure.

Combination chemotherapy

Modified triple therapy with Mtx–FA, Act-D and cyclophosphamide has been the preferred combination drug protocol at the NETDC (Berkowitz et al, 1984a). However, triple therapy is inadequate as an initial treatment in metastatic patients with a high-risk prognostic score (score >8) (DuBeshter et al, 1987). Triple therapy induced remission in only five (45%) of 11 patients with a high-risk score.

Etoposide (VP16) has been demonstrated to be a new effective antitumour agent in GTT. Primary oral etoposide induced complete sustained remission in 56 (93.3%) of 60 patients with non-metastatic or low-risk metastatic GTT (Wong et al, 1986). Bagshawe (1984) has recently reported an 83% remission rate in patients with a high-risk score using a new combination chemotherapy which includes etoposide. This new regimen includes etoposide, Mtx, Act-D, cyclophosphamide and vincristine, and may be currently the preferred primary therapy for patients with a high-risk score. The optimal combination drug regimen will most likely include Mtx, Act-D and etoposide, and perhaps other agents, administered in the most dose-intensive manner.

Patients who require combination chemotherapy must be treated intensively to achieve remission. We administer combination chemotherapy as frequently as toxicity permits until the patient attains normal hCG levels.

After the patient achieves normal hCG values, additional chemotherapy is administered to reduce the risk of relapse.

SUBSEQUENT PREGNANCIES

After molar pregnancy

Patients with molar pregnancies can anticipate normal reproduction in the future (Berkowitz et al, 1987a). Patients with complete moles who were managed at the NETDC had a total of 1048 later pregnancies between June 1965 and December 1986, which resulted in 723 (69.0%) full-term live births, 81 (7.7%) premature deliveries, seven (0.6%) ectopics and six (0.6%) stillbirths (Table 8). First-trimester spontaneous abortion occurred

Table 8. Subsequent pregnancies in patients with complete mole (NETDC June 1965–December 1986).

Outcome	Number of pregnancies (%)
Term delivery	723 (69.0)
Stillbirth	6 (0.6)
Premature delivery	81 (7.7)
Spontaneous abortion	
1st trimester	174 (16.6)
2nd trimester	17 (1.6)
Therapeutic abortion	26 (2.6)
Ectopic	7 (0.6)
Repeat mole	14 (1.3)
Total number of pregnancies	1048
	Number of deliveries (%)
Congenital malformations	34/810 (4.2)
Primary caesarean sections	29/205 (14.1)*

* January 1979–December 1986.

in 174 (16.6%) pregnancies, and major and minor congenital anomalies were detected in only 34 (4.2%) infants. Primary caesarean section was performed in only 29 (14.1%) of 205 subsequent full-term and premature births between January 1979 and December 1986.

When a patient has had a molar pregnancy, however, she *is* at increased risk of developing molar disease in subsequent conceptions. Eleven (1:150) of our patients have had at least two consecutive molar gestations. Three of our patients who had repetitive molar pregnancies were later able to attain a normal full-term pregnancy.

It seems prudent, therefore, to obtain an ultrasound in the first trimester of any subsequent pregnancy to confirm normal gestational development. Furthermore, to exclude trophoblastic mischief, the placenta or products of conception from later pregnancies should undergo thorough pathological review, and an hCG measurement should be obtained six weeks after the completion of any future pregnancy.

Limited information is available concerning subsequent pregnancies in patients with partial mole. However, preliminary data indicates that their later reproductive outcome is consistent with the favourable experience of patients with complete mole (Berkowitz et al, 1987a).

After GTT

Data from the NETDC, National Cancer Institute and Charing Cross Hospital demonstrate that patients with GTT, who are successfully treated with chemotherapy, can anticipate normal reproduction in the future (Berkowitz et al, 1987a; Van Thiel et al, 1970; Walden and Bagshawe, 1976). Patients who had received chemotherapy for GTT at the NETDC had 324 subsequent pregnancies between June 1965 and December 1986. These later gestations resulted in 227 (70.0%) full-term live births, 14 (4.3%) premature deliveries, three (0.9%) ectopics, and six (1.8%) stillbirths (Table 9). First-trimester spontaneous abortion occurred in 51 (15.8%)

Table 9. Subsequent pregnancies in patients with gestational trophoblastic tumours (NETDC June 1965–December 1986).

Outcome	Number of pregnancies (%)
Term delivery	227 (70.0)
Stillbirth	6 (1.8)
Premature delivery	14 (4.3)
Spontaneous abortion	
1st trimester	51 (15.8)
2nd trimester	7 (2.2)
Therapeutic abortion	15 (4.7)
Ectopic pregnancy	3 (0.9)
Repeat molar pregnancy	1 (0.3)
Total number of pregnancies	324
	Number of deliveries (%)
Congenital malformations	5/247 (2.0)
Primary caesarean sections	20/141 (14.3)*

* January 1979–December 1986.

pregnancies, and major and minor congenital malformations were detected in only 5 (2.0%) infants. It is particularly reassuring that the incidence of congenital anomalies is not increased. Primary caesarean section was performed in only 20 (14.3%) of 141 later full-term and premature deliveries between January 1979 and December 1986. The subsequent pregnancies in these patients have no increased risk of complications during either the prenatal or intrapartum period.

IMMUNOLOGICAL STUDIES OF GESTATIONAL TROPHOBLASTIC DISEASE

Gestational trophoblastic tumours are unique immunologically and biologically because they express paternal antigens. The remarkable curability of GTT has been attributed in part to the maternal host's immunological response to the trophoblastic tumour.

HLA antigen expression and complete mole

Yamashita et al (1981b) demonstrated that molar tissue contains paternal HLA antigens. The localization of HLA antigens in molar chorionic villi is the same as in normal placental chorionic villi. While class I MHC antigens are detectable on molar villous stromal cells and extravillous trophoblast, class I MHC antigens are detectable in neither villous trophoblast nor villous fluid (Berkowitz et al, 1983a, 1984b). Class I HLA antigens were detectable on extravillous trophoblast using four different antibodies to monomorphic determinants, but not with antibodies to the appropriate polymorphic HLA-A or -B type (Sunderland et al, 1985a). Therefore, HLA antigens expressed by molar extravillous trophoblast may be similar to those expressed by normal placental extravillous trophoblast and could be modified MHC antigens (Sunderland et al, 1981; Ellis et al, 1986).

The maternal host with a complete mole may become sensitized to paternal HLA antigens. Lawler et al (1974) have reported anti-HLA antibodies in the sera of primigravid women following a molar pregnancy. Four of 31 primigravid women with complete mole had anti-HLA antibodies specific for their partner's HLA specificities. Furthermore, circulating antigen–antibody complexes in patients with complete mole have been shown to contain paternal HLA antigen (Lahey et al, 1984).

Trophoblast–leukocyte common antigens and complete mole

Trophoblast–leukocyte common (TLX) antigens are polymorphic antigens expressed on all trophoblast populations throughout normal pregnancy (McIntyre et al, 1983; Bulmer and Johnson, 1985). The TLX antigen system has been attributed an important role in regulating fetal–maternal immunological interactions. Paternal TLX antigens expressed on trophoblast may be expected to elicit a maternal immune response. Importantly, TLX antigens are also expressed on molar villous trophoblast and may contribute to the immunogenicity of a complete mole (Berkowitz et al, 1986c).

Maternal immune response and complete molar pregnancy

Because all chromosomes are of paternal origin in complete hydatidiform mole, this tissue is a complete allograft. Complete mole might, therefore, be expected to induce a vigorous maternal immunological response.

The molar implantation site is an area of intimate contact between maternal and molar tissues. The molar implantation site has, therefore, been studied to detect possible host humoral or cellular immune response.

Implantation sites from complete moles were examined by direct immunofluorescence for the deposition of immunoglobulin and complement (Berkowitz et al, 1982b). None of the ten patients with their first molar pregnancy had

GESTATIONAL TROPHOBLASTIC DISEASE

detectable immunoglobulin or complement deposition at the implantation site. Similarly, circulating immune complex levels were in normal range in 27 of 31 patients with complete mole at the time of uterine evacuation (Berkowitz et al, 1983b). Complete moles do not appear to induce a vigorous host humoral immune response at the time of clinical presentation.

Patients with complete mole may develop a humoral immune response with the passage of time after molar evacuation. Eighteen patients with complete mole were followed with serial circulating immune complex levels after uterine evacuation (Berkowitz et al, 1983b). All eighteen patients developed increased immune complex levels as they approached gonadotrophin remission. Immune complex values remained elevated from 6 to 16 weeks (mean = 11.5 weeks) and then declined to initial values. Lawler and Fisher (1987) tested the sera of patients with complete mole for HLA antibodies both at the time of evacuation and at the time of treatment for post-molar persistent GTT. While only two of 14 patients had HLA antibodies at evacuation, ten patients developed HLA antibodies when they required treatment for post-molar persistent disease.

Cellular infiltration at the molar implantation site has been investigated using monoclonal antibodies that recognize lymphocyte subsets and macrophages (Kabawat et al, 1985). As compared with implantation sites in normal pregnancy of the same gestational age, molar implantation sites had a fivefold increased infiltration of T cells. These T cells were predominantly (75%) T4-positive, Leu3a-positive cells (helper/inducer T cells) which tended to aggregate around implantation site blood vessels. The immunopathology of the molar implantation site will be reviewed in further detail in Chapter 8.

HLA antigen expression and gestational choriocarcinoma

The development and progression of GTT may be favoured by histocompatibility between the patient and her partner. Trophoblastic tissues which express paternal antigens might not be immunogenic in the maternal host if the patient and her partner were histocompatible. The intensity of the host's immunological response may depend upon the immunogenicity of the tumour. Morgensen et al (1969) reported that histocompatibility between patients and their partners was more common than expected at certain HLA specificities in patients with metastatic GTT. Furthermore, Tomoda et al (1976) observed increased histocompatibility between patients and their partners in drug-resistant choriocarcinoma. The development and rapid progression of poor-prognosis GTT may be facilitated by patient–partner (host–tumour) histocompatibility.

Histocompatibility between patients and their partners, however, does not appear to be a prerequisite for the development and persistence of GTT. We have studied the frequency distribution of HLA-A, -B, -C (54 specificities) and -DR (7 specificities) in 29 patients with gestational choriocarcinoma and their partners (Berkowitz et al, 1981c). There was no abnormal HLA antigen sharing between patients and their partners and the HLA antigen frequency was normal in both groups. Most patients were not histocompatible with their partners and their frequency of histocompatibility did not differ from control couples. Mittal et al (1975) and Yamashita et al (1981a) also noted no increase in HLA-compatible couples among patients with GTT.

Several investigations indicate that gestational choriocarcinoma cells express class I HLA antigens. A subpopulation of trophoblast cells in gestational choriocarcinoma has been shown to express class I HLA antigen in immunohistochemical studies (Sunderland et al, 1985b). Anti-HLA antibodies specific for paternal HLA specificities have been detected in the sera of patients with choriocarcinoma (Shaw et al, 1979).

The BeWo human choriocarcinoma cell line has shown to synthesize class I HLA antigens in vitro (Trowsdale et al, 1980). The expression of surface HLA-A, -B, -C antigen by choriocarcinoma cell lines has been demonstrated to be rate-limited by the amount of HLA-A, -B, -C mRNA and not by β_2-microglobulin mRNA which is present in excess (Kawata et al, 1984).

The expression of HLA antigens by human gestational choriocarcinoma cells has been investigated in the presence of phytohemagglutinin-activated lymphocyte culture supernatants (PHA-ALCS) and high doses of γ-interferon (Anderson and Berkowitz, 1985). There was a marked increase in surface expression of class I HLA antigens in BeWo choriocarcinoma cell cultures following a 7 day exposure to PHA-ALCS or high doses of γ-interferon. All BeWo cultures were negative for class II HLA antigens in these assays and another choriocarcinoma cell line, Jar, did not demonstrate class I or II HLA expression under any of the experimental conditions. Enhancement of HLA expression in trophoblast cells may have clinical and biological significance. Rapidly progressing and drug-resistant choriocarcinoma may be of the non-HLA inducible type. The enhanced expression of HLA by choriocarcinoma cells could provide a more vigorous stimulus for maternal immunologic response and thereby contribute to tumour regression. Modulation of antigen expression by choriocarcinoma cells may be of therapeutic benefit.

Class II MHC (HLA-DR) antigens have not been detected in choriocarcinoma tissues or cell lines in immunohistochemical studies. However, Takahashi et al (1987) have observed by Northern blot analysis the presence of HLA-DR mRNA in the human choriocarcinoma cell line GCH-1. The GCH-1 choriocarcinoma cell line transcribed both the α- and β-chain of HLA-DR mRNAs. It is not known whether HLA-DR is present on the surface of GCH-1 cells or whether it is the same as HLA-DR which is present in normal lymphocytes.

Cytokines and gestational choriocarcinoma

The prognosis of patients with gestational choriocarcinoma has been correlated with the intensity of lymphocytic infiltration at the tumour–host interface. Ito et al (1981) observed that 26 (81%) of 32 patients survived when the lymphocytic reaction was marked. However, only 22 (35%) of 61 patients were cured when the lymphocytic reaction was mild. Deligdisch et al (1978) also noted that six of seven patients who died from choriocarcinoma had no lymphocytic infiltration at the tumour–host interface.

Lymphocytes and macrophages, on activation, produce soluble factors known as lymphokines and monokines, respectively, which promote and regulate immune responses. Some of the factors such as γ-interferon and tumour necrosis factor are cytotoxic to tumour cells. Lymphokines, monokines and cytokines (mediators produced by both macrophages and lymphocytes) are now available in purified form because of advances in recombinant DNA technology and biochemistry, thereby enabling a systematic study of the effects of these factors on trophoblast cells. Recent studies have indicated that recombinant γ-interferon, tumour necrosis factor, and colony-stimulating factor preparations reduce proliferation of JEG-3 human choriocarcinoma cells in vitro over a wide dosage range (Berkowitz et al, 1988). Immunologically active cells may promote the regression of choriocarcinoma through the release of lymphokines and monokines. Furthermore, lymphokines and monokines individually or in combination may be useful in the treatment of gestational choriocarcinoma.

REFERENCES

Amir SM, Osathanondh R, Berkowitz RS & Goldstein DP (1984) Human chorionic gonadotropin and thyroid function in patients with hydatidiform mole. *American Journal of Obstetrics and Gynecology* **150:** 723–728.

Anderson DJ & Berkowitz RS (1985) Gamma-interferon enhances expression of Class I MHC antigens in the weakly HLA-positive human choriocarcinoma cell line Be Wo but does not induce MHC expression in the HLA-negative choriocarcinoma cell line, Jar. *Journal of Immunology* **135:** 2498–2501.

Athanassiou A, Begent RHJ, Newlands ES et al (1983) Central nervous system metastasis of choriocarcinoma: 23 years experience at the Charing Cross Hospital. *Cancer* **52:** 1728–1735.

Bagshawe KD (1976) Risks and prognostic factors in trophoblastic neoplasia. *Cancer* **38:** 1373–1385.

Bagshawe KD (1984) Treatment of high-risk choriocarcinoma. *Journal of Reproductive Medicine* **29:** 813–820.

Bagshawe KD & Harland S (1976) Immunodiagnosis and monitoring of gonadotropin-producing metastases in the central nervous system. *Cancer* **38:** 112–118.

Begent RHJ, Searle F & Stanway G (1980) Radioimmunolocalization of tumors by external scintigraphy after administration of ^{131}I antibody to human chorionic gonadotropin: Preliminary communication. *Journal of Royal Society of Medicine* **73:** 624.

Berkowitz RS & Goldstein DP (1981) Pathogenesis of gestational trophoblastic neoplasms. *Pathobiology Annual* **11:** 391–411.

Berkowitz RS & Goldstein DP (1986) Management of molar pregnancy and gestational trophoblastic tumors. In Knapp RC & Berkowitz RS (eds) *Gynecologic Oncology*, pp 425–443. New York: MacMillan.

Berkowitz RS, Goldstein DP, Jones MA, Marean AR & Bernstein MR (1981a) Methotrexate with citrovorum factor rescue—reduced chemotherapy toxicity in the management of gestational trophoblastic neoplasms. *Cancer* **45:** 423–426.

Berkowitz RS, Goldstein DP, Marean AR & Bernstein MR (1981b) Oral contraceptives and postmolar trophoblastic disease. *Obstetrics and Gynecology* **58:** 474–478.

Berkowitz RS, Hornig-Rohan J, Martin-Aloscr S et al (1981c) HLA antigen frequency distribution in patients with gestational choriocarcinoma and their husbands. *Placenta* **3** (supplement): 263–267.

Berkowitz RS, Goldstein DP & Bernstein MR (1982a) Methotrexate with citrovorum factor rescue as primary therapy for gestational trophoblastic disease. *Cancer* **50:** 2024–2027.

Berkowitz RS, Mostoufizadeh M, Kabawat SE, Goldstein DP & Driscoll SG (1982b) Immuno-pathologic study of the implantation site of molar pregnancy. *American Journal of Obstetrics and Gynecology* 144: 925–930.
Berkowitz RS, Anderson DJ, Hunter NJ & Goldstein DP (1983a) Distribution of major histocompatibility (HLA) antigens in chorionic villi of molar pregnancy. *American Journal of Obstetrics and Gynecology* 146: 221–222.
Berkowitz RS, Lahey SJ, Rodrick ML et al (1983b) Circulating immune complex levels in patients with molar pregnancy. *Obstetrics and Gynecology* 61: 165–168.
Berkowitz RS, Goldstein DP & Bernstein MR (1984a) Modified triple chemotherapy in the management of high-risk metastatic gestational trophoblastic tumors. *Gynecologic Oncology* 19: 173–181.
Berkowitz RS, Hoch EJ, Goldstein DP & Anderson DJ (1984b) Histocompatibility antigens (HLA-A,B,C) are not detectable in molar villous fluid. *Gynecologic Oncology* 19: 74–78.
Berkowitz RS, Goldstein DP & Bernstein MR (1986a) Ten years experience with methotrexate and folinic acid as primary therapy for gestational trophoblastic disease. *Gynecologic Oncology* 23: 111–118.
Berkowitz RS, Goldstein DP & Bernstein MR (1986b) Natural history of partial molar pregnancy. *Obstetrics and Gynecology* 66: 677–681.
Berkowitz RS, Umpierre SA, Johnson PM, McIntyre JA & Anderson DJ (1986c) Expression of trophoblast–leukocyte common antigens and placental-type alkaline phosphatase in complete molar pregnancy. *American Journal of Obstetrics and Gynecology* 155: 443–446.
Berkowitz RS, Goldstein DP, Bernstein MR & Sablinska B (1987a) Subsequent pregnancy outcome in patients with molar pregnancy and gestational trophoblastic tumors. *Journal of Reproductive Medicine* 32: 680–684.
Berkowitz RS, Goldstein DP, DuBeshter B & Bernstein MR (1987b) Management of complete molar pregnancy. *Journal of Reproductive Medicine* 32: 634–639.
Berkowitz RS, Hill JA, Kurtz CB & Anderson DJ (1988) Effects of products of activated leukocytes (Lymphokines and monokines) on the growth of malignant trophoblast cells in vitro. *American Journal of Obstetrics and Gynecology* 158: 199–203.
Bulmer JN & Johnson PM (1985) Antigen expression by trophoblast populations in the human placenta and their possible immunobiological relevance. *Placenta* 6: 127–140.
Cole L (1986) O-linked oligosaccharides on normal and neoplastic trophoblast proteins: A) HCG. *Proceedings of Third World Congress on Gestational Trophoblastic Neoplasms*, p 1.
Curry SL, Hammond CB, Tyrey L, Creasman WT & Parker RT (1975) Hydatidiform mole—Diagnosis, management and long-term follow-up of 347 patients. *American Journal of Obstetrics and Gynecology* 45: 1–8.
Deligdisch L, Driscoll SG & Goldstein DP (1978) Gestational trophoblastic neoplasms: morphologic correlates of therapeutic response. *American Journal of Obstetrics and Gynecology* 130: 801–806.
Depue RH, Bernstein L, Ross RK, Judd HL & Henderson BE (1987) Hyperemesis gravidarum in relation to estradiol levels, pregnancy outcome, and other maternal factors: A sero-epidemiologic study. *American Journal of Obstetrics and Gynecology* 156: 1137–1141.
DuBeshter B, Berkowitz RS, Goldstein DP, Cramer DW & Bernstein MR (1987) Metastatic gestational trophoblastic disease: Experience at the New England Trophoblastic Disease Center, 1965–1985. *Obstetrics and Gynecology* 69: 390–395.
Ellis SA, Sargent IL, Redman CWG & McMichael AJ (1986) Evidence for a novel HLA antigen found on human extravillous trophoblast and a choriocarcinoma cell line. *Immunology* 59: 595–601.
Goldstein DP & Berkowitz RS (1982) *Gestational Trophoblastic Neoplasms—Clinical Principles of Diagnosis and Management*, pp 1–301. Philadelphia: WB Saunders.
Hammond CB, Weed JC Jr & Currie JL (1980) The role of operation in the current therapy of gestational trophoblastic disease. *American Journal of Obstetrics and Gynecology* 136: 844–856.
Hankins G, Wendel GD, Snyder RR & Cunningham FG (1987) Trophoblastic embolization during molar evacuation—Central hemodynamic observations. *Obstetrics and Gynecology* 69: 368–372.
Ito S, Sekine T, Komuro N et al (1981) Histologic stromal reaction of the host with gestational choriocarcinoma and its relation to clinical stage classification and prognosis. *American Journal of Obstetrics and Gynecology* 140: 781–786.

Kabawat S, Mostoufizadeh M, Berkowitz RS et al (1985) Implantation site in complete molar pregnancy: a study of immunologically competent cells with monoclonal antibodies. *American Journal of Obstetrics and Gynaecology* 152: 97–99.

Kajii T & Ohama K (1977) Androgenetic origin of hydatidiform mole. *Nature* 268: 633–634.

Kawata M, Parnes JR & Herzenberg LA (1984) Transcriptional control of HLA-ABC antigen in human placental cytotrophoblast isolated using trophoblast and HLA-specific monoclonal antibodies and the fluorescence-activated cell sorter. *Journal of Experimental Medicine* 160: 633–651.

Kim DS, Moon H, Kim KT, Moon YJ & Hwang YY (1986) Effects of prophylactic chemotherapy for persistent trophoblastic disease in patients with complete hydatidiform mole. *Obstetrics and Gynecology* 67: 690–694.

Kohorn EI, McGinn RC, Bernard J et al (1978) Pulmonary embolization of trophoblastic tissue in molar pregnancy. *Obstetrics and Gynecology* 51: 16–20.

Lahey SJ, Steele G Jr, Berkowitz RS et al (1984) Identification of material with paternal HLA antigen immunoreactivity from purported circulating immune complexes in patients with gestational trophoblastic neoplasia. *Journal of National Cancer Institute* 72: 983–990.

Lawler SD, Klouda PT & Bagshawe KD (1974) Immunogenicity of molar pregnancies in the HLA system. *American Journal of Obstetrics and Gynecology* 120: 857–861.

Lawler SD & Fisher RA (1987) Immunogenicity of hydatidiform mole. *Placenta* 8: 195–199.

McIntyre JA, Faulk WP, Verhulst SJ et al (1983) Human trophoblast–lymphocyte cross-reactive (TLX) antigens define a new alloantigen system. *Science* 222: 1135–1138.

Mittal KK, Kachru RB & Brewer JI (1975) The HL-A and ABO antigens in trophoblastic disease. *Tissue Antigens* 6: 57–69.

Montz FJ, Schlaerth JB & Morrow CP (1987) Natural history of theca lutein cysts. *Gynecologic Oncology* 26: 414.

Morgensen B, Kissmeyer-Nielsen F & Hauge M (1969) Histocompatibility antigens on the HL-A locus in gestational choriocarcinoma. *Transplantation Proceedings* 1: 76–80.

Morrow P, Nakamura R, Schlaerth J, Gaddis O, Jr & Eddy G (1985) The influence of oral contraceptives on the postmolar human chorionic regression curve. *American Journal of Obstetrics and Gynecology* 151: 906–914.

Mutch DG, Soper JT, Baker ME et al (1986) Role of computed axial tomography of the chest in staging patients with nonmetastatic gestational trophoblastic disease. *Obstetrics and Gynecology* 68: 348–352.

Nisula BC & Taliadouros GS (1980) Thyroid function in gestational trophoblastic neoplasia—Evidence that the thyrotropic activity of chorionic gonadotropin mediates the thyrotoxicosis of choriocarcinoma. *American Journal of Obstetrics and Gynecology* 138: 77–85.

Osathanondh R, Goldstein DP & Pastorfide GB (1975) Actinomycin D as the primary agent for gestational trophoblastic disease. *Cancer* 36: 863–866.

Osathanondh R, Berkowitz RS, deCholnoky C et al (1986) Hormonal measurements in patients with theca lutein cysts and gestational trophoblastic disease. *Journal of Reproductive Medicine* 31: 179–182.

Ozturk M, Berkowitz R, Goldstein D, Bellet D & Wands JR (1988) Differential production of human chorionic gonadotropin and free subunits in non-pregnant subjects, during normal pregnancy and in gestational trophoblastic disease. *American Journal of Obstetrics and Gynecology* 158: 193–198.

Pattillo RA, Sasaki S, Katayama KP et al (1981) Genesis of 46, XY hydatidiform mole. *American Journal of Obstetrics and Gynecology* 141: 104–105.

Romero R, Horgan JG, Kohorn EI et al (1985) New criteria for the diagnosis of gestational trophoblastic disease. *Obstetrics and Gynecology* 66: 553–558.

Shaw ARE, Dasgupta MK, Kovithavongs T et al (1979) Humoral and cellular immunity to paternal antigens in trophoblast neoplasia. *International Journal of Cancer* 24: 586–593.

Stone M, Dent J, Kardana A & Bagshawe K (1976) Relationship of oral contraception to development of trophoblastic tumor after evacuation of a hydatidiform mole. *British Journal of Obstetrics and Gynaecology* 83: 913–916.

Sunderland CA, Redman CWG & Stirrat GM (1981) HLA-A,B,C antigens are expressed on non-villous trophoblast of the early human placenta. *Journal of Immunology* 127: 2614–2615.

Sunderland CA, Redman CWG & Stirrat GM (1985a) Characterization and localization of HLA antigens on hydatidiform mole. *American Journal of Obstetrics and Gynecology* 151: 130–135.

Sunderland CA, Sasagawa M, Kanazawa K, Stirrat GM & Takeuchi S (1985b) An immuno-histochemical study of HLA antigen expression by gestational choriocarcinoma. *British Journal of Cancer* **51**: 809–814.

Surti U, Szulman AE & O'Brien S (1979) Complete (classic) hydatidiform mole with 46, XY karyotype of paternal origin. *Human Genetics* **51**: 153–155.

Surwit EA & Hammond CB (1980) Treatment of metastatic trophoblastic disease with poor prognosis. *Obstetrics and Gynecology* **55**: 565–570.

Szulman AE & Surti U (1978a) The syndromes of hydatidiform mole: I. Cytogenetic and morphologic correlations. *American Journal of Obstetrics and Gynecology* **131**: 665–771.

Szulman AE & Surti U (1978b) The syndromes of hydatidiform mole: II. Morphologic evolution of the complete and partial mole. *American Journal of Obstetrics and Gynecology* **132**: 20–27.

Szulman AE & Surti U (1982) The clinicopathologic profile of the partial hydatidiform mole. *Obstetrics and Gynecology* **59**: 597–602.

Takahashi H, Adachi S, Yoshiya N et al (1987) Expression of HLA-DR molecules in human gestational choriocarcinoma cell lines and malignant cell lines. *Placenta* **8**: 293–298.

Tomoda Y, Fuma M, Saiki N, Ishizuka N & Akaza T (1976) Immunologic studies in patients with trophoblastic neoplasia. *American Journal of Obstetrics and Gynecology* **126**: 661–667.

Trowsdale J, Travers P, Bodmer WF & Pattillo RA (1980) Expression of HLA-ABC and beta-2 microglobulin antigens in human choriocarcinoma cell lines. *Journal of Experimental Medicine* **152**: 11S–17S.

Van Thiel DH, Ross GT & Lipsett MB (1970) Pregnancies after chemotherapy of trophoblastic neoplasms. *Science* **169**: 1326–1327.

Walden PAM & Bagshawe KD (1976) Reproductive performance of women successfully treated for gestational trophoblastic tumors. *American Journal of Obstetrics and Gynecology* **125**: 1108–1114.

Weed JC Jr & Hammond CB (1980) Cerebral metastatic choriocarcinoma: Intensive therapy and prognosis. *Obstetrics and Gynecology* **55**: 89–94.

Wong LC, Choo YC & Ma HK (1986) Primary oral etoposide therapy in gestational trophoblastic disease, an update. *Cancer* **58**: 14–17.

Yamashita K, Wake N, Araki T, Ichinoe K & Makoto K (1979) Human lymphocyte antigen expression in hydatidiform mole: Androgenesis following fertilization by a haploid sperm. *American Journal of Obstetrics and Gynecology* **135**: 597–600.

Yamashita K, Ishikawa M, Shimizu T & Kuroda M (1981a) HLA-antigens in husband–wife pairs with trophoblastic tumor. *Gynecologic Oncology* **12**: 68–74.

Yamashita K, Wake N, Araki T, Ichinoe K & Kuroda M (1981b) A further HLA study of hydatidiform moles. *Gynecologic Oncology* **11**: 23–28.

Yordan EL Jr, Schlaerth J, Gaddis O & Morrow CP (1987) Radiation therapy in the management of gestational choriocarcinoma metastatic to the central nervous system. *Obstetrics and Gynecology* **69**: 627–630.

7

Autoimmunity and pregnancy

PAMELA V. TAYLOR

Perceptions of both autoimmune disease and immunological factors associated with pregnancy have changed a great deal in recent years. Ability to respond to self antigens, and maternal immune interaction with the fetus, are now recognized as normal features. The relationship between these two processes is complex. This chapter discusses the generation of autoimmunity, its effect on the reproductive process, and interrelationships between autoimmunity and pregnancy in a number of individual diseases.

AUTOIMMUNITY

The immune system has the potential for recognizing and responding to an enormous range of antigenic determinants. This depends upon the activities of T and B lymphocytes, which are equipped with receptors for a correspondingly diverse repertoire of antigenic specificities. These will inevitably include some that are directed towards antigens present on the body's own cells and tissues. The potential for such self-recognition may well be an important component of immune functions in general. Small amounts of autoantibodies in normal subjects may facilitate removal of metabolic and catabolic products by opsonization. Furthermore, immune function seems to involve both recognition of cell-surface antigens encoded by the major histocompatibility complex (MHC) and anti-idiotypic responses against self idiotypes, the latter being antigenic determinants provided by the hypervariable regions of immunoglobulins (Jerne et al, 1982). Naturally occurring autoantibodies may also serve to prevent the initiation of a damaging autoimmune response by binding to self-mimicking epitopes on microbes.

Factors which influence potential autoreactivity probably include an absence of T helper cells, so that no assistance is given to autoreactive B cells in producing the relevant antibody. This functional deletion of T cell help is effective from an early stage of development. Operation of the T suppressor cell system may provide a back-up, particularly in relation to antigens encountered after the neonatal period. The outcome of these controlling factors is maintenance throughout life of the lack of response to self tissues which, coupled with responsiveness to foreign antigens, is fundamental to the normal working of the immune system.

Since these immunoregulatory mechanisms exist, it is axiomatic that they may sometimes break down. Tipping the balance into pathological expression of self-reactivity may be associated with various genetic and immunological abnormalities, combined with exogenous factors, and differing from one individual to another. Genetic predisposition is crucial to the development of autoimmunity. Autoimmune disease tends to occur within families and there is a high rate of concordance in identical twins. Virtually all autoimmune diseases show an association with some or other MHC specificity, particularly the DR3 and B8 antigens. Other genes that may be involved include those for complement components and immunoglobulin allotypes.

Abnormal immunological parameters are demonstrable in many autoimmune conditions, although it may be difficult to know whether these are causative or a consequence of the disease. Pathogenesis is almost always related to autoantibody production, but the primary defect may be located in the cellular arm of immunity. This probably involves a bypass of the normal requirement for T cell help to potentially autoreactive B cells or a deletion of suppressor T cells. Alterations in the function and number of immunoregulatory T cells are commonly associated with autoimmune disease. An alternative mechanism provides an explanation for the occurrence of highly specific antibodies, such as those directed to the acetylcholine receptor in myasthenia gravis, and involves the production of antibodies directed towards the idiotype. Rabbits immunized to produce antibodies against a synthetic agonist of the acetylcholine receptor also produce anti-idiotypic antibodies directed against homologous structures both on the anti-agonist antibodies and on the acetylcholine receptors. These anti-idiotypes are able to function as anti-receptor antibodies and are associated with a myasthenia-like syndrome.

Exogenous factors influence expression of autoreactivity, and the most likely candidates are viruses. Their involvement at various levels in the autoimmune process would explain the persistence of the stimulus and the chronic nature of autoimmune diseases, but solid evidence for viral involvement is lacking. An important influence upon the expression, rather than the induction, of autoimmunity is provided by the organs and tissues ultimately affected by the disease. These may not function merely as quiescent targets but may be modified by drugs, viruses or chemical degradation to become immunogenic. Alternatively, antigens may become accessible to the body's immune system by being unmasked in some way or brought out from seclusion within a cell or organ, or tissues may acquire new specificities at certain times, for example at puberty or in old age. Changes in cells related to MHC antigen expression may occur, allowing cells to function as antigen-presenting cells by expression of class II MHC antigens.

Finally, physiological factors must be involved in the production of autoimmunity. The ageing process may be accompanied by a decreased ability of the immune system to function normally, thus allowing the induction of autoreactivity. Many autoimmune disorders have a greater prevalence, and younger age-onset, in women than men. This suggests an effect of hormones, but the mechanism is unknown. The importance of this apparent hormonal effect to the clinician is that immunological disease occurs frequently in women in their reproductive years. Whatever the mechanisms of auto-immunity are, the result of this complex network of causative factors is ultimately the appearance of abnormal antibodies and the development of disease. This ranges from diseases in which the antibodies are directed against single organs, commonly the thyroid, adrenals, stomach and pancreas, to those in which the target antigens are widespread and the lesions corre-spondingly disseminated, involving the skin, kidney, joints and muscles. The diseases covered in this chapter are shown in Table 1, classified by their degree

Table 1. Spectrum of autoimmune diseases of importance in pregnancy.

Organ-specific	Hashimoto's thyroiditis
↑	Graves' disease
	Pernicious anaemia
	Type 1 diabetes mellitus
	Myasthenia gravis
	Autoimmune haemolytic anaemia
	Autoimmune thrombocytopenic purpura
	Sjögren's syndrome
	Rheumatoid arthritis
	Dermatomyositis
↓	Scleroderma
Non organ-specific	Systemic lupus erythematosus

of organ-specificity. Overlaps exist at both ends of this spectrum. For a fuller discussion of autoimmune processes the reader is referred to Smith and Steinberg (1983), Shoenfeld and Schwartz (1984), Male (1986) and MacKay et al (1986).

AUTOIMMUNITY AND THE REPRODUCTIVE PROCESS

Immunological effects are clearly important at many levels in the repro-ductive process, including fertilization, implantation and the development of the feto-placental unit. All these processes involve considerable modi-fication of the immune system. The occurrence of an autoimmune disease in a women in her reproductive years represents the superimposition of a pathological alteration of immunoregulatory mechanisms related to auto-immunity upon a physiological modulation of her immune status associated with the reproductive process. It is not surprising that the interaction between these two processes culminates in a complex set of events which may be difficult to unravel in terms of cause and effect. There are two aspects of this interactive relationship: (i) the influence of the reproductive process on the natural history of the disease and (ii) the effect of the disease on the outcome of reproduction. Scott (1966) first examined the possibility that observations of effects related to both these aspects would give important insights into the mechanisms and modes of treatment of immunological disease.

Expression of such disease may be influenced by endocrinological, haematological and immunological alterations associated with the ovarian cycle and administration of cyclic steroid preparations as well as by pregnancy. Effects of pregnancy on autoimmune diseases vary considerably but, in general, there is a tendency to remission or stabilization during late pregnancy followed by post-partum relapse. Observations of this nature in rheumatoid arthritis led to the discovery of cortisone and its introduction into clinical therapeutics. Practical management of some autoimmune disorders is made more difficult by the fact that levels of hormone-binding globulins increase under the influence of oestrogens, obscuring the significance of hormone estimations in assessment of disease. Assays of protein-bound thyroxine, for example, become unreliable in patients with autoimmune thyroid disease during pregnancy.

AUTOIMMUNITY AND THE MATERNO–FETAL MODEL

The evolution of viviparity has culminated in a complex symbiotic relationship between mother and fetus involving many immunological compromises. The placental barrier holding the fetal and maternal circulations separate allows only minor and infrequent interchange of blood, mostly at parturition. Antibody transfer is almost entirely a function of the intact placenta, and is highly specific for immunoglobulin G; no other class of maternal antibody gains access to the fetus.

Where there is an autoimmune disease in the mother, gestation may be accompanied by various circulating autoantibodies. Those antibodies which are IgG will cross the placenta and may produce disease in the baby if the relevant target antigen is present. This materno–fetal model (Figure 1)

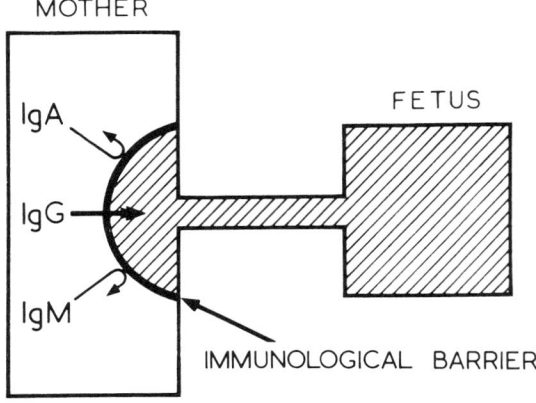

Figure 1. The materno–fetal model: only maternal IgG antibodies cross the immunological barrier provided by the placenta and gain access to the fetus.

provides a unique, naturally occurring, experimental system which has been extremely valuable in gaining an understanding of the pathogenic process in many autoimmune diseases. Neonatal disease will regress within three months, in keeping with the time course of catabolism of maternal IgG. The female preponderance of the maternal disease is not observed in affected infants. Genetic differences may explain the differential appearance of disease in dizygotic twins. Clinical features may occur in the baby of a mother who is in remission, has occult disease, or is asymptomatic due to therapy.

How do the placentally-transferred autoantibodies produce pathogenic effects? Antibody may bind to cellular receptors, as in Graves' disease, activate complement and effector cells, as in autoimmune haemolytic anaemia, or form circulating immune complexes that become deposited at various sites, as in systemic lupus erythematosus (SLE). Secondary effector functions of antibodies are shown in Table 2. It is of interest that subclasses displayed by various connective tissue disease autoantibodies are predominantly IgG1 and IgG3 (Rubin et al, 1986).

Interactions between pregnancy and autoimmunity have been the subject of various reviews (El-Roeiy and Shoenfeld, 1985; Gleicher, 1986).

Table 2. Some properties of human antibody classes and subclasses.

	IgG1	IgG2	IgG3	IgG4	IgM	IgA	IgD	IgE
Placental transfer	+	±	+	+	−	−	−	−
Complement fixation	++	+	+++	−	+++	−	−	−
Binding to mononuclear cells	+	−	+	−	−	−	−	?
Binding to neutrophils	+	−	+	+	−	+	−	−
Binding to platelets	+	+	+	+	−	−	−	?
Binding to mast cells	−	−	−	?	−	−	−	+++

ORGAN-SPECIFIC AUTOIMMUNITY

Autoimmune thyroid disease

The thyroid is the endocrine gland responsible for secreting two hormones, thyroxine (tetra-iodothyronine; T4) and tri-iodothyronine (T3), necessary for growth, development and metabolism. Disordered function of the thyroid gives rise to a spectrum of diseases in which clinical entities can be broadly defined: Graves' disease, Hashimoto's thyroiditis and primary myxoedema, representing separate manifestations of the same pathological process. They are more frequent in females than males and are associated with HLA-A8 and Dw3. The interrelationship of these disorders is complex (Brown et al, 1978), as is their association with pregnancy (Scott, 1977; Davies and Weiss, 1981; Levy, 1982).

Effects of autoimmune thyroid disease on the fetus must be assessed in the context of altered thyroid function in pregnancy. Maternal basal metabolic rate is elevated due to the presence of the feto–placental unit. Thyroid-stimulating hormone (TSH) levels are not altered during pregnancy, but T3 and T4 are elevated because of an oestrogen-stimulated increase in thyroid hormone-binding globulin. Protein-bound iodine and T3 resin uptake will, therefore, be increased and assessment of thyroid function may be best achieved during pregnancy by measuring urinary T3 and T4. Since TSH does not cross the placenta, the maternal and fetal thyroid systems function independently. Maternal free T3 and T4 cross the placenta only very slowly, but anti-thyroid drugs cross freely and depress fetal thyroid function. Development of the fetal thyroid is such that iodine is accumulated and thyroglobulin synthesized from early in the second trimester. Placental trophoblast itself produces a thyrotrophic hormone, human chorionic thyrotrophin.

Graves' disease

In normal individuals production of thyroglobulin, which is subsequently hydrolysed to yield thyroxine, is under the control of TSH secreted by the pituitary gland. The hormone binds to specific receptors on the surface of thyroid cells and activates them, via the adenylate cyclase channels, to synthesize and secrete thyroglobulin (Figure 2a). This process is mimicked in some individuals by the action of IgG autoantibodies which bind with the TSH receptor (Figure 2b). Since action of the antibody is not subject to hormone feedback control, the thyroid cells continue to produce thyroglobulin over long periods and the antibodies are called long-acting thyroid stimulating antibodies (LATS). These antibodies were first detected in the animal system used for assaying TSH. Injection of plasma from patients with Graves' disease into mice and assay of the release of labelled iodine from the thyroid gland revealed a different time-course compared with effect of TSH; one of delayed onset and longer duration (Adams and Purves, 1956). Another antibody affecting thyroid function was demonstrated subsequently by the same group (Adams and Kennedy, 1967). Protein isolated from human thyroid cell membranes, probably the TSH receptor, blocks the action of LATS on the thyroid cells (Figure 2c). However, when sera from some Graves' disease patients is injected together with this protein and the LATS, it prevents inhibition of the LATS by competing with it for the thyroid protein (Figure 2d). This second antibody, referred to as LATS-protector (LATS-P), binds only to human and not to mouse thyroid. LATS-P was subsequently shown to have thyroid-stimulating activity in man (Adams et al, 1974).

Other autoantibodies have subsequently been described using different bioassay systems and, in general, the relationships of these various autoantibodies is not certain. It is quite clear, however, that there is a whole family of autoantibodies affecting thyroid function. These range from the thyroid-stimulating immunoglobulins (TSI) discussed above, to thyroid-binding inhibiting immunoglobulins (TBII) which block TSH-binding to thyroid cells. Functional effects vary correspondingly from hyper- to hypothyroidism. Antibodies to thyroglobulin and thyroid microsomal antigens may also be present but their pathogenic significance is unclear. Graves' ophthalmopathy, which sometimes occurs in the absence of thyroid

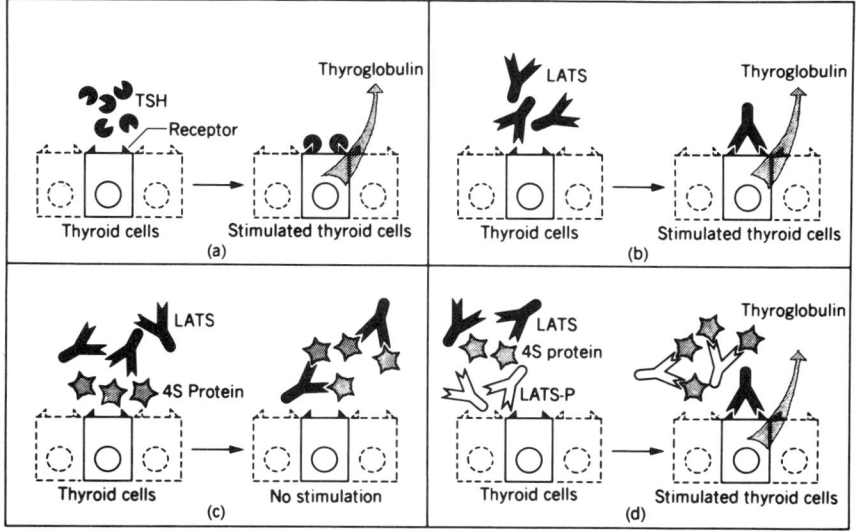

Figure 2. Action of hormones and antibodies on the thyroid. (a) Stimulation of thyroid cells by TSH. (b) Stimulation of thyroid cells by LATS. (c) Blocking of LATS by protein. (d) Competitive inhibition of LATS-protein binding by LATS-P. From Klein (1982).

disease, may be due to autoantibody reactive with orbital antigens; these have been defined using monoclonal antibodies (Kodama et al, 1982).

Support for an aetiological role of TSI in Graves' disease comes from their correlation with the disease and from the neonatal effects (see below). LATS is highly specific for Graves' disease but is not found in a considerable proportion of such patients and, when present, the levels do not correlate with the degree of thyrotoxicosis. Adams et al (1974) showed that LATS-P, measured by determining the degree to which the test serum protected a standard LATS serum from being neutralized by a standard thyroid extract, was present in 90% of 50 consecutive untreated patients with Graves' disease. Furthermore, serum levels of the antibody were highly correlated with thyroid ^{131}I uptake rate. A receptor assay for TSH using human thyroid and ^{125}I-labelled TSH was used by Smith and Hall (1974) to measure the inhibition of binding by immunoglobulins from Graves' patients. This was positive for 22 of 25 patients, the reaction being species-specific and probably due to LATS-P immunoglobulins. It now seems evident that some type of TSI is present in almost all cases of Graves' disease, with no overlap in the TSI activity levels between normal controls and patients with untreated Graves' disease (Mukhtar et al, 1975).

Participation of cellular mechanisms are indicated by lymphocytic infiltration of the thyroid, elevated T:B cell ratios and in vitro production of lymphokines in response to thyroid antigens. A primary pathogenic role of T lymphocytes has been proposed (Volpé et al, 1974), as has the operation of a T cell suppressor defect (Davis and Platzer, 1986).

Neonatal thyrotoxicosis

The occurrence of a self-limiting form of the disease in babies of mothers with Graves' disease, first described by White (1912), provides strong evidence for a causative role for TSI. Earlier reports showed an incomplete correlation between presence of LATS and neonatal thyrotoxicosis (Maisey and Stimmler, 1972; Nutt et al, 1974). Munro et al (1978) measured TSI during 96 pregnancies in 93 women with Graves' disease; the twelve infants with definite neonatal thyrotoxicosis were born to mothers with high serum levels of LATS-P. Measurement of LATS-P was thought to provide a method of predicting neonatal thyrotoxicosis with a critical level of 20 units per ml, the antibody being assayed by inhibition of binding of a standard LATS preparation by human thyroid extract. An assay using adenylate cyclase stimulation of human thyroid showed high concentrations of TSI in eight mothers of ten hyperthyroid infants when 20 pregnancies were followed in 17 women with Graves' disease or a previous child with neonatal hyperthyroidism (Zakarija and McKenzie, 1983). There was a decline in TSI concentrations in many patients and occurrence of neonatal disease was correlated with maternal TSI levels remaining high during the third trimester.

Two of the mothers in the study of Zakarija and McKenzie (1983) had hypothyroidism related to Hashimoto's disease. Similarly, a LATS-negative mother reported by Thomson and Riley (1966) had hypothyroidism associated with goitre and exopthalmos, and LATS-P was subsequently demonstrated in the patient's serum when the technique became available. More recently, blocking antibodies inhibiting binding of TSH to the thyroid have been recognized as causing temporary neonatal hypothyroidism by preventing normal thyroid stimulation by the infant's TSH (Matsura et al, 1980). Differential effects on the fetal and neonatal thymus exerted by stimulating and blocking antibodies, with the titres and affinities possibly changing as pregnancy proceeds, would lead to fluctuating thyroid function and a progression from hypo- to hyperthyroidism.

In summary, it seems that TSI cause neonatal Graves' disease and are also the mechanism of the adult disease process. Relative importance of the individual TSI's is not known, but LATS-P seems to be the prime candidate. The clinical relevance is that serum concentrations of TSI should be measured in the third trimester of pregnancy in all women with a history of autoimmune thyroid disease, using a convenient and widely available assay such as inhibition of TSH binding to solubilized TSH receptors (Shewring and Smith, 1982). This is particularly important since it is not possible to predict the likelihood of neonatal thyrotoxicosis from the maternal clinical status. The general adoption of standardized assays for TSI based on an immortalized line of rat thymocytes has been recommended (Bottazzo and Doniach, 1986). These allow measurement of several parameters of thyroid stimulation, e.g. radioiodine uptake, TSH receptor binding and thyroid cell growth.

Pregnancy associations and management in Graves' disease

Graves' disease complicates between one in 1000 and one in 3000 pregnancies; next to diabetes, it is the commonest endocrine or metabolic disease in pregnancy. Treatment of the pregnant patient is by appropriate dosage of anti-thyroid drugs adjusted to keep the mother marginally hyperthyroid with the aim of preventing transplacental TSI affecting the fetal thyroid and, at the same time, avoiding thyroid suppression. Propylthiouracil in daily doses of 200 mg or less has been found satisfactory, although mild hypothyroidism has occasionally been detected in the newborn. If high levels of maternal TSI are demonstrated, anti-thyroid treatment may be necessary in clinically asymptomatic or euthyroid women. Carbimazole decreases levels of TSI (McGregor et al, 1980) and may be the preferred treatment in pregnancy, particularly perhaps where fetal involvement is indicated by sustained fetal tachycardia in the antenatal period.

Features of transferred thyrotoxicosis and treatment

Signs of Graves' disease are not confined to the neonatal period. Fetal tachycardia, retarded intrauterine growth and stillbirth are all possible effects of intrauterine Graves' disease. The incidence of the neonatal disease is of the order of 5% of babies of mothers with Graves' disease. Several factors may account for this lack of concordance with maternal disease. Maternal TSI may not be maintained at the critical level until the third trimester or there may be variations in placental transfer related to IgG subclass; the fetal thymus may be refractory to stimulation in general or its susceptibility might be related to genetic factors.

The neonatal presentation is of an underweight, fractious baby with tachycardia, tachypnoea, goitre, possible exophathalmia and diarrhoea. Transferred maternal autoantibodies responsible for these affects can come from a mother after she has had thyroidectomy or treatment with radioiodine, so neonatal disease may occur in babies of mothers with normal or depressed thyroid function. This emphasizes the importance of TSI measurements during pregnancy in women who have had thyroid disease. Neonatal effects may be delayed in onset by placental transfer of anti-thyroid drugs administered to the mother or of maternal IgG that blocks binding of TSH to the fetal thyroid (Zakarija and McKenzie, 1983). Such autoantibodies (see above) may cause transient hypothyroidism associated with elevated levels of TSH; detection of the antibody can prevent inappropriate long-term thyroxine replacement therapy. Duration of untreated neonatal thyroid disease is generally less than three months—the survival time of the transferred IgG. Severity of transient Graves' disease in the newborn varies; mortality is of the order of 25%, generally associated with heart failure. Treatment is by appropriate dosage of anti-thyroid drugs which can generally be stopped gradually after eight to ten weeks.

Hashimoto's disease (autoimmune thyroiditis)

This disease is characterized by an inflammatory response in the thyroid with destruction of the normal architecture, leading to goitre formation and hypothyroidism. Autoantibodies are produced to thyroglobulin, microsomal antigens and thyroid cell surface antigens. It occurs most often in women between 30 and 50 years of age, and is rarely encountered in association with pregnancy. The pregnant patient is treated by thyroid replacement therapy so as to maintain her in a slightly hyperthyroid state.

Post-partum thyroiditis

There is a decrease in several thyroid-associated autoantibodies during pregnancy followed by a rise post-partum (Amino et al, 1978). This is associated with amelioration of disease in the latter half of pregnancy and exacerbation after delivery. Similar changes in levels of antibody occur in the course of normal pregnancy (Armiento et al, 1980) and post-partum thyroid disease has been found in 9% of 238 women in the United States (Turney et al, 1982). The disease is characterized by goitre with and without hyperthyroidism, later progressing to hypothyroidism, and high titres of thyroid microsomal antibodies at three to four months. Euthyroidism is generally re-established within five to ten months with occasional persistence of goitre. This transient condition may herald a later onset of frank autoimmune thyroid disease, and it has been suggested that screening for thyroid microsomal antibodies should be performed as part of the routine antenatal screen (McGregor et al, 1984). An enzyme-linked immunoassay has been used to confirm an association between thyroid microsomal antibodies of IgG 1 subclass and hypothyroidism (Thompson et al, 1986).

Myasthenia gravis

Myasthenia gravis is a chronic muscle disease characterized by weakness and increased fatiguability of striated muscle. The muscles involved may be of a particular group (e.g. ocular, limb or respiratory) or generalized, and involvement may be asymmetrical (e.g. unilateral ptosis). Clinical features are variable, as is the natural history of the disease (Engel, 1979). The disorder has a female preponderance of two to one, with a peak age onset during the third decade; in this group there is an association with HLA-B8 and DRw3.

An autoimmune basis for myasthenia gravis was proposed independently by Simpson and by Nastuk et al in 1960. The hypothesis of Simpson was based largely upon the observation of a neonatal form of the disease. Validation of the theory in recent years has been facilitated by the discovery of Chang and Lee (1962) of a snake toxin, α-bungarotoxin, that blocks acetylcholine-induced depolarization at the neuromuscular junction. Irreversible binding of the toxin to acetylcholine receptors (AChR) made possible the study of AChR in normal and affected muscle, and their isolation from the electric organs of electric eels. Injection of these purified AChR into rabbits caused a myasthenia-like condition with death from respiratory paralysis (Patrick and Lindstrom, 1973), prompting a search for AChR antibody (see Vincent 1980 for review). Radioimmunoassay of α-bungarotoxin-labelled AChR isolated from human muscle has been performed. The labelled receptors are incubated with patient's serum, the IgG fraction precipitated and the ^{125}I-labelled toxin AChR–IgG complexes in the precipitate are counted (Monnier and Fulpius, 1977). This assay gives positive results in 87 to 93% of patients with myasthenia gravis, depending on the source of AChR. Range of antibody titres is not closely correlated with clinical status, but this has been related to ability of autoantibody to degrade and block AChR in vitro (Drachman et al, 1982). Analyses with monoclonal antibodies to AChR have defined different antigenic sites on the receptor and routine assays may not detect the relevant antibody (Gomez and Richman, 1983). Recently, the heterogeneity of anti-AChR, as well as the determinants to which it binds, have been demonstrated by Vincent et al (1987). An autoantibody that binds to end-plate determinants other than AChR has also been found (Mossman et al, 1986).

Thymic hyperplasia occurs in 65% of myasthenic patients, associated with germinal centres and increased numbers of lymphocytes and plasma cells, and thymomas in 10 to 15%. Thymectomy has been used for decades to alleviate the disease, and the role of the thymus in pathogenesis has recently been assessed by Berrih-Aknin et al (1987). The gland contains muscle-like (myoid) cells bearing AChR and thymic cells have been shown to enhance production of AChR antibody to autologous blood lymphocytes (Newsom-Davis et al, 1981). Thymic B cells transformed by the Epstein–Barr virus produce a monoclonal antibody to AChR that induces a myasthenia-like syndrome in rats (Kamo et al, 1982). Antibody production by the thymus accounts for only 5% of serum levels so that these are not greatly affected by thymectomy.

Although there are problems related to measurement of the relevant antibody, evidence points to myasthenia being caused by an antibody to AChR. Attempts to demonstrate cellular responses have generally failed (see Behan et al, 1975) and all the structural, biochemical and electrophysiological abnormalities of myasthenia can be induced by passive monoclonal antibody to AChR (Gomez and Richman, 1987). Production of neuromuscular block may be due to complement-dependent lysis (Engel et al, 1977), removal of AChR from the membrane (Drachman et al, 1982) or direct blocking of AChR function (Vincent and Newsom-Davis, 1979).

Neonatal myasthenia gravis

The occurrence of a transient neonatal form of myasthenia gravis gave an early clue to the autoimmune nature of the disease (Simpson, 1960) and provides cogent support for an autoantibody being the causative factor. Many reports of neonatal myasthenia are recorded (see Namba et al, 1970 for review). More recently, cases have been assessed in relation to presence of AChR antibodies (Keesey et al, 1977, Ohta et al, 1981). Neonatal disease is associated with transplacental passage of AChR antibodies, but disease may not occur in their presence and severity is not correlated with antibody titre. Genetic susceptibility, inhibition of antibody by α-fetoprotein (Brenner et al, 1980) or heterogeneity of AChR antibodies (see above) may all be crucial factors.

An interesting study by Lefvert and Osterman (1983) showed that the half-life of AChR antibody was three to 11 days in unaffected infants compared with 42 and 91 days in two affected children (Figure 3). Inhibition of binding of antibody from mothers and infants to AChR by an ^{125}I-labelled anti-idiotypic antibody revealed idiotypic differences between the mother and the affected babies. This emphasizes that there may be a fetal contribution to pathogenesis and also raises the prospect of using anti-idiotypic antibody as a form of immunotherapy. It has been shown that experimental myasthenia in chickens can be both prevented and abrogated with anti-idiotypes (Souroujon et al, 1986).

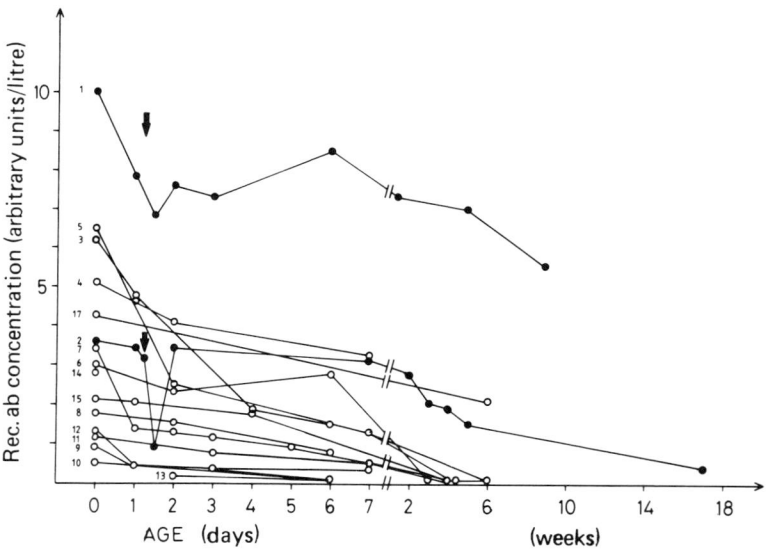

Figure 3. Time course of receptor antibody (Rec.ab) concentrations (arbitrary units) in infants with neonatal myasthenia (●——●) and in normal children (○——○) of mothers with myasthenia gravis. Exchange transfusions are marked with arrows. From Lefvert & Osterman (1983).

Pregnancy associations and management in myasthenia gravis

The incidence of myasthenia gravis in pregnancy is of the order of one in 20 000. Clinical and immunological features in relation to pregnancy have been reviewed by J. S. Scott (1977), Jones (1979) and Fennell and Ringel (1987). The course of the disease is variable; two thirds of patients remain stable or improve in the second and third trimester and worsen post-partum, while the remainder have exacerbation of disease during pregnancy. These features are not altered by therapeutic abortion. The overall relapse rate does not appear to be affected by pregnancy but dosage of anticholinesterase may require frequent adjustment. Anticholinesterase drugs cross the placenta, although no congenital malformations have been attributed to them. Corticosteroid therapy is associated with a slightly elevated incidence of cleft lip and palate, although the overall rate of fetal malformation is the same as in the normal population. Thymectomy, while not impossible, is best avoided during pregnancy. The temporary reversal of symptoms afforded by plasmapheresis is useful in pregnancy crises since it does not cause any significant risk to the fetus. Labour generally proceeds normally since the uterus is composed of smooth muscle and contraction is independent of AChR. Myasthenic patients are abnormally sensitive to drugs and central nervous system depressants should be used with caution. The use of forceps to shorten the second stage is recommended to spare unnecessary voluntary muscle effort. There is no contraindication to breast feeding.

Features of neonatal myasthenia gravis and treatment

The incidence of the neonatal disease is 12 to 19% in babies of myasthenic mothers (Plauché, 1983). Clinical features include generalized muscle hypotonia, weakness of sucking, respiratory difficulties, absent Moro reflex, feeble cry and facial paresis. Onset is from several hours up to a few days after birth, possibly related to placental transfer of anticholinesterase preparations given to the mother. The mean duration of the neonatal syndrome is three weeks but it may persist for up to two months. Before the widespread availability of neonatal intensive case units, the mortality rate was as high as 11%.

Since it is impossible to predict occurrence of neonatal myasthenia, it is essential that its potential development should be borne in mind. Failure to establish respiration by intubation and ventilation in affected infants may otherwise be wrongly attributed to irreversible brain damage and attempts abandoned. Diagnosis of neonatal myasthenia can be established if improvement occurs following subcutaneous injection of a short-acting anticholinesterase, such as edrophonium chloride (0.1–0.2 mg). Management includes control of nasopharyngeal secretions, nasogastric feeding, and intubation and ventilation if necessary. Cholinesterase inhibitors should not be used excessively since they increase secretions and further obstruct the airway. The dosage is adjusted on an individual basis and with regard to the rapid natural regression of the disease in the first few weeks of life; 0.1 mg neostigmine or 0.15 mg pyridostigmine intramuscularly or subcutaneously are suitable as initial doses. Plasmapheresis may be necessary in severe cases.

Autoimmune thrombocytopenic purpura (ATP)

This insidious disease is characterized by the destruction of circulating platelets by autoantibodies, resulting in thrombocytopenia. It has a female preponderance of about 3:1 and the peak incidence is between 20 and 40 years of age. Data on genetic predisposition are conflicting; associations with HLA-B8, -B12 and -DR2 have been reported. It is sometimes associated with other autoimmune disorders, particularly SLE and autoimmune haemolytic anaemia. Previously known as 'idiopathic' thrombocytopenic purpura, it is firmly established as an autoimmune disorder. A key observation was the occurrence of a transient neonatal form of the disease (Epstein et al, 1950). Harrington confirmed the humoral basis by passive transfer of thrombocytopenia to himself using patient's plasma (Harrington et al, 1951).

The existence of an anti-platelet factor was subsequently demonstrated using a variety of assays (see Karpatkin, 1985 for review) and its IgG nature established. The indirect assays characteristically detect anti-platelet antibody in approximately 30 to 65% of patients with ATP and levels do not correlate with severity of thrombocytopenia. Later, assays were developed for the quantitative detection of membrane-bound platelet-associated IgG (PA-IgG) utilizing inhibition of complement-mediated red blood cell lysis (Dixon et al, 1975), solid-phase radioimmunoassay (Hymes et al, 1979), radiolabelled monoclonal anti-human IgG (Lobuglio et al, 1983) and enzyme-linked immunosorbent assay (Lynch et al, 1985). Such techniques detect between 1 and 11 ng of non-specific IgG on 10^6 normal platelets, and an increase on platelets from patients with ATP of four to thirteenfold. Tests are characteristically positive in more than 92% of cases of ATP and PA-IgG levels correlate with severity of disease. PA-IgG includes all four subclasses of IgG at concentrations proportional to those in serum IgG in normal subjects. Platelet-associated IgM has also been found, sometimes in the absence of PA-IgG (Hegde et al, 1985), emphasizing the possible pathological significance of IgM in these cases. Current technology does not distinguish between platelet-associated immunoglobulin and immunoglobulin-antigen complexes bound to the platelet Fc receptor. However, immune complexes are probably not involved in ATP (Kiefel et al, 1986); an analysis of platelet antigen by Western blotting has revealed multiple binding sites for specific antibodies (Lynch and Howe, 1986).

Platelet destruction by phagocytosis occurs particularly in the spleen and sometimes in the liver, especially in association with high levels of anti-platelet antibody, leading to thrombocytopenia even in splenectomized patients. Platelet lysis by platelet antibodies and complement may occur; this has been demonstrated in vitro (Tsubakio et al, 1986). Platelet survival is reduced to less than 10% of the normal 10-day life span and is inversely related to levels of PA-IgG. Megakaryocytes are increased in number, volume and immaturity and there is evidence of intravascular thrombocytolysis and abnormal platelet function. Clinical features may appear when the platelet count is insufficient to support haemostasis, generally less than 30 000 per mm³ for purpura to occur and less than 10 000 to 50 000 per mm³ for haemorrhage.

The diagnosis of ATP is generally one of exclusion of other causes of thrombocytopenia, augmented by the application of a quantitative assay for PA-IgG. This test will also distinguish between ATP and the rare maternal isoimmunization by platelets as a result of blood transfusions or pregnancy, analogous to Rh-isoimmunization. Such distinction has practical importance with regard to treatment of neonatal thrombocytopenia (see below).

Neonatal thrombocytopenia

Just as occurrence of a transient neonatal disorder provided strong evidence of the immunological nature of ATP, so the birth of an affected child adds confirmation to a diagnosis of maternal ATP. Development of transient thrombocytopenia in the child is associated with transfer of anti-platelet antibodies (Table 3). There is an extensive literature on the occurrence of neonatal autoimmune thrombocytopenia (Heys, 1966; Karpatkin et al, 1972; Kelton, 1983). Although a correlation between platelet counts of mother and child was reported (Territo et al, 1973), more recent findings show that maternal PA-IgG is not predictive of fetal platelet count (J. R. Scott et al, 1980). This may be due to unequal distribution of maternal IgG in mother and infant (see Table 3) or differential transfer of IgG subclasses across the placenta. Affinity of the maternal antibody may be different for mother's and infant's platelets. Alternatively, the reticuloendothelial system of the child may operate differently, affecting platelet destruction.

Table 3. Maternal and neonatal serum antiplatelet antibody detected in auto-immune neonatal thrombocytopenia. From Karpatkin (1985).

Platelet antibody titre		Platelet count/mm^3		
Mother	Infant	Mother	Infant	Past history of ATP
1:8	1:16	49 000	43 000	No
1:32	1:32	162 000	100 000	No
1:48	1:40	10 000	56 000	Yes
1:32	1:40	Not done	38 000	No
1:20	1:16	Low	100 000	Yes
1:8	1:32	114 000	18 000	No
1:68	Not done	Low	60 000	Yes
1:20	0	39 000	32 000	Yes
1:8	0	65 000	60 000	Yes

Pregnancy associations and management in ATP

ATP is commonly encountered in the pregnant patient and obstetric aspects have been extensively reviewed (Jones, 1979; Levy, 1982; Kelton, 1983). There is no consistent effect of pregnancy on the course of ATP in terms of maternal platelet count. Management is essentially similar to that of the non-pregnant patient, i.e. blocking or removing the major site of platelet destruction. Corticosteroid administration reduces splenic sequestration of platelets and may suppress splenic autoantibody production. Its use in pregnancy has drastically reduced maternal risk, and 10 to 20 mg prednisone per day for one to two weeks before and during delivery may result in significantly higher neonatal platelet counts (Karpatkin et al, 1981). There is a marginal increase in the risk of fetal malformation and growth retardation with the use of steroids. Splenectomy, which has a reported response rate of 50 to 92%, can be performed with relative safety during pregnancy.

Patients refractory to corticosteroids and splenectomy are sometimes treated with azathioprine; this carries a very small risk of teratogenicity. Other forms of treatment are plasmapheresis, which achieves a rapid improvement in platelet count, and the intravenous administration of high dose γ-globulin. The recommended dose of immunoglobulin is 400 mg per kg for five consecutive days. This may have its effect by reticuloendothelial blockage and/or inhibition of antibody binding to platelets, or by anti-idiotypic suppression of autoantibody. Administration of intravenous γ-globulin before delivery has been reported to result in placental transfer of the γ-globulin and a normal neonatal platelet count. Such treatment is not always effective, however, in the prevention of neonatal thrombocytopenia (Davies et al, 1986).

Maternal mortality and morbidity in ATP are now rare, the main risk being from haemorrhage at the time of labour and delivery. Problems are associated with tears and incisions rather than with the placental site, where control of blood loss depends on contraction of the myometrium and with intracranial haemorrhage. Assisted vaginal delivery, or caesarean section if difficulty is anticipated, are indicated. The main fetal risk is from intracranial bleeding at the time of delivery. Difficulties with predicting neonatal thrombocytopenia from maternal factors have led to attempts to monitor the fetal platelet count by scalp blood samples obtained as early as possible during labour. Delivery by caesarean section has been advocated if the count is less than 50 000 per mm^3 (J. R. Scott et al, 1980).

Features of neonatal thrombocytopenia and treatment

The incidence of neonatal thrombocytopenia is 60% in babies of mothers with ATP; overt purpura develops in 20% and the overall perinatal mortality rate is of the order of 15%, intracranial haemorrhage being a common autopsy finding. Neonatal thrombocytopenia may occur when the mother is clinically cured of ATP by splenectomy, since antiplatelet antibodies will still be present and can cross the placenta to cause platelet sequestration in the baby's spleen. Onset of a lowered infant platelet count may be delayed for 12 to 24 hours, possibly because of immaturity of the reticuloendothelial system. The duration of thrombocytopenia averages three to four weeks, but can be three months.

Although most affected infants require no treatment, this may be necessary if cord blood specimens show severely depressed platelet counts. Corticosteroids are used to reduce antibody binding and platelet sequestration: 12 mg intravenous hydrocortisone 12 hourly for two to three days, followed by oral prednisolone 1 mg per kg per day. Platelet transfusion may be needed: two platelet packs over six to eight hours. In more severe cases, exchange transfusion may be required. In the isoimmune type of neonatal thrombocytopenia, the baby requires treatment with maternal platelets. All these measures are secondary in importance to the obstetric prevention of intracranial haemorrhage at the time of delivery (see above). Breast feeding should be avoided.

Autoimmune haemolytic anaemia

In autoimmune haemolytic disease, both immunoglobulin and complement components can be demonstrated coating the erythrocytes. Autoantibodies are present which cause complement-mediated lysis of the erythrocytes or adherence to macrophages, resulting in reduction of erythrocyte numbers to a varying extent. The anti-erythrocyte antibodies are either IgG antibodies directed at the Rh antigens or cold agglutinins, mostly IgM, directed at the I or i blood group antigens. Other antigens may be involved since leucopenia and thrombocytopenia sometimes also occur. Autoimmune haemolytic disease occurs mainly in young females and so is therefore of obstetric interest. It tends to worsen during pregnancy and remit after delivery, possibly related to passage of fetal red cells across the placenta or to changes in macrophage function and accelerated red cell destruction.

Risks to the fetus are hypoxia due to maternal anaemia and haemolysis due to transplacental maternal anti-erythrocyte IgG. Occurrence of still-birth or severe neonatal anaemia has been estimated at 35 to 40% (Chaplin et al, 1975). Haemoglobin and reticulocyte levels should be monitored throughout pregnancy and anti-erythrocyte antibody assessed by the direct Coombs' test, i.e. erythrocyte agglutination using xenogeneic antisera to human immunoglobulins. In severe cases, administration of corticosteroids may be effective in maintaining haemoglobulin levels above 10 g/dl, otherwise blood transfusion and premature delivery may be required. Plasmapheresis and splenectomy may be indicated in some cases. If high levels of maternal anti-erythrocyte antibody are present, fetal haemolysis should be assessed by spectrophotometric analysis of amniotic fluid. Management is then conducted on the same basis as with rhesus isoimmunization.

Type 1 diabetes mellitus

In recent years this has come to be regarded as a chronic autoimmune disease (Eisenbarth, 1986). There is an established pattern of genetic susceptibility together with triggering factors, such as drugs and viruses, particularly congenital rubella, and the subsequent production of auto-antibodies to various antigens including thyroglobulin, thyroid microsomes, single-stranded DNA, insulin and islet cells. Appearance of antibodies to insulin and islet cells may precede overt diabetes by years, by which time islet-cell antibody has generally disappeared. Although these antibodies have prognostic value, and despite the fact that islet-cell antibody reacts with the cell surface to inhibit insulin secretion, β cell destruction may be a function of T cells rather than antibody. Two lines of evidence are pertinent: transfer of the disease in the non-obese diabetic mouse model by splenocytes (Wicker et al, 1986) and the lack of transplacental antibody effects. Although infants of diabetic mothers do suffer from metabolic disturbance, a transient transferred neonatal form of the disorder has not been described in babies of affected mothers. Interestingly, transient neonatal diabetes has been described in the babies of mothers who have no history of diabetes (see J. S. Scott, 1966). The neonatal presentation in these cases has been of an undernourished baby who fails to thrive and develops dehydration. On confirmation of the diagnosis by blood glucose estimation, treatment is by insulin and carbohydrate control. The condition remits within three months of birth so that the pattern is entirely in keeping with a causative transplacental factor. Since the islet-cell and insulin antibodies precede overt disease and then disappear, it may be that only women in a prediabetic asymptomatic stage are liable to give birth to affected babies. Transplacental antibody may act in conjunction with fetal T cell factors.

Pernicious anaemia

In pernicious anaemia, there is an autoantibody that inhibits the uptake of dietary vitamin B12. This is normally transported across the intestinal mucosa after forming a complex with a protein, intrinsic factor, synthesized by the parietal cells in the gastric mucosa. Plasma cells in the gastric mucosa of patients with the disease secrete IgA autoantibodies to intrinsic factor which combine with it to block its role as carrier for the B12 vitamin. Pernicious anaemia is rarely seen in association with pregnancy because of its age distribution (usually after 40 years) and because it is specifically associated with infertility. However, pregnancy observations on lack of effect in babies of mothers with pernicious anaemia have given support to the idea that circulating IgG antibodies to intrinsic factor are not pathogenic. It is of interest that breast-fed infants have been observed to develop megaloblastic anaemia. This may be due to IgA anti-intrinsic factor antibodies being present in colostrum or milk and passing directly into the gastrointestinal tract.

NON ORGAN-SPECIFIC DISEASE

Systemic lupus erythematosus

Systemic lupus erythematosus (SLE), the prototype autoimmune disease, is a syndrome characterized by a very wide range of immunological abnormalities. SLE can be regarded as part of a spectrum of disordered immunity and is closely related to a number of other autoimmune disorders, such as rheumatoid arthritis and Sjögren's syndrome (see below). There is involvement of multiple organ systems; the joints, skin, kidney, central nervous system, synovial membranes, lungs, heart and skeletal muscles are all susceptible to the disease process. As suspicion of it as a cause of otherwise unexplained signs and symptoms become commoner, it is diagnosed with increasing frequency in its milder forms. Criteria for the classification of SLE, described by the American Rheumatism Association, have been revised in recent years (Tan et al, 1982). There is a high female preponderance of nine to one, particularly in the reproductive years, and an association with HLA-DRw2 and -DRw3.

Genesis of disease in relation to both human and murine SLE has been discussed by Smith and Steinberg (1983). A complex set of factors, which may differ in individual patients, culminates in B cell hyperactivity and production of autoantibodies to a variety of non organ-specific antigens. These include double-stranded DNA, single-stranded DNA, histones, non-histone nuclear proteins and RNA–protein complexes (Sm, U1-RNP, Ro [SS-A], La [SS-B] and Ma), together with cell-surface structures and phospholipids. Shoenfeld et al (1983) suggested that this serological diversity is partly due to binding to a common antigenic structure, a phosphate ester, that recurs in various molecules. An antibody may be detected as an anti-nuclear or anti-DNA antibody, a biological false–positive test for syphilis or as a lupus anticoagulant (see below), depending on the assay used. These findings raise questions as to the primary antigenic stimulus in SLE as well as the immunological target. Further evidence for a restricted family of germ-line genes being involved comes from the report of cross-reactive idiotypes in lupus autoantibodies (Isenberg et al, 1984).

Tissue damage may be related to immune complex deposition, reaction of antinuclear antibodies with antigen bound to basement membranes, and direct binding of antibodies to their target antigens. The pathogenic role of anti-DNA has recently been assessed (Bach et al, 1986).

Neonatal lupus erythematosus (NLE)

Initial observations on the lack of fetal effects, despite the transplacental passage of some autoantibodies, established that anti-nuclear factor and lupus erythematosus factor were irrelevant to pathogenesis. This gave rise to the assumption that all the autoantibodies were epiphenomena, but subsequently it became clear that neonatal sequelae could result from maternal SLE. These range from transient neonatal discoid lupus to a severe systemic disorder characterized by anaemia, thrombocytopenia, generalized skin lesions and congenital complete heart block (CCHB). The lesion associated with CCHB is permanent, due to fibrosis of parts of the specialized conducting tissue of the heart. Reports of neonatal lupus erythematosus have been reviewed by Provost et al (1987).

Several groups have found anti-Ro (SS-A)/La (SS-B) in association with NLE (Kephart et al, 1981; Weston et al, 1982), and these autoantibodies have now been identified in 100% of mothers of babies with CCHB and in all affected infants within the first three months of life (Taylor et al, 1988). They are detected by a variety of assays, including immunofluorescence, immuno-diffusion, immunoblots, radioimmunoassay and enzyme-immunosorbent assays. The Ro (SS-A) and La (SS-B) particles are composed of RNA and an antigenic protein component. There is a molecular association between Ro (SS-A) and La (SS-B), and the relevant autoantibodies often coexist in patients' sera (Deng et al, 1985). These interesting antibodies have been used as probes to study events related to cellular metabolism: La (SS-B) may have a functional role related to ribosomal RNA synthesis and Ro (SS-A) may participate in translation of mRNA. It is relevant in the context of NLE that Wolin and Steitz (1983) found Ro (SS-A) to be tenfold more abundant in brain and heart than in other tissues. There is evidence that Ro (SS-A) antibody is the pathogenic agent in both skin lesions (Lee et al, 1986) and the kidney in lupus nephritis (Maddison and Reichlin, 1979). NLE does not always occur when anti-Ro (SS-A)/La (SS-B) are present. Fetal outcome is not correlated with maternal antibody titre and the genetic association with production of Ro (SS-A) antibody (HLA-A1, B8, DR3, MB2 and MT2) is not seen in NLE. Fetal immune responses may be relevant; IgM and IgA, as well as IgG, immunoglobulins are deposited in affected hearts (Litsey et al, 1985; Taylor et al, 1986a) and neonates may produce anti-DNA of different idiotype to the maternal idiotype (El-Roeiy et al, unpublished data; see El-Roeiy and Schoenfeld, 1985).

NLE is associated with presence of antibody rather than presence or type of maternal disease. Many mothers of babies with CCHB have other varieties of connective tissue disease (CTD), such as rheumatoid arthritis, 'mixed' CTD and Sjögren's syndrome, and many are asymptomatic (J. S. Scott et al, 1983). This emphasizes two important points: (i) the definition of CTD by antibody profiles (see J. S. Scott and Taylor, 1985), including clinical subsets like ANA-negative, Ro (SS-A) antibody-positive patients with subacute cutaneous disease, and (ii) the fact that birth of a child with CCHB is a marker for future development of CTD in clinically asymptomatic women (Esscher and Scott, 1979).

The clinical relevance is that pregnant women with any form of CTD should have an autoantibody screen performed including the ribonucleoprotein antibodies. Anti-Ro (SS-A)/La (SS-B) can be screened using indirect immunofluorescence on Hep-2 cells and counterimmunoelectrophoresis, and specific identification achieved by double immunodiffusion, Western blots or enzyme-immunosorbent assay, depending on laboratory facilities. Since many anti-Ro (SS-A) positive women are clinically normal, they will not be identified antenatally. Inclusion of autoantibody measurements in the routine antenatal screen depends upon the development of convenient diagnostic tests, such as that devised by Whittingham et al (1987) to detect La (SS-B) antibody using an enzyme-immunosorbent assay and human recombinant La nucleoprotein as the antigen. Although fetal outcome cannot be predicted, a positive anti-Ro (SS-A)/La (SS-B) test will alert the obstetrician to the possible development of NLE.

Pregnancy associations and management in SLE

In addition to possible NLE, there is an overall increased rate of pregnancy loss in SLE, as well as intrauterine growth retardation and pre-term delivery. There is an extensive literature on the interaction between SLE and pregnancy (El-Roeiy and Shoenfeld, 1985; Lockshin et al, 1987). Twelve series reported since 1975 have been reviewed by Branch (1987). Overall pregnancy loss ranged from 11 to 46%. The rate of spontaneous abortion (prior to 20 weeks gestation) was 0 to 35%, and fetal death (after 10 weeks gestation) occurred in 0 to 29% of pregnancies. The primary pathology seems to be at the level of the placenta; decidual vasculopathy characterized by fibrinoid necrosis has been described.

Some of this pregnancy loss may be related to presence of autoantibody. Anti-phospholipid antibodies have been particularly implicated and are discussed in the next section. Ro (SS-A) antibody seems to operate in reproductive failure as well as development of NLE (Maddison et al, 1984). A retrospective study suggested that black patients with SLE were at increased risk of fetal wastage if they possessed Ro (SS-A) antibody (Watson et al, 1985). A similar study by Ramsey-Goldman et al (1986) revealed no such association, apart from risk of CCHB. A preliminary prospective study showed that prevalence of various anti-nuclear antibodies, including Ro (SS-A) antibody, was elevated in unexplained spontaneous recurrent abortion compared with normal pregnancy and other types of reproductive failure (Taylor et al, 1986b). These findings raise the question of whether some types of pregnancy loss are treatable by immunotherapy (see also lupus anticoagulant).

The frequency of SLE in pregnancy is about one in 1500. Severe renal or cardiac disease, or primary pulmonary hypertension, are the main contra-indications to pregnancy, which ideally should be timed to occur during remission. There is often exacerbation of disease, particularly in the first half of pregnancy and in the puerperium. The effects are variable and patient management must be individualized (J. S. Scott, 1979). Prediction of flare-up may to some extent be made by measuring anti-DNA antibody, comple-ment levels and acute phase proteins. Treatment of mild disease is by non-steroidal anti-inflammatory or anti-malarial drugs. More severe disease is treated by corticosteroids, azathioprine or plasmapheresis. Steroid dosage over 55 mg cortisol per day, or its equivalent, may interfere with fetal monitoring by oestriol measurement. Severe renal and vascular effects associated with SLE may be mistaken for pre-eclampsia.

Presence of CCHB can be detected antenatally by a sustained fetal bradycardia of 60 to 70 beats per minute. Such early detection will facilitate the early institution of pacemaker therapy, if required, after delivery of the infant. Caesarean section may not be necessary, particularly if continuous fetal pH monitoring is used during labour. Corticosteroid supplementation should be given during labour and delivery, as necessary, and steroid therapy continued for at least two months post-partum. Breast-feeding is not contraindicated, except possibly in corticosteroid-treated mothers.

The possibility of affecting fetal outcome by reducing or suppressing maternal autoantibody levels has been addressed in a few cases. Successful pregnancies have been reported following steroid therapy and plasma exchange (Barclay et al, 1987; Buyon et al, 1987). Similar treatment commenced after 22 weeks gestation was ineffective in reversal of CCHB (Herreman and Galezowski, 1985). Despite the lack of systematic data because of the difficulty of conducting a clinical trial of such therapy, early institution of steroid therapy supplemented by plasma exchange might be justified in anti-Ro (SS-A)/La (SS-B)-positive women with a history of unexplained recurrent abortion and/or previous children with CCHB.

Features of NLE and treatment

Risk of NLE in infants born to mothers with Ro (SS-A)/La (SS-B) anti-bodies has been calculated as 7 to 38% (Lockshin et al, 1987). Risk of CCHB is much lower, probably less than 5%; the incidence of CCHB is one in 20 000 births.

Clinical features of NLE include cutaneous lesions, CCHB and thrombocytopenia. The skin disease is characterized by annular, erythematous, oedematous lesions which are present at birth or develop within the first month of life, often after exposure to sunlight. Healing occurs generally within six months leaving no sequelae. Thrombocytopenia occurs in approximately 10 to 20% of infants with NLE and occasionally a petechial dermatitis may be the dominant clinical feature.

CCHB has been detected as early as 16 weeks gestation and is a permanent defect, associated with destruction or entrapment of the sinoatrial node, atrioventricular node and/or bundle of His by fibrosis. The current post-delivery mortality rate for babies with CCHB is approximately 25%. Most babies surviving the neonatal period have a reasonable prognosis since the cardiac fibrosis is apparently non-progressive. Cases must be assessed individually as to the necessity for pacemaker therapy.

Lupus anticoagulant: the anti-phospholipid syndrome

Lupus anticoagulant was the name assigned by Feinstein and Rapaport (1972) to factors causing inhibition of blood coagulation, first described by Conley and Hartmann (1952). Lupus anticoagulants are immunoglobulins (IgG and/or IgM) which interfere with phospholipid-dependent coagulation tests without inhibiting the activity of specific coagulation factors. They occur in approximately 24% of patients with SLE, to varying extents in other autoimmune disorders, and also in individuals with no sign of disease. There is a clinical association of these immunoglobulins with thrombosis, thrombocytopenia and recurrent fetal death.

The lupus anticoagulant is an antiphospholipid antibody, probably directed at phosphodiester-linked phosphate groups. It acts at the level of the prothrombin converter complex of the clotting cascade (Figure 4) by binding with the phospholipid portion of the complex (Thiagarajan et al, 1980). This feature allows its detection in patients' plasma by causing prolongation of the activated partial thromboplastin time (APTT), the Russell viper venom time (RVVT) and, less often, the prothrombin time. All these coagulation tests reflect the conversion of prothrombin to thrombin by factor Xa, and they are all phospholipid-dependent. Coagulation factor deficiency is excluded by retesting the plasma after admixture with an equal volume of normal plasma; clotting times will not correct to normal if lupus anticoagulant is present. Sometimes the clotting time is further prolonged indicating a lupus cofactor which allows full expression of lupus anticoagulant activity (Shapiro and Thiagarajan, 1982). The kaolin clotting time (KCT), with no added phospholipid, and the dilute tissue thromboplastin time, are claimed to be more sensitive. There is disagreement about the best assay to use; most laboratories identify 85% or more patients with lupus anticoagulant using APTT, but the RVVT may have a stronger association with thrombotic events. Standardization of coagulation tests is difficult; pre-analytical variables including plasma storage and preparation are involved, as well as analytical variables such as reference reagents and plasmas. Laboratory procedure should consist of screening

DUNNE Martina.

300370

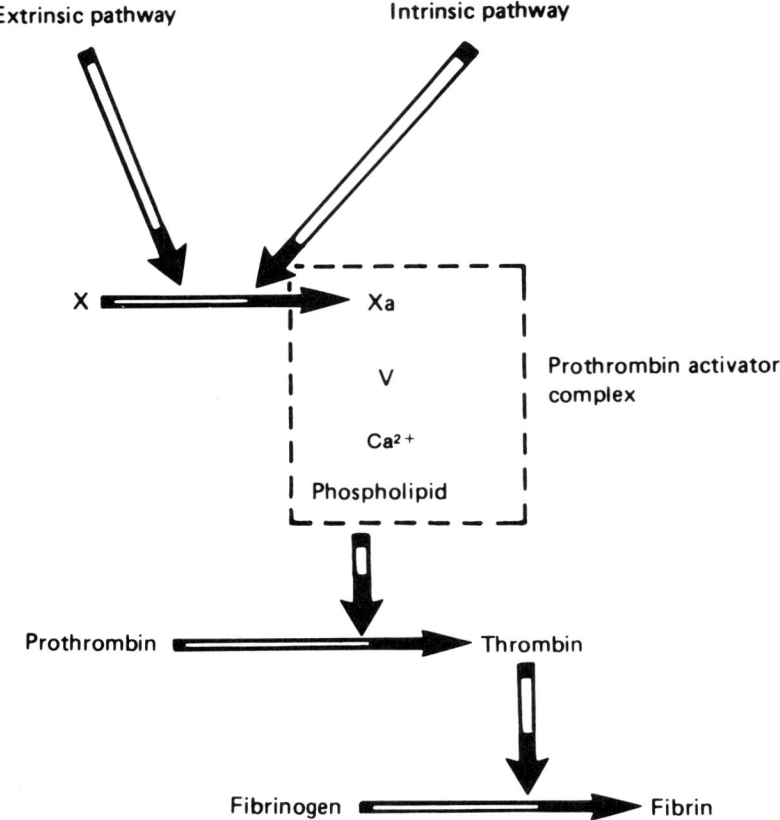

Figure 4. The lupus anticoagulant acts at the level of the prothrombin activatory complex. It is believed to bind the phospholipid portion of the complex and so delay the conversion of prothrombin to thrombin. From Harris et al (1985a).

with the APTT and RVVT, testing for inhibitors using mixing studies, and confirmatory assays with both decreased (KCT, dilute APTT) and increased (platelet neutralization test) phospholipid.

In contrast to its effects in vitro, the prominent clinical association is with thrombosis. Carreras and Vermylen (1982) reviewed 211 patients with lupus anticoagulant, of whom 28.9% had arterial or venous thrombosis. A later review by Lechner and Pabinger-Fasching (1985) found that 32.8% of 259 patients with the antibody developed thrombosis. Since thrombotic events occur in 8 to 12% of patients with SLE in the absence of lupus anticoagulant, its presence seems a serious risk factor for thrombosis. There is also a strong correlation with pregnancy loss. Of 242 reported cases of untreated pregnancies in 65 women with lupus anticoagulant, 91% were lost as spontaneous abortions or fetal deaths (see Branch, 1987). A frequent finding is extensive infarction and necrosis of the placenta. Intrauterine fetal death tends to occur in the second trimester and there are only six published cases of untreated women with lupus anticoagulant who had a live infant.

The mode of action of lupus anticoagulant is unknown. It may bind to phospholipids in endothelial cell membranes and decrease prostacyclin production by blocking arachidonic acid release (Carreras and Vermylen, 1982). The antagonist, thromboxane, would then predominate and cause vasoconstriction, platelet aggregation and intravascular thrombosis. Other postulated mechanisms have invoked interference with antithrombin III activity (Cosgriff and Martin, 1981) or prekallikrein activity (Sanfelippo and Drayna, 1982), the latter linking lupus anticoagulant to defective intra-vascular fibrin removal. Recently, Cariou et al (1986) demonstrated that thrombin-mediated activation of protein C is inhibited by endothelial cells in the presence of lupus anticoagulant. Protein C is a circulating inhibitor of several coagulation factors. Another possibility is that lupus anticoagulant may activate platelets by binding membrane phospholipids, initiating platelet aggregation and thrombosis. Finally, anti-idiotypic antibody to lupus anticoagulant may be involved, the anti-idiotype acting as an internal image of negatively-charged phospholipids and promoting the activation of clotting factors.

Different behaviour patterns in the coagulation tests emphasize that these may not detect identical antibodies. Development of a solid-phase radio-immunoassay (Harris et al, 1983) and an enzyme-immunosorbent assay (Gharavi et al, 1987) were important advances in this respect, giving specific, reproducible and quantitative tests which can be applied to stored sera. Although cardiolipin is used as the antigen, antibodies detected probably bind all negatively-charged phospholipids and these could equally well be used as antigens. On this basis the term 'anti-phospholipid' antibody seems preferable to 'anti-cardiolipin'. The anti-cardiolipin and lupus anti-coagulant tests clearly detect a similar antibody, but possibly not an identical one (Branch et al, 1987). Antibodies detected by both tests are probably responsible for some of the biological false-positive results seen in standard tests for syphilis, now primarily of historic interest in detection of anti-phospholipid antibodies. The cross-reactions between anti-DNA and anti-cardiolipin activities, demonstrated in several studies, have not been con-firmed by Harris et al (1985b). Smeenk et al (1987) explain this discrepancy in terms of antibody activity. In a study using patients' sera and a panel of monoclonal anti-DNA antibodies, anti-DNA of low avidity cross-reacted with anti-cardiolipin whereas those of high avidity did not.

Anti-cardiolipin antibodies of all three main immunoglobulin classes have been detected in 40 to 60% of patients with SLE. They have also been found in a variety of cutaneous and neurological syndromes, as well as non-specific infections and hypergammaglobulinaemic conditions (see Sontheimer 1987 for review). The strongest correlation between anti-cardiolipin antibody and the clinical disorders with which lupus anticoagulant is associated is with the IgG isotype. High levels of IgG anti-cardiolipin antibody may occur in individuals with no SLE or defined autoimmune disorder, who suffer a high prevalence of thrombosis, fetal loss, thrombocytopenia and Coombs' positivity (Harris et al, 1986). This has been described as the 'anti-phospholipid syndrome'. Associations between anti-cardiolipin antibody and unexplained habitual abortion was not confirmed by Petri et al (1987), but many patients in this study were tested when not pregnant. A prospective study of women with SLE showed that anti-cardiolipin antibody strongly predicted fetal distress or death (Lockshin et al, 1985).

Demonstration of these clinical associations raises the question of whether patients with anti-phospholipid antibodies are potentially treatable by suppression of the antibodies. Patients with lupus anticoagulant have been treated during pregnancy with prednisone and aspirin, with subsequent delivery of live infants (Lubbe et al, 1983; Branch et al, 1985). Reduction in pregnancy loss rate was significant, although not always correlated with suppression of lupus anticoagulant (Branch et al, 1985). Unlike lupus anti-coagulant activity, levels of anti-cardiolipin antibody are not greatly affected by corticosteroids. When patients with either lupus anticoagulant or anti-cardiolipin antibody were grouped together, corticosteroid therapy was still associated with a fetal mortality rate of over 50% (Lockshin et al, 1987). Although prednisone and aspirin appear to improve fetal survival, such treatment maintained over several months may cause serious maternal and fetal side effects. Randomized, prospective, controlled trials are currently being initiated with both treated and untreated groups receiving the same antenatal care (Harris, 1988). Until such data is known, it is very difficult to make recommendations about treatment. Patients with a history of pregnancy loss should be tested, on at least two occasions separated by several weeks, for both lupus anticoagulant and anti-cardiolipin antibody. A sustained positive lupus anticoagulant test and/or moderate to high titre (more than 5 to 6 standard deviations above the mean) IgG anti-cardiolipin antibody may justify inclusion in a trial of prednisone and aspirin. In any event, monitoring patients for anti-cardiolipin antibodies is useful in predicting both fetal distress, which will facilitate obstetric management, and potential thrombotic episodes, which are preventable by prolonged anticoagulant therapy. Finally, patients with high levels of anti-phospholipid antibodies, whether or not they have a history of fetal loss, should be followed prospectively to gain an insight into the clinical consequences of these antibodies.

Rheumatoid arthritis, Sjögren's syndrome, dermatomyositis and scleroderma

These diseases have many similarities to SLE and represent gradations in the variety and severity of system involvement within the group of systemic rheumatic diseases. Rheumatoid arthritis, mixed connective tissue disease (MCTD), Sjögren's syndrome and scleroderma do not show the diversity of involvement characteristic of SLE, and dermato/polymyositis are even more limited, mainly affecting the skin and muscle. Rheumatoid arthritis tends to improve during pregnancy (see above). An increased rate of pregnancy loss has been reported in several of these disorders. In scleroderma, the stillbirth rate in one study was 3.5% and the spontaneous abortion rate 30% (Slate and Graham, 1968). An overall pregnancy loss of nearly 70%, including a

23% fetal death rate, was found in MCTD by Kaufman and Kitridou (1982). Dermato/polymyositis has also been associated with an increased rate of fetal death (Bauer et al, 1979).

Autoantibody profiles characterizing these disorders include autoantibodies to non-histone nuclear proteins and RNA-protein complexes, some of which are 'marker' antibodies, for example Scl-70 antibody in scleroderma and Jo-1 antibody in polymyositis. Other autoantibodies have wider distributions, such as U1-RNP and Ro (SS-A) antibodies, and it is in relation to these that transient neonatal effects may occur. Thus, the manifestations of NLE and CCHB may occur in the infants of mothers with these types of connective tissue disease (J. S. Scott et al, 1983). In addition, anti-phospholipid antibodies may play a role in the effects of these diseases on the outcome of pregnancy.

SUMMARY

The generation of autoimmune disease results from a breakdown of the regulatory mechanisms keeping the normal autoreactive potential of the immune system in check. Such a breakdown may be related to a spectrum of immune, genetic, environmental and endogenous factors. Gestation involves many immunological and physiological alterations to the maternal system so that pregnancy may have a profound effect on the natural history of autoimmune disease in the mother. Conversely, since immunological factors operate at many levels in the reproductive process, autoimmunity may influence fertility, pregnancy and fetal well-being.

Transport of maternal IgG autoantibodies across the placenta during pregnancy may give rise to a neonatal form of maternal autoimmune disease if the relevant antigen is present in the fetus. The neonatal disease will be transient, provided no irreversible damage occurs, and disappear as the maternal antibodies are catabolized. Such neonatal effects have been observed in a range of organ-specific and non organ-specific diseases, and have often been crucial in confirming an autoimmune basis for the disorder. Whatever the nature of the primary defect, the materno–fetal model has contributed to our understanding of pathogenesis and established that this is related to antibody effects in many diseases. Characterization of placentally transferred autoantibodies has given useful information concerning the relationships between individual autoimmune diseases. Recent observations have suggested that there may be a fetal immune contribution to expression of neonatal disease.

In a clinical setting, measurement of maternal autoantibodies is useful in assessing the likelihood of neonatal involvement, facilitating obstetric and paediatric management. Birth of an affected infant to a mother with no clinical history may alert the clinician to potential development of maternal autoimmune disease. Characterization of pathogenic autoantibodies opens up the possibility of treatment of severe forms of neonatal disease by immunosuppression of the relevant antibody, and also provides a means of monitoring such treatment.

Finally, obstetricians are in a position to make important contributions to the scientific understanding of autoimmunity. Pregnancy observations in the context of maternal autoimmune disease will be of continuing value in the elucidation of immunopathogenic mechanisms and the influence of maternal and fetal genetic factors in the disease process.

REFERENCES

Adams DD & Purves HD (1956) Abnormal response in the assay of thyrotrophin. *University of Otago Medical School Proceedings* **34:** 11.

Adams DD & Kennedy TH (1967) Occurrence in thyrotoxicosis of a gammaglobulin which protects LATS from neutralization by an extract of thyroid gland. *Journal of Clinical Endocrinology* **27:** 173–177.

Adams DD, Kennedy TH & Stewart RDH (1974) Correlation between long-acting thyroid stimulator protector level and thyroid ^{131}I uptake in thyrotoxicosis. *British Medical Journal* **2:** 199–201.

Amino N, Kuro R, Tanizawa O et al (1978) Changes in serum anti-thyroid antibodies during and after pregnancy in autoimmune thyroid diseases. *Clinical and Experimental Immunology* **31:** 30–37.

Armiento M, Salabe H, Vetrano G et al (1980) Decrease of thyroid antibodies during pregnancy. *Journal of Endocrinological Investigation* **4:** 437–438.

Bach JF, Jacob L, Feutren G & Tron F (1986) The questionable role of anti-DNA antibodies in the pathogenesis of systemic lupus erythematosus. *Annals of the New York Academy of Sciences* **475:** 231–240.

Barclay CS, French MAH, Ross LD & Sokol RJ (1987) Successful pregnancy following steroid therapy and plasma exchange in a woman with anti-Ro (SS-A) antibodies. Case Report. *British Journal of Obstetrics and Gynaecology* **94:** 369–371.

Bauer KA, Siegler M & Lindheimer MA (1979) Polymyositis complicating pregnancy. *Archives of Internal Medicine* **139:** 449.

Behan WHH, Behan PO & Simpson JA (1975) Absence of cellular hypersensitivity to muscle and thymic antigens in myasthenia gravis. *Journal of Neurology and Neurosurgical Psychiatry* **38:** 1039–1047.

Berrih-Aknin S, Morel E, Raimond F et al (1987) The role of the thymus in myasthenia gravis: Immunohistological and immunological studies in 115 cases. *Annals of the New York Academy of Sciences* **505:** 50–70.

Bottazzo GF & Doniach D (1986) Autoimmune thyroid disease. *Annual Review in Medicine* **37:** 353–359.

Branch DW (1987) Immunologic disease and fetal death. *Clinical Obstetrics and Gynaecology* **30:** 295–311.

Branch DW, Scott JR, Kochenour NK & Hershgold E (1985) Obstetric complications associated with the lupus anticoagulant. *New England Journal of Medicine* **313:** 1322–1326.

Branch DW, Rote NS, Dostal DA & Scott JR (1987) Association of lupus anticoagulant with antibody against phosphatidylserine. *Clinical Immunology and Immunopathology* **42:** 63–75.

Brenner T, Beyth Y & Abramsky O (1980) Inhibitory effect of alpha fetoprotein on binding of myasthenia gravis antibody to acetylcholine receptors. *Proceedings of the National Academy of Science (USA)* **77:** 3635–3639.

Brown J, Solomon DH, Beall GN et al (1978) Autoimmune thyroid diseases—Graves' and Hashimoto's. *Annals of Internal Medicine* **88:** 379–391.

Buyon JP, Swersky SH, Fox HE et al (1987) Intrauterine therapy for presumptive fetal myocarditis with acquired heart block due to systemic lupus erythematosus. *Arthritis and Rheumatism* **30:** 44–49.

Cariou R, Tobelem G, Soria C & Caen J (1986) Inhibition of protein C activation by endothelial cells in the presence of lupus anticoagulant. *New England Journal of Medicine* **314:** 1193–1194.

Carreras LO & Vermylen JG (1982) Lupus anticoagulant and thrombosis; possible role of inhibition of prostacyclin formation. *Thrombosis and Haemostasis* **48:** 38–40.

Chang CE & Lee CY (1962) Isolation of neurotoxins from the venom of bungarus multicinctus and their modes of neuromuscular blocking action. *Archives de Internationale Pharmacodynamie et de Therapie* **144:** 241–257.

Chaplin H, Cohen R, Bloomberg G et al (1975) Pregnancy and idiopathic haemolytic anaemia: a prospective study during 6 months gestation and 3 months post-partum. *British Journal of Haematology* **24:** 219–229.

Conley CL & Hartmann RC (1952) A hemorrhagic disorder caused by circulating anticoagulant in patients with disseminated lupus erythematosus. *Journal of Clinical Investigation* **31:** 621–622.

Cosgriff TM & Martin BA (1981) Low functional and high antigenic anti-thrombin III level in a patient with the lupus anticoagulant and recurrent thrombosis. *Arthritis and Rheumatism* **24:** 94–96.

Davies TF & Platzer M (1986) The T cell suppressor defect in autoimmune thyroiditis: evidence for a high set 'autoimmunostat'. *Clinical and Experimental Immunology* **63:** 73–79.

Davies TF & Weiss I (1981) Autoimmune thyroid disease and pregnancy. *American Journal of Reproductive Immunology* **i:** 187–192.

Davies SV, Murray JA, Gee H & Giles H (1986) Transplacental effect of high-dose immunoglobulin in idiopathic thrombocytopenia (ITP). *Lancet* **i:** 1098–1099.

Deng JS, Sontheimer RD & Gilliam JN (1985) Molecular characteristics of SS-B/La and SS-A/Ro cellular antigens. *Journal of Investigative Dermatology* **84:** 86–90.

Dixon R, Rosse W & Ebbert L (1975) Quantitative determination of antibody in idiopathic thrombocytopenic purpura. *New England Journal of Medicine* **292:** 230–236.

Drachman DB, Adams RN, Josifek LF & Self SG (1982) Functional activities of autoantibodies to acetylcholine receptors and the clinical severity of myasthenia gravis. *New England Journal of Medicine* **307:** 769–775.

Eisenbarth GS (1986) Type 1 diabetes mellitus: A chronic autoimmune disease. *New England Journal of Medicine* **314:** 1360–1368.

El-Roeiy A & Shoenfeld Y (1985) Autoimmunity and pregnancy. *American Journal of Reproductive Immunology and Microbiology* **9:** 25–32.

Engel AG (1979) Myasthenia gravis. In Winken PJ & Bruyn GW (eds) *Handbook of Clinical Neurology*, pp 95–145. Amsterdam: North-Holland.

Epstein RD, Lozner EL, Coffey TS et al (1950) Congenital thrombocytopenia purpura. Purpura hemorrhagica in pregnancy and in the newborn. *American Journal of Medicine* **9:** 44.

Esscher E & Scott JS (1979) Congenital heart block and maternal systemic lupus erythematosus. *British Medical Journal* **i:** 1235–1238.

Feinstein DI & Rapaport SI (1972) Acquired inhibitors of blood coagulation. In Spaet TH (ed.) *Progress in Hemostasis and Thrombosis*, p 75. New York: Grune and Stratton.

Fennell DF & Ringel SP (1987) Myasthenia gravis and pregnancy. *Obstetrical and Gynecological Survey* **41:** 414–421.

Gharavi AE, Harris EN, Asherson RA & Hughes GRV (1987) Isotype distribution and phospholipid specificity in the anti-phospholipid syndrome. *Annals of Rheumatic Diseases* **46:** 1–6.

Gleicher N (1986) Pregnancy and autoimmunity. *Acta Haematologica* **76:** 68–77.

Gomez CM & Richman DP (1983) Anti-acetylcholine receptor antibodies directed against the α-bungarotoxin binding site induce a unique form of experimental myasthenia. *Proceedings of the National Academy of Science USA* **80:** 4089–4093.

Gomez CM & Richman DP (1987) Chronic experimental autoimmune myasthenia gravis induced by monoclonal antibody to acetylcholine receptor: Biochemical and electrophysiologic criteria. *Journal of Immunology* **139:** 73–76.

Harrington WJ, Minnich V, Hollingsworth JW (1951) Demonstration of a thrombocytopenic factor on the blood of patients with thrombocytopenic purpura. *Journal of Laboratory and Clinical Medicine* **38:** 1.

Harris EN (1988) Protocol for international co-operative clinical and laboratory study of patients with anti-phospholipid antibodies and fetal loss. *Anti-phospholipid antibodies*. Abstracts of the Third International Conference, 1988; Kingston (in press).

Harris EN, Gharavi AE, Boey ML et al (1983) Anticardiolipin antibodies: detection by radioimmunoassay and association with thrombosis in systemic lupus erythematosus. *Lancet* **ii:** 1211–1214.

Harris EN, Gharavi AE & Hughes GRV (1985a) Antiphospholipid Antibodies. *Clinics in Rheumatic Diseases* **11:** 596.

Harris EN, Gharavi AE, Tincani A et al (1985b) Affinity-purified anti-cardiolipin and anti-DNA antibodies. *Journal of Clinical and Laboratory Immunology* **17:** 155–162.

Harris EN, Chan, JKH, Asherson RA et al (1986) Thrombosis, recurrent fetal loss, and thrombocytopenia. *Archives of Internal Medicine* **146:** 2153–2156.

Hegde UM, Balls S, Zuiable A & Roter BLT (1985) Platelet associated immunoglobulins (PAIgG and PAIgM) in autoimmune thrombocytopenia. *British Journal of Haematology* **59:** 221–226.

Herreman G & Galezowski N (1985) Maternal connective tissue disease and congenital heart block. *New England Journal of Medicine* **312:** 1329.

Heys RF (1966) Child bearing and idiopathic thrombocytopenia purpura. *Journal of Obstetrics and Gynaecology of the British Commonwealth* **73:** 205–214.

Hymes K, Shulman S & Karpatkin S (1979) A solid phase radioimmunoassay for bound anti-platelet antibody. Studies on 45 patients with autoimmune platelet disorders. *Journal of Laboratory and Clinical Medicine* **94:** 639.

Isenberg DA, Shoenfeld Y & Madaio MP (1984) Anti-DNA antibody idiotypes in SLE. *Lancet* **2:** 417–422.

Jerne NK, Roland J & Cazenave PA (1982) Recurrent idiotypes and internal images. *EMBO Journal* **1:** 1823.

Jones WR (1979) Tissue-specific autoimmune diseases in pregnancy. *Clinics in Obstetrics and Gynaecology* **6:** 473–491.

Kamo I, Furakawa S & Tada A (1982) Monoclonal antibody to acetylcholine receptor: cell line established from the thymus of patient with myasthenia gravis. *Science* **215:** 995–997.

Karpatkin S (1985) Autoimmune thrombocytopenic purpura. *Seminars in Hematology* **22**(4): 260–288.

Karpatkin S, Strick N, Karpatkin MH & Siskind GW (1972) Cumulative experience on the detection of anti-platelet antibody in 234 patients with idiopathic thrombocytopenic purpura, systemic lupus erythematosis and other clinical disorders. *American Journal of Medicine* **52:** 776–785.

Karpatkin M, Porges RF & Karpatkin S (1981) Platelet counts in infants of women with autoimmune thrombocytopenia. Effect of steroid administration to the mother. *New England Journal of Medicine* **305:** 736–939.

Kaufman RL & Kitridou RC (1982) Pregnancy in mixed connective tissue disease: Comparison with systemic lupus erythematosus. *Journal of Rheumatology* **9:** 549–555.

Keesey J, Lindstrom J, Cokely H et al (1977) Anti-acetylcholine receptor antibody in neonatal myasthenia gravis. *New England Journal of Medicine* **296:** 55.

Kelton JG (1983) Management of the pregnant patient with idiopathic thrombocytopenic purpura. *Annals Internal Medicine* **99:** 796–800.

Kephart DC, Hood AF & Provost TT (1981) Neonatal lupus erythematosus: new serologic findings. *Journal of Investigative Dermatology* **77:** 331–333.

Kiefel V, Spaeth P, Mueller-Eckhardt C (1986) Immune thrombocytopenic purpura: auto-immune or immune complex disease? *British Journal of Haematology* **64:** 57–68.

Klein J (1982) *Immunology: The Science of Self-Nonself Discrimination*, p 652. New York: John Wiley.

Kodama K, Sikorska M, Bandy-Dafoe P, Bayly R & Wall JR (1982) Demonstration of a circulating autoantibody against a soluble eye-muscle antigen in Graves' ophthalmopathy. *Lancet* **ii:** 1353–1356.

Lechner K & Pabinger-Fasching I (1985) Lupus anticoagulants and thrombosis. A study of 25 cases and review of the literature. *Haemostasia* **15:** 254–262.

Lee LA, Coulter S, North D et al (1986) An animal model for studying transplacental passage in tissue deposition of antibody in neonatal lupus. *Journal of Investigative Dermatology* **86:** A488.

Lefvert AK & Osterman PO (1983) Newborn infants to myasthenic mothers: A clinical study and an investigation of acetylcholine receptor antibodies in 17 children. *Neurology* **33:** 133–138.

Levy DL (1982) Fetal–neonatal involvement in maternal autoimmune disease. *Obstetrical and Gynaecological Survey* **37**(supplement): 122–127.

Litsey SE, Noonan JA, O'Connor WN, Cottrill CM & Mitchell B (1985) Maternal connective tissue disease and congenital heart block: demonstration of immunoglobulin in cardiac tissue. *New England Journal of Medicine* **312**: 98–100.

LoBuglio AF, Court WS, Vincour L et al (1983) Immune thrombocytopenic purpura. Use of a ^{125}I-labelled anti-human IgG monoclonal antibody to quantify platelet bound IgG. *New England Journal of Medicine* **309**: 459–463.

Lockshin MD, Druzin ML, Goei S et al (1985) Antibody to cardiolipin as a predictor of fetal distress or death in pregnant patients with systemic lupus erythematosus. *New England Journal of Medicine* **313**: 152–156.

Lockshin MD, Qamar T & Druzin ML (1987) Hazards of lupus pregnancy. *Journal of Rheumatology* **14** (supplement 13): 214–217.

Lubbe WF, Palmer SJ, Butler WS & Liggins GC (1983) Fetal survival after prednisone suppression of maternal lupus-anticoagulant. *Lancet* **i**: 1361–1363.

Lynch DM & Howe SE (1986) Antigenic determinants in idiopathic thrombocytopenic purpura. *British Journal of Haematology* **63**: 301–308.

Lynch DM, Lynch JM & Howe SE (1985) A quantitative ELISA procedure for the measurement of membrane-bound platelet-associated IgG (PAIgG). *American Journal of Clinical Pathology* **83**: 331–336.

McGregor AM, Peterson MM, McLachlan SM et al (1980) Carbimazole and the autoimmune response in Graves' disease. *New England Journal of Medicine* **303**: 302–307.

McGregor AM, Hall R & Richards C (1984) Autoimmune thyroid disease and pregnancy. *British Medical Journal* **288**: 1780–1781.

Mackay IR, Frazer IH, McNeilage LJ & Whittingham S (1986) Auto-epitopes and autoimmune diseases. *Annals of the New York Academy of Sciences* **475**: 59–65.

Maddison PJ & Reichlin M (1979) Deposition of antibodies to a soluble cytoplasmic antigen in the kidneys of patients with systemic lupus erythematosus. *Arthritis and Rheumatism* **22**: 858–863.

Maddison PJ, Taylor PV, Tompkins DS & Scott JS (1984) False positive VDRL and anti-Ro antibodies related to pregnancy outcome. *Lancet* **i**: 108–109.

Maisey MN & Stimmler L (1972) The role of long acting thyroid stimulator in neonatal thyrotoxicosis. *Clinical Endocrinology* **i**: 81–90.

Male DK (1986) Idiotypes and autoimmunity. *Clinical and Experimental Immunology* **65**: 1–9.

Matsura N, Yamada Y, Nohara Y et al (1980) Familial neonatal transient hypothyroidism due to maternal TSH-Binding inhibitor immunoglobulins. *New England Journal of Medicine* **303**: 738–741.

Monnier VM & Fulpius BW (1977) A radioimmunoassay for the quantitative evaluation of anti-human acetylcholine receptor antibodies in myasthenia gravis. *Clinical and Experimental Immunology* **29**: 16–22.

Mossman S, Vincent A & Newsom-Davis J (1986) Myasthenia gravis without acetylcholine-receptor antibody: a distinct disease entity. *Lancet* **i**: 116–119.

Mukhtar ED, Smith BR, Pyle GA et al (1975) Relation of thyroid-stimulating immuno-globulins to thyroid function and effects of surgery, radioiodine and anti-thyroid drugs. *Lancet* **i**: 713–715.

Munro DS, Dirmikis SM, Humphries H et al (1978) The role of thyroid stimulating immuno-globulins of Graves' disease in neonatal thyrotoxicosis. *British Journal of Obstetrics and Gynaecology* **85**: 837–843.

Namba T, Brown SB & Grob D (1970) Neonatal myasthenia gravis: report of two cases and review of the literature. *Paediatrics* **45**: 488–504.

Nastuk WL, Plescia OJ & Osserman KE (1960) Changes in serum complement activity in patients with myasthenia gravis. *Proceedings of the Society for Experimental Biology and Medicine* **105**: 177–184.

Newsom-Davies J, Willcox N & Calder L (1981) Thymus cells in myasthenia gravis selectively enhance production of anti-acetylcholine-receptor antibody by autologous blood lympho-cytes. *New England Journal of Medicine* **305**: 1313–1318.

Nutt J, Clark F & Welch RG (1974) Neonatal hyperthyroidism and long-acting thyroid stimulator protector. *British Medical Journal* **4**: 695–696.

Ohta M, Matsubara MS, Hayash K et al (1981) Acetylcholine receptor antibodies in infants of mothers with myasthenia gravis. *Neurology* **31:** 1019–1022.

Patrick J & Lindstrom J (1973) Autoimmune response to acetylcholine receptor. *Science* **180:** 871–872.

Petri M, Golbus M, Anderson R et al (1987) Antinuclear antibody, lupus anticoagulant, and anti cardiolipin antibody in women with idiopathic habitual abortion. *Arthritis and Rheumatism* **30:** 601–606.

Plauché WC (1983) Myasthenia Gravis. *Clinical Obstetrics and Gynaecology* **26:** 592–598.

Provost TT, Watson R, Gaither KK & Harley JB (1987) The neonatal lupus erythematosus syndrome. *Journal of Rheumatology* **14** (supplement 13): 199–205.

Ramsey-Goldman R, Hom D, Deng JS et al (1986) Anti-SS-A antibodies and fetal outcome in maternal systemic lupus erythematosus. *Arthritis and Rheumatism* **29:** 1269–1273.

Rubin RL, Tang FL, Chan E et al (1986) IgG subclasses of autoantibodies in systemic lupus erythematosus, Sjögren's syndrome, and drug-induced autoimmunity. *Journal of Immunology* **137:** 2528–2534.

Sanfelippo MJ & Drayna CJ (1982) Prekallikrein inhibition associated with the lupus anti-coagulant: a mechanism of thrombosis. *American Journal of Clinical Pathology* **77:** 275–279.

Scott JR, Cruikshank DP, Kochenoor NK et al (1980) Fetal platelet counts in the obstetric management of immunologic thrombocytopenic purpura. *American Journal of Obstetrics and Gynaecology* **136:** 495–499.

Scott JS (1966) Immunological diseases and pregnancy. *British Medical Journal* **i:** 1559–1567.

Scott JS (1977) Immunological diseases in pregnancy. *Progress in Allergy* **23:** 321–366.

Scott JS (1979) Systemic lupus erythematosus and allied disorders in pregnancy. *Clinics in Obstetrics and Gynaecology* **6:** 461–471.

Scott JS & Taylor PV (1985) Pregnancy and the connective tissue diseases. In Tuffanelli DL & Rowell NR (eds) *Seminars in Dermatology: Connective Tissue Disease*, pp 126–135. New York: Thieme-Stratton.

Scott JS, Maddison PJ, Taylor PV et al (1983) Connective-tissue disease, antibodies to ribonucleoprotein, and congenital heart block. *New England Journal of Medicine* **309:** 209–212.

Shapiro S & Thiagarajan P (1982) Lupus anticoagulants. *Progress in Hemostasis and Thrombosis* **6:** 263–285.

Shewring G & Smith BR (1982) An improved radioreceptor assay for TSH receptor antibodies. *Clinical Endocrinology* **17:** 409–417.

Shoenfeld Y & Schwartz RS (1984) Immunologic and genetic factors in autoimmune diseases. *New England Journal of Medicine* **311:** 1019–1028.

Shoenfeld Y, Rauch J, Massicote H, Datta SK & Schwartz JA (1983) Polyspecificity of monoclonal lupus autoantibodies produced by human–human hybridoma. *New England Journal of Medicine* **308:** 414–420.

Simpson JA (1960) Myasthenia gravis a new hypothesis. *Scottish Medical Journal* **5:** 419–436.

Slate WG & Graham AR (1968) Scleroderma and pregnancy. *American Journal of Obstetrics and Gynaecology* **101:** 335–341.

Smeenk RJT, Lucassen WAM & Swaak TJG (1987) Is anticardiolipin activity a cross-reaction of anti-DNA or a separate entity? *Arthritis and Rheumatism* **30:** 607–617.

Smith BR & Hall R (1974) Thyroid—stimulating immunoglobulins in Graves' disease. *Lancet* **ii:** 427–431.

Smith H & Steinberg AD (1983) Autoimmunity—A Perspective. *Annual Reviews in Immunology* **I:** 175–210.

Sontheimer RD (1987) The anticardiolipin syndrome. A new way to slice an old pie, or a new pie to slice? *Archives of Dermatology* **123:** 590–595.

Souroujon MC, Pachner AR & Fuchs S (1986) The treatment of passively transferred experimental myasthenia with anti-idiotypic antibodies. *Neurology* **36:** 622–625.

Tan EM, Cohen AS, Fries JF et al (1982) The 1982 revised criteria for the classification of systemic lupus erythematosis. *Arthritis and Rheumatism* **25:** 1271–1277.

Taylor PV, Scott JS, Gerlis LM, Esscher E & Scott O (1986a) Maternal antibodies against fetal cardiac antigens in congenital complete heart block. *New England Journal of Medicine* **315:** 667–672.

Taylor PV, Campbell JM, Jackson SM & Scott JS (1986b) The role of maternal autoimmunity in reproductive failure. Abstracts of the 3rd International Conference of Reproductive Immunology, Toronto, 1986, *Journal of Reproductive Immunology* (June supplement): 146.

Taylor PV, Taylor KF, Norman A, Griffiths S & Scott JS (1988) Prevalence of maternal Ro (SS-A) and La (SS-B) autoantibodies in relation to congenital heart block. *British Journal of Rheumatology* **27:** 128–132.

Territo M, Finklestein J, Oh W et al (1973) Management of autoimmune thrombocytopenia in pregnancy and the neonate. *Obstetrics and Gynaecology* **41:** 579.

Thiagarajan P, Shapiro SS & De Marco L (1980) Monoclonal immunoglobulin M coagulation inhibitor with phospholipid specificity—mechanism of a lupus anticoagulant. *Journal of Clinical Investigation* **66:** 397–405.

Thomson JA & Riley ID (1966) Neonatal thyrotoxicosis associated with maternal hypothyroidism. *Lancet* **i:** 635–636.

Thompson PM, Clark F & McLachlan SM (1986) Association between thyroid microsomal antibodies of subclass IgG 1 and hypothyroidism in autoimmune postpartum thyroiditis. *Clinical and Experimental Immunology* **63:** 80–86.

Tsubakio T, Tani P, Curd JG & McMillan R (1986) Complement activation in vitro by antiplatelet antibodies in chronic immune thrombocytopenic purpura. *British Journal of Haematology* **63:** 293–300.

Turney S, Nikolai T, Roberts R (1982) The prevalence and clinical course of post-partum lymphocytic thyroiditis. *Proceedings of 63rd Annual Meeting of the American Endocrine Society*, San Francisco (abstract 557).

Vincent A (1980) Immunology of acetylcholine receptors in relation to myasthenia gravis. *Physiological Reviews* **60**(3): 756–824.

Vincent A & Newsom-Davies J (1979) Alpha-bungarotoxin and anti-acetylcholine receptor antibody binding to human acetylcholine receptor. In Ceccarelli B & Clementi F (eds) *Advances in Cytopharmacology. Neurotoxins—Tools in Neurobiology*, pp 267–278. New York: Raven.

Vincent A, Whiting PJ, Schluep M et al (1987) Antibody heterogeneity and specificity in myasthenia gravis. *Annals of the New York Academy of Sciences* **505:** 106–120.

Volpé R, Farid NR, Westarp C (1974) The pathogenesis of Graves' disease and Hashimoto's thyroiditis. *Clinical Endocrinology* **3:** 239–261.

Watson RM, Braunstein BL, Watson AJ et al (1985) Fetal wastage in women with anti-Ro (SS-A) antibody. *Journal of Rheumatology* **13:** 90–94.

Weston WL, Harmon C, Peebles C et al (1982) A serological marker for neonatal lupus erythematosus. *British Journal of Dermatology* **107:** 377–382.

White C (1912) A foetus with congenital hereditary Graves' disease. *Journal of Obstetrics and Gynaecology of the British Commonwealth* **21:** 231–233.

Whittingham S, McNeilage LJ, Naselli G et al (1987) Serological diagnosis of primary Sjögren's syndrome by means of human recombinant La (SS-B) as nuclear antigen. *Lancet* **i:** 1–3.

Wicker LS, Miller BJ & Mullen Y (1986) Transfer of autoimmune diabetes mellitus with splenocytes from nonobese diabetic (NOD) mice. *Diabetes* **35:** 855–860.

Wolin SL & Steitz JA (1983) The Ro small cytoplenic ribonucleoproteins: Identification of the antigenic protein and its binding site on the Ro RNAs. *Proceedings of the National Academy of Science (USA)* **81:** 1996–2000.

Zakarija M & McKenzie JM (1983) Pregnancy-associated changes in the thyroid-stimulating antibody of Graves' disease and the relationship to neonatal hyperthyroidism. *Journal of Clinical Endocrinology and Metabolism* **57:** 1036–1040.

8

Immunopathology of pregnancy

JUDITH N. BULMER

The placenta has been proposed as a prime target for immune-mediated attack. However, despite suggestions that pregnancy disorders such as pre-eclampsia and spontaneous abortion may have an immunological basis, studies of placental tissues have so far failed to provide unequivocal evidence of immune damage. The substantial recent advances in elucidation of materno-fetal immune interactions in normal uteroplacental tissues may, nevertheless, provide a basis for more fruitful study of placental immunopathology. Thus, before consideration of abnormalities, local uterine materno-fetal relationships in normal pregnancy will be discussed.

NORMAL PREGNANCY

Fetal trophoblast

Morphological aspects

The chorionic villi forming the definitive placenta are composed of a fetal mesenchymal core covered by an inner cytotrophoblast and an outer syncytio-trophoblast layer. In early pregnancy, cytotrophoblast proliferates from the tips of the villi to form cytotrophoblast columns which extend laterally to form a shell of cytotrophoblast covering the endometrial surface (Boyd and Hamilton, 1970). Interstitial trophoblast invades maternal decidua and inner myometrium, individual cytotrophoblast cells fusing to form tropho-blast giant cells. Endovascular trophoblast migrates retrogradely up spiral arteries in two waves replacing the endothelium and reaching terminal segments of the radial arteries by 16–20 weeks' gestation (Robertson, 1976; Pijnenborg et al, 1980). Loss of musculoelastic tissue, deposition of fibrinoid and progressive distension convert the artery into a dilated fibrinoid tube with perivascular trophoblast embedded within its wall.

Invasion of maternal uterine tissues and vessels by extravillous tropho-blast appears essential for normal placental development, and deficient vascular invasion by fetal trophoblast has been implicated as an important aetiological factor in pre-eclampsia and growth retardation.

MHC antigen expression by trophoblast

Class I and class II major histocompatibility complex (MHC) antigens are of fundamental importance for immune recognition, cytotoxicity and regulation. The fetus inherits paternal MHC antigens and fetal trophoblast forms several interfaces with potentially immunocompetent maternal cells in blood and decidua; thus, expression of MHC antigens by trophoblast has been of immense interest.

It is now generally accepted that chorionic villous trophoblast fails to express class I or class II MHC antigens (Sunderland et al, 1981a; Galbraith et al, 1981; Bulmer and Johnson, 1985a) (Figure 1). In contrast, villous

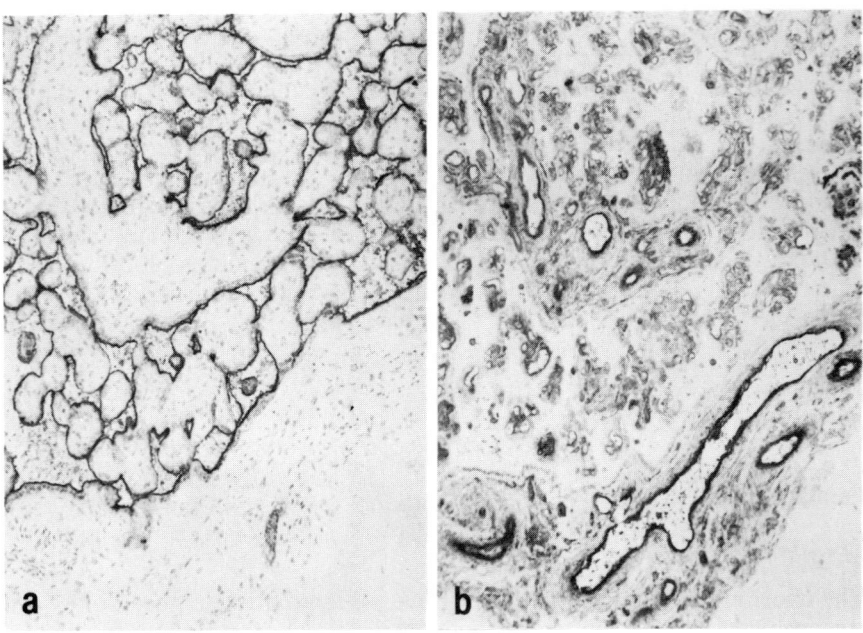

Figure 1. Serial cryostat sections of term placenta labelled with (a) H317 (placental alkaline phosphatase), (b) W6/32 (class I MHC). Villous trophoblast is H317-positive but class I MHC-negative, whereas villous stroma with fetal stem vessels is class I HLA-positive, × 75.

stromal cells do express fetal class I MHC antigens and a substantial proportion of stromal macrophages are also class II MHC-positive (Sutton et al, 1983, 1986; Bulmer and Johnson, 1984; Redman et al, 1984; Bulmer et al, 1988a). Villous trophoblast thus forms an extensive HLA-negative layer separating HLA-bearing fetal stromal cells from maternal lymphocytes and monocytes in intervillous spaces. Regulation of class I MHC antigen expression on villous trophoblast appears to be at the level of gene transcription with low levels of detectable class I MHC heavy chain mRNA (Kawata et al, 1984).

Interferons appear to play a key role in regulation of MHC antigen expression (Halloran et al, 1986) and detection of high interferon levels in human placental tissues (Chard et al, 1986; Duc-Goiran et al, 1986) has stimulated attempts to induce or upregulate trophoblast MHC antigens with γ-interferon and other lymphokines (reviewed by Head et al, 1987). Affinity-purified γ-interferon was reported to increase class I MHC antigen expression on the weakly HLA-positive BeWo choriocarcinoma line but had no effect on the class I MHC-negative Jar line (Anderson and Berkowitz, 1985; Hunt et al, 1987), suggesting that a degree of constitutive expression may be necessary for modulation of MHC antigens on choriocarcinoma cells. In normal human placental tissues, MHC-negative villous trophoblast was not induced to express class I MHC antigens by γ-interferon (Hunt et al, 1987). In the murine system, however, γ-interferon enhanced expression on mid-gestation spongiotrophoblast (Zuckerman and Head, 1986; Head et al, 1987) and apparent *de novo* induction of MHC antigens was reported in early post-implantation ectoplacental cone (Drake et al, 1987). Methylation of DNA cytosine residues has been proposed as a mechanism of permanent inacti-vation of eukaryotic genes (Doerfler, 1983), and there is evidence that gene methylation leads to irreversible down-regulation of MHC antigens in the Jar choriocarcinoma line (Alberti and Herzenberg, 1986). The mechanisms whereby MHC gene expression is switched off in normal HLA-negative villous trophoblast remain to be established but may be of importance in protection of the feto-placental unit.

In contrast, extravillous trophoblast in maternal uterine tissues and cytotrophoblast columns, and on the maternal aspect of the chorion laeve does express a class I MHC antigen (Sunderland et al, 1981b; Hsi et al, 1984; Redman et al, 1984; Wells et al, 1984; Bulmer and Johnson, 1985a). There is no convincing evidence of class II MHC antigen expression by trophoblast (Redman, 1983). Class I MHC antigen on extravillous trophoblast reacts with W6/32, a monoclonal antibody directed against monomorphic (framework) determinants (Sunderland et al, 1981b) but fails to label with 61.D2, which has similar specificity (Hsi et al, 1984; Wells et al, 1984). W6/32-positive trophoblast also does not express polymorphic determinants specific for the fetal HLA type (Redman et al, 1984). The nature of this class I HLA antigen has been a source of speculation. The class I MHC antigen expressed on trophoblast isolated from chorion laeve and on the BeWo choriocarcinoma line has been shown to possess a 40–41 kD heavy chain (Ellis et al, 1986; Stern et al, 1986c). The precise characterization of the antigen is awaited, but could be a human *Qa* analogue: murine *Qa* gene products show a smaller heavy chain than classical class I MHC antigens (see Lew et al, 1986). There are indications in humans for existence of class I MHC-like gene products exhibiting reduced polymorphism and limited tissue distribution (van Leeuwen et al, 1985; Lew et al, 1986) and cloning has revealed class I MHC genes not defined serologically (Jordan et al, 1985). Furthermore, multiparous human sera have been shown to contain anti-bodies to non HLA-A,-B,-C structures considered as possible human *Qa* analogues (Gazit et al, 1984; van Leeuwen et al, 1985).

Expression of a class I MHC antigen by trophoblast populations in intimate contact with maternal tissues implies a function, and induction of specific suppression of maternal anti-fetal cytotoxic responses has been hypothesized (Stern et al, 1986a). Mechanisms of regulation, and function, of MHC antigen expression by villous and extravillous trophoblast are unknown. Hypothetically, failure of regulation or defective function could lead to abnormal materno-fetal interactions and pregnancy pathology: no such abnormalities have so far been demonstrated.

Trophoblast antigens

The syncytiotrophoblast microvillous plasma membrane (StMPM) forms a major interface between fetal tissues and maternal blood. Biochemical analyses of isolated StMPM preparations have identified more than 50 associated protein subunits, most of which are integral membrane proteins (reviewed by Whyte, 1983; Webb et al, 1985; Whyte et al, 1985). Characterization of trophoblast membrane antigens with heteroantisera was rapidly superseded by development of murine trophoblast-reactive monoclonal antibodies (mAbs) (Johnson et al, 1981; Lipinski et al, 1981; Sunderland et al, 1981c). Despite early enthusiasm and subsequent development of numerous mAbs raised by immunization with early and term placental tissues, absolute specificity for trophoblast has been elusive after thorough testing of normal adult tissues (Johnson and Bulmer, 1985a; Anderson et al, 1987). Nevertheless, trophoblast-reactive mAbs have allowed immunohistochemical characterization of anatomically and functionally diverse trophoblast populations. Investigations of secretory products (Gosseye and Fox, 1984; Kurman et al, 1984a) and lectin-binding properties (Lalani et al, 1987) have further highlighted the heterogeneity of villous and extravillous trophoblast.

Heterogeneity of fetal trophoblast. Reactivities of various mAbs with anatomically defined trophoblast subtypes are given in Table 1. As well as mAbs raised to trophoblast, markers of other structures including receptors and cytokeratins are reactive with trophoblast. The heterogeneous expression of class I MHC has been discussed, but other antigens also show differing expression between villous and extravillous trophoblast populations.

Most mAbs raised to trophoblast are reactive with villous syncytiotrophoblast, since StMPM often formed the immunogen. Some determinants, including receptor structures, are expressed predominantly by villous syncytiotrophoblast (see Bulmer and Johnson, 1985a; Anderson et al, 1987). Other antigens common to all or most villous and extravillous trophoblast populations often show tissue cross-reactivities (Figure 2): H316, for example, is directed against a trophoblast–leukocyte common antigen but also reacts with endometrial gland epithelium and endothelial cells (Bulmer et al, 1984, 1986; Bulmer and Johnson, 1985a). Similarly, markers of low molecular weight cytokeratins, which are widely available and of value for distinguishing trophoblast from maternal cells in the placental bed, also react with endometrial glands (Bulmer et al, 1986, 1988c). In a recent WHO workshop, only two mAbs showed widespread reactivity with all trophoblast populations and minimal cross-reactivity with non-trophoblastic cells (Anderson et al, 1987).

Table 1. Antigenic heterogeneity of trophoblast.

	Villous sT	Villous cT	cT column/shell	Interstitial cT	Endovascular cT	Amniochorion	Gland epithelium
TLX / Low MW CK }	+	+	+	+	+	+	+
PLAP	+	−	±	±	−	±	−
NDOG1	+	−	+	−	−	−	−
FDO161G	+	+	+	+	+	+	−
HMFG1 / EMA }	−	−	−	± rare	−	±	+
W6/32 / β$_2$M }	−	−	+	+	+	±	−
61.D2	−	−	−	−	−	−	−
Trf-R	+	−	+	−	−	+	+
hCG / SP1 }	+	−	±	±	±	−	−
hPL	+	−	±	±	±	−	−

sT, syncytiotrophoblast; cT, cytotrophoblast; Low MW CK, low molecular weight cytokeratin; PLAP, placental-type alkaline phosphatase; Trf-R, transferrin receptor; hCG, human chorionic gonadotrophin; hPL, human placental lactogen; SP1, pregnancy-specific β1-glycoprotein; β$_2$M, β$_2$-microglobulin. **REFERENCES:** Anderson et al (1987); Bulmer and Johnson (1985a); Bulmer et al (1986); Gosseye and Fox (1984); Hsi et al (1984); Kurman et al (1984a); Redman et al (1984); Wells et al (1984).

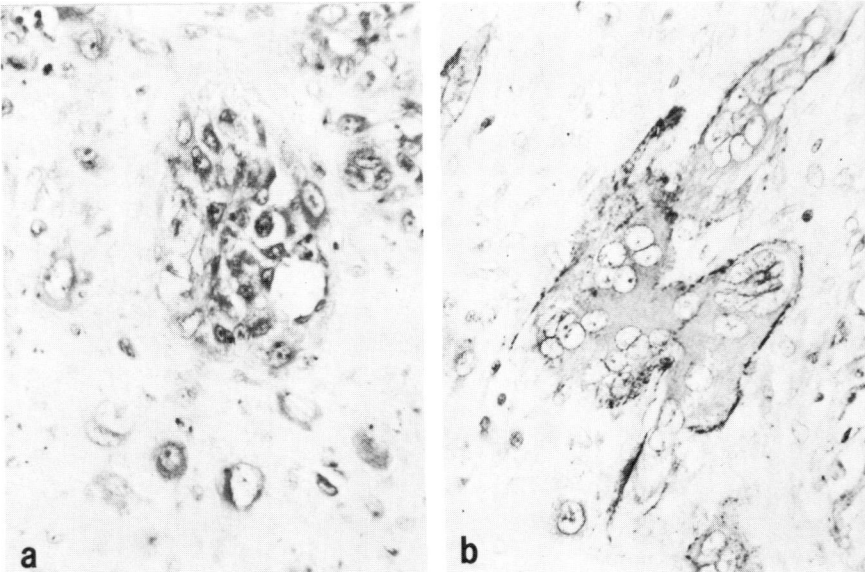

Figure 2. Paraffin-embedded sections of first trimester placental bed tissues labelled with H316 (TLX antigen) showing reactivity with (a) endovascular and perivascular trophoblast, × 175. (b) Trophoblast giant cells, × 195.

The antigenic heterogeneity of morphologically indistinguishable tropho-blast populations can be highlighted by immunohistology (Bulmer and Johnson, 1985a). In amniochorion, for example, at least three trophoblast phenotypes may be distinguished by their reactivity with H316, low molecular weight cytokeratin markers, HMFG1 (an epithelial membrane antigen), H317 (placental alkaline phosphatase) and W6/32 (class I MHC) (Bulmer and Johnson, 1985a). Similar antigenically distinct trophoblast subpopulations may be defined in the placental bed (Bulmer et al, 1986). Trophoblast antigens also vary according to gestational age: for example, HMFG1 labels a small population of placental bed trophoblast in the third trimester but not in early pregnancy, and placental alkaline phosphatase (PLAP) is detectable in tissue sections only in the second and third trimesters (Bulmer and Johnson, 1985a; Bulmer et al, 1986).

NDOG1, raised against term StMPM (Sunderland et al, 1981c), appears to recognize hyaluronic acid which plays a role in developmental systems allowing efficient cell migration (Comper and Laurent, 1978). Localization of granular NDOG1 reactivity to the cytotrophoblast columns and shell (Figure 3) from which cells migrate into uterine tissues may suggest a similar role in early pregnancy (Sunderland et al, 1985b). However, despite the develop-ment of numerous trophoblast-reactive mAbs with varying reaction patterns, the functional significance of the phenotypic heterogeneity exhibited by morphologically indistinguishable trophoblast at any one site and between different sites remains largely elusive.

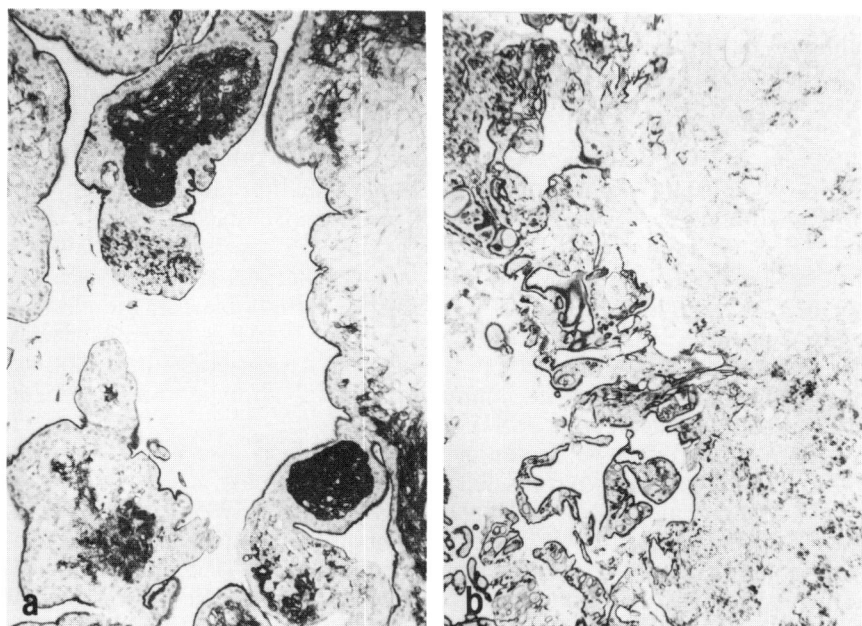

Figure 3. Paraffin-embedded sections stained with NDOG1 (hyaluronic acid). (a) A six-week pregnancy with staining of villous syncytiotrophoblast and stroma, and granular reactivity with cytotrophoblast columns, × 70. (b) Granular reactivity at the implantation site in an ectopic tubal pregnancy, × 45.

Trophoblast–leukocyte common antigens. The concept of an antigen system common to trophoblast and maternal immunocompetent cells is attractive. Faulk et al (1978) described a trophoblast–leukocyte cross-reactive (TLX) antigen system with heteroantisera which inhibited in vitro mixed lymphocyte reactions (McIntyre and Faulk, 1979) and identified non-HLA polymorphic determinants when tested on lymphocyte panels (McIntyre et al, 1983). Further support for a TLX system was provided by two mAbs, H310 and H316 (Johnson et al, 1981; Johnson, 1981): H316 reacts with villous and extravillous trophoblast throughout gestation (Figure 2), as well as with peripheral blood lymphocytes, monocytes, polymorphonuclear leukocytes and, weakly, with platelets (Bulmer et al, 1984, 1986; Bulmer and Johnson, 1985a). The antigen recognized by H316 shows molecular weight heterogeneity (55–65 kD) between individual trophoblast membrane preparations (Stern et al, 1986b).

The expression of a TLX antigen by all trophoblast cells in the placental bed would allow participation in local intrauterine materno-fetal interactions. Detection of a TLX system led to the hypothesis that recognition of non-self TLX antigens leads to a protective maternal immune response underpinning successful pregnancy, whilst recognition of self TLX antigens in association with trophoblast-specific antigens causes early abortion

(Faulk et al, 1978; Faulk and McIntyre, 1981). Support for trophoblast alloimmunization in normal pregnancy may be taken from studies of blocking factors in pregnancy and from observations on women suffering recurrent spontaneous abortions (see Johnson et al, 1987).

Placental alkaline phosphatase. Placental alkaline phosphatase (PLAP) forms a significant proportion of trophoblast membrane protein in term placenta (Jones and Fox, 1976; Doellgast and Benirschke, 1979). It is expressed predominantly after the first trimester, appearing initially on syncytial sprouts. Extravillous trophoblast populations are largely PLAP-negative, although a substantial proportion of trophoblast in the chorion laeve is positive (Bulmer and Johnson, 1985a). PLAP is the most clearly documented example of genetic polymorphism expressed by a trophoblast membrane protein, although immunity to fetal allotypes has not been documented (Johnson et al, 1987).

PLAP is an oncodevelopmental protein which is also expressed by a variety of human tumour cells, including testis, breast, cervix and ovary (McLaughlin et al, 1982, 1987; McDicken et al, 1983, 1985; Epenetos et al, 1984; Sunderland et al, 1984). The function of PLAP on placental syncytiotrophoblast is unknown: it has been suggested that PLAP could act as a cell surface modulator of trophoblast growth and differentiation after the first half of pregnancy (Bulmer and Johnson, 1985a), serving a similar function on tumour cells. Study of PLAP expression in abnormal pregnancy and trophoblast tumours may thus be worthwhile.

Trophoblast membrane receptors

The trophoblast membrane is involved in recognition and transport processes, and specific receptor structures have been localized to syncytiotrophoblast membrane (reviewed by Wild, 1983): these include receptors for insulin and insulin-like growth factors, receptors for the Fc portion of IgG, epidermal growth factor (EGF) receptors and transferrin (Trf) receptors, amongst others. Specific membrane receptors for insulin and insulin-like growth factors may be important in growth, development and cellular metabolic control.

Transferrin (Trf) receptors have been localized to villous syncytiotrophoblast both by transferrin binding and with mAbs (Galbraith et al, 1980a; Johnson and Molloy, 1983; Johnson, 1984). Several mAbs raised by immunization with syncytiotrophoblast membrane have been found to be directed against Trf receptor (Yeh et al, 1987). Syncytiotrophoblastic Trf receptor is most likely to be involved in iron transport to the fetus, but immunobiological roles have also been proposed (Johnson, 1984) including restriction of available iron in the intervillous spaces with consequent impairment of maternal lymphocyte proliferation. Trf receptor has also been localized to the proximal portion of cytotrophoblast columns and the fetal aspect of the cytotrophoblast shell in first trimester placental tissues, which are zones of maximal proliferative activity as evidenced also by a high mitotic rate and labelling with the proliferation-associated marker Ki67

(Wislocki and Bennett, 1943; Bulmer, unpublished data). The reactivity raises the possibility of a role for transferrin in trophoblast proliferation in early pregnancy.

Retroviruses and oncogenes in trophoblast

Trophoblast oncogene expression has recently been reviewed (Adamson, 1987). The retrovirus-related sequence *erv-1* is expressed as a 75 kD protein in the human placental syncytiotrophoblast (Suni et al, 1984), retrovirus structural protein p30 has been localized to the same site (Wahlstrom et al, 1984) and retrovirus-like particles have been detected in human trophoblast by electron microscopy (Dirksen and Levy, 1977).

High levels of c-*fos* and c-*fms* transcripts have been detected in full-term human placenta, amnion and chorion (Muller et al, 1983), but no localization is available. In situ hybridization has been used to localize c-*sis* and c-*myc* to villous cytotrophoblast and cytotrophoblast columns and shell in early pregnancy (Pfeifer-Ohlsson et al, 1984; Goustin et al, 1985), sites of maximal proliferative activity. The β-chain of platelet-derived growth factor (PDGF) is encoded by c-*sis*: PDGF and other mitogens activate c-*myc* and c-*fos*, and detection of c-*sis* in trophoblast in early pregnancy may indicate autocrine growth regulation by placental control of oncogene expression (Goustin et al, 1985). Further evidence of autocrine growth regulation may be seen in expression by placental syncytiotrophoblast of EGF receptor (Richards et al, 1983; Magid et al, 1985), a product of the c-*erb*-B oncogene. EGF receptor binds both EGF and transforming growth factor (TGF α), thereby activating several cellular processes (Adamson, 1987). TGFα is detectable in term human placentae, but the source is unknown (Stromberg et al, 1982). Placental EGF receptors may play a selective role in allowing maternal EGF to pass into the fetal circulation, but EGF receptor expression may also be important in regulating placental development by binding of maternal EGF or autocrine placental TGF (Adamson, 1987).

Expression of oncogenes and growth factors and their receptors represents a potentially fruitful area for future investigations. If their role is indeed concerned with control of growth and differentiation, comparison of normal pregnancy with abnormalities of trophoblast proliferation, such as hydatidiform mole and choriocarcinoma, may be worthwhile.

Trophoblast hormones

Many hormones and proteins, including human chorionic gonadotrophin (hCG), human placental lactogen (hPL) and pregnancy specific β_1-glycoprotein (SP1), are produced by the placenta although the site of synthesis of many pregnancy proteins is disputed (reviewed in Pattillo et al, 1983; Bohn et al, 1983). Immunohistochemical techniques have recently been employed to localize hCG, hPL and SP1 in normal and abnormal placental tissues (Kurman et al, 1984a,b; Gosseye and Fox, 1984; Chemnitz et al, 1984; Earl et al, 1986, 1987a). In normal pregnancy, hCG, hPL and SP1 were localized to villous syncytiotrophoblast throughout gestation, although the staining intensity varied with gestational age. Both SP1 and hCG were detected in only occasional interstitial cytotrophoblast in decidua and spiral arteries, whereas hPL was present in most interstitial extravillous trophoblast, labelling being particularly prominent in deeper decidua and myometrium. Endovascular trophoblast was consistently hPL-positive (Gosseye and Fox, 1984; Kurman et al, 1984a).

Kurman et al (1984a,b) distinguished 'intermediate trophoblast' as a type of trophoblast intermediate between syncytiotrophoblast and cytotrophoblast with specific biochemical, morphological and functional features: intermediate trophoblast was located overlying chorionic villi, in trophoblast columns and shell and in the placental bed, and consistently contained hPL whilst hCG and SP1 were occasionally detected. It was proposed that this form of trophoblast may be particularly important for implantation and establishment of the uteroplacental circulation. Despite other suggestions for an intermediate type of trophoblast, this concept has not yet been widely accepted.

Lysosomal enzymes in trophoblast

Histochemical techniques have been widely used to characterize the enzyme content of trophoblast (reviewed in Contractor, 1983). More recently, proteases and protease inhibitors have been localized in the placenta by immunohistology. Alpha$_2$-macroglobulin (α_2M) has been shown to bind to isolated StMPM preparations, and radiobinding and inhibition studies indicate binding to surface protease (Johnson et al, 1985). Alpha$_2$-macroglobulin inhibits a wide variety of endoproteases: it was suggested that by binding to trophoblast it may modulate trophoblast invasiveness and degradative potential (Johnson et al, 1985), but α_2M was not investigated in the invasive extravillous trophoblast populations. A similar role for α_2M in the regulation of proteolysis in cell invasion was suggested by Saksela et al (1981), who noted absence of α_2M in invasive moles and choriocarcinomas. Alpha$_1$-antitrypsin (α_1AT) and α_1-antichymotrypsin (α_1ACT) have been localized to villous syncytiotrophoblast throughout pregnancy by immunohistology (Braunhut et al, 1984; Bulmer, unpublished data), but reports of localization in extravillous trophoblast are limited. In our own studies, we have noted α_1AT and α_1ACT in endovascular trophoblast, but very rarely in interstitial populations (Bulmer, unpublished data). This observation suggests that endovascular trophoblast may possess specific properties equipping it for vascular invasion.

Lymphokines in the placenta

Various cytokines can be isolated from the human placenta (see Toder et al, 1987; Duc-Goiran et al, 1986). Endogenous α and β interferon (IFN) have been detected in human placentas (Chard et al, 1986; Duc-Goiran et al, 1986), as well as unusual IFNs of varying molecular weights (Duc-Goiran et al, 1986). Placental blood extract shows higher IFN levels than amniotic fluid extract, suggesting an origin within the placenta (Duc-Goiran et al, 1986). In a recent immunohistological study employing a polyclonal antibody, α-IFN was localized to term villous syncytiotrophoblast (Howatson et al, 1988). There are no data published regarding localization of other placental IFNs.

There is evidence for suppression of the effects of interleukin-2 (IL-2) in human and murine decidua (Clark et al, 1986). Decidual lymphocytes do not respond to IL-2 (Toder et al, 1987; Ritson and Bulmer, unpublished data) and IL-2 receptor-bearing lymphocytes are deficient in human decidua (Bulmer and Johnson, 1986; Khong, 1987). Toder et al (1987) suggested that local immunosuppression could account for inhibition of both IL-2 production and IL-2 receptor expression by decidual lymphocytes. IL-2-like material has recently been localized to human villous syncytiotrophoblast using three anti-IL-2 heteroantisera and one mAb (15.2), although a second mAb to human IL-2 gave no reaction (Soubiran et al, 1987). These results are unconfirmed and difficult to explain.

Human placenta is a good source of colony stimulating factors (CSFs): their localization in placenta is not known but it has been claimed that both adherent and non-adherent placental cells produce CSF (Toder et al, 1987). Toder et al (1987) found human placental CSF capable of stimulating both decidua and trophoblast in a dose-dependent fashion. Interleukin-1 is also produced in large quantities in human placenta, primarily from the mononuclear phagocytes within the villous stroma (Flynn, 1984). Placental lymphokines represent a relatively new area of investigation. Localization of their site of origin in normal and abnormal pregnancy is a promising area for future studies.

Extraembryonic fetal mesenchymal cells

Hofbauer cells are placental mononuclear phagocytes and can be identified in early and term placental tissues (Fox and Kharkongor, 1969) and in amniotic mesenchyme, where they often appear distorted (Hoyes, 1975). Attention was redirected towards Hofbauer cells by the observation of class II MHC-bearing cells in chorionic villous stroma and amniotic mesenchyme (Jenkins et al, 1983; Sutton et al, 1983). Their irregular shape and high levels of class II MHC antigen expression suggested that they may represent a specialized dendritic antigen-presenting cell but enzyme histochemistry was more indicative of a 'classical' phagocytic macrophage (Nehemiah et al, 1981; Sutton et al, 1983; Bulmer and Johnson, 1984), and this has been supported by subsequent immunohistochemical studies (Sutton et al, 1986).

Macrophages in chorionic villous stroma and amniotic mesenchyme have a similar antigenic phenotype, although a higher proportion in the amnion are class II MHC-positive (Bulmer et al, 1988a). They express CD45, CD14 and CD4 differentiation antigens, but not CD11b or CD11c (Bulmer and Johnson, 1984; Sutton et al, 1986; Bulmer, unpublished data). A proportion express the CD1 antigen present on cortical thymocytes and epidermal Langerhans cells, CD1-positive cells being commoner in early placental tissues (Sutton et al, 1986). Although Fcγ and C3b receptors have been detected in cell suspensions and tissues (Wood, 1980; Loke et al, 1982), neither has been demonstrated by immunohistology.

The in vivo function of fetal macrophages in extraembryonic tissues is obscure. Expression of class II MHC gene products, and their position at an interface between maternal and fetal tissues, suggests a role in normal placental immunobiology and they are able to act as stimulators in a mixed lymphocyte reaction (Hunt et al, 1984). However, placental macrophages are also capable of immune and non-immune phagocytosis (Wood, 1980; Loke et al, 1982) and acid phosphatase and non-specific esterase activity suggest a phagocytic role (Nehemiah et al, 1981; Bulmer and Johnson, 1984). Further studies are necessary to determine the function of these fetal macrophages in vivo. Investigation of their phenotype and distribution in abnormal placentae may facilitate elucidation of their role in normal pregnancy.

Maternal decidua

Decidual leukocytes

Appreciation of the extent of trophoblastic invasion, and demonstration of class I MHC antigens on extravillous trophoblast, focused attention on decidualized endometrium. Regulation of trophoblast proliferation and invasion may be an inherent autocrine property of trophoblast but could also be influenced by maternal cellular responses in decidua.

The complexity of human decidua was appreciated by light and electron microscopy (Tekelioglu-Uysal et al, 1975; Pijnenborg et al, 1980) but has also been highlighted by immunohistological studies. As well as 'true' decidualized endometrial stromal cells many leukocytes have been identified (Figure 4) (Bulmer and Sunderland, 1983, 1984; Bulmer and Johnson, 1984, 1985b, 1986; Bulmer et al, 1986, 1987b; Kabawat et al, 1985a; Khong, 1987). Leukocyte common antigen-bearing (CD45+) cells form up to 50% of cells in decidua and in the first trimester up to 40% are lymphoid cells. The majority of decidual lymphocytes have an unusual phenotype: they express the T cell differentiation antigens CD2, CD7 and CD38, but are CD3, CD4, CD5, CD8 and interleukin 2-receptor (CD25)-negative (Bulmer and Sunderland, 1984; Bulmer and Johnson, 1986; Bulmer et al, 1987b,c). The distribution of these phenotypically unusual decidual lymphocytes, aggregated around vessels and glands, together with their prominence in early pregnancy, suggested that they are the so-called 'endometrial stromal granulocytes' (EGs), also known as Körnchenzellen or 'K' cells (Dallenbach-Hellweg, 1981). These cells are characterized by their phloxinophilic cytoplasmic granules and are prominent in late secretory phase endometrium and in the first trimester of pregnancy. They were previously thought to derive from endometrial stromal cells and secrete relaxin (Dallenbach-Hellweg, 1981). Initial immunohistological studies were performed on snap-frozen tissues in which the granules characteristic of EGs failed to survive. Subsequent studies of decidual cell suspensions and imprints and of formalin-fixed paraffin-embedded sections have provided convincing evidence that EGs are granulated lymphoid cells (Bulmer et al, 1987a). Although their lineage and function is not fully established, the term 'endometrial granulocyte' or 'K

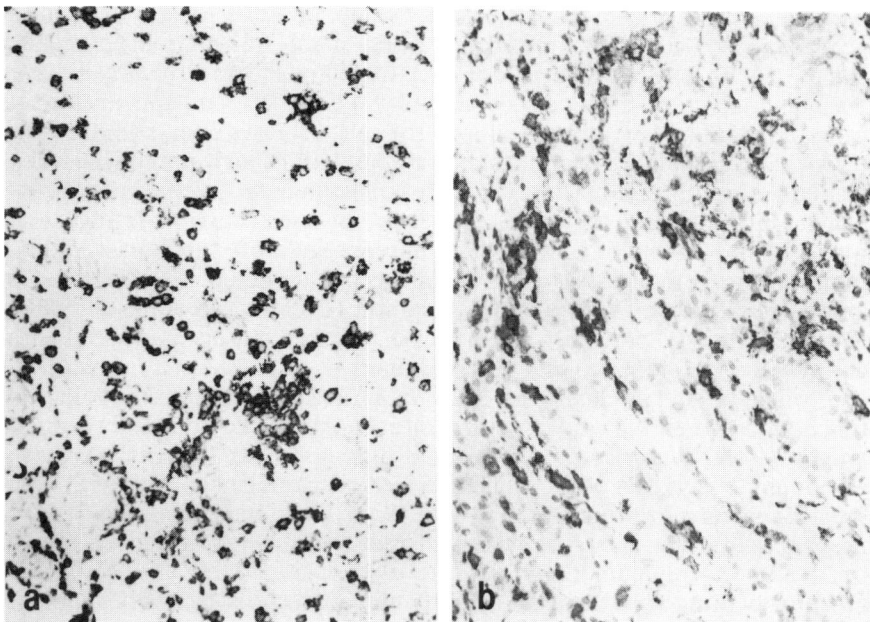

Figure 4. (a) Cryostat section of first trimester decidua labelled for leukocyte common antigen showing numerous leukocytes in decidua, × 85. (b) Cryostat section of implantation site from a partial molar pregnancy labelled with DA6.231 (class II MHC), × 105. Note numerous positive macrophages, many of which are closely associated with trophoblast.

cell' is clearly inappropriate, misleading and confusing.

Decidual granulated lymphocytes resemble natural killer (NK) cells at light and electron microscopic levels (Neighbour et al, 1982; Bulmer, 1985), but do not express the 'classical' NK cell markers leu 7, CD16 or CD11b (Bulmer and Sunderland, 1984; Ritson and Bulmer, 1987a). They do, however, label intensely with NKH1, which is directed against large granular lymphocytes (LGL) including NK cells (Ritson and Bulmer, 1987a).

Suppressor activity in murine decidua has been attributed to a small granulated lymphocyte which secretes a soluble factor blocking lymphocyte response to interleukin-2 (IL-2) (Clark et al, 1986). Human decidua has been reported to contain 'small' and 'large' suppressor cells, but neither has been fully characterized (Daya et al, 1985). The association of suppression in mouse decidua with a granulated lymphocyte suggested that granulated lymphocytes in human decidua may be natural suppressor cells, another functional group of LGLs. Current evidence does not support this hypothesis: semi-purified granulated lymphocytes from first trimester human decidua show lower levels of suppression of mitogen-induced lymphocyte proliferation than unfractionated decidual cell suspensions. Semi-purified decidual LGL do, however, consistently exhibit low but significant killing in a K562 chromium release assay (Ritson and Bulmer, unpublished data). An NK cell subset in peripheral blood has a similar phenotype (CD16−, NKH1++) and is also a poor effector in the same assay (Lanier et al, 1986). It is difficult to propose an in vivo role for an NK cell in the placental bed in normal pregnancy and there is no histological evidence of cytotoxicity. However, NK cells have been demonstrated in murine decidua (Croy et al, 1985) and appear distinct from the granulated lymphoid suppressor cells (Slapsys et al, 1986).

Decidual granulated lymphocytes are abundant in early pregnancy when trophoblast proliferation and invasion is maximal and when many pregnancies fail. Although they may perform a vital role in early placentation, it would be reasonable to assume that immunoregulatory function would be required throughout gestation. Macrophages are abundant in decidua basalis and decidua parietalis throughout gestation (Bulmer and Johnson, 1984; Kabawat et al, 1985a; Khong, 1987) and are often closely associated with extravillous trophoblast (Figure 4) (Bulmer et al, 1988b). Expression of determinants such as class II MHC and CD11c suggests an immunological function, but their enzyme content indicates phagocytic potential (Bulmer and Johnson, 1984; Bulmer et al, 1987c). Suppressor activity has been attributed to secretion of prostaglandin E_2 by decidual macrophages in both mouse and human pregnancy (Tawfik et al, 1986; Lala et al, 1986), and pregnancy loss in indomethacin-treated mice has been forwarded to support this as an in vivo phenomenon (Lala et al, 1986). Class II MHC and fibronectin receptor-bearing adherent cells in early human decidua, possibly dendritic cells or macrophages, have been shown to possess antigen-presenting capacity (Oksenberg et al, 1986). The relation, if any, between macrophages mediating suppression and those capable of antigen presentation is not known.

Decidualized endometrial stromal cells have also been claimed to derive ultimately from bone marrow and to mediate immunosuppression (Lala et al, 1986). Endometrial gland epithelial cells are also capable of suppressor activity. The function of phenotypically characterized potentially immuno-competent cells in human decidua remains disputed. Conversely, decidual suppression and antigen-presenting capacity have been well documented but the cells responsible have not been well characterized. If cells within decidua are vital for maintenance of the feto-placental unit and suppression of any maternal anti-fetal response, their investigation in abnormal pregnancy would be worthwhile.

Endometrial glands

Endometrial glands in early pregnancy are often associated with a prominent mononuclear cell response and at light microscope level only isolated fragments may be apparent after the first trimester (Pijnenborg et al, 1980). Endometrial epithelial cells share antigens with trophoblast and in early pregnancy appear to decrease expression of class I MHC antigens (Johnson and Bulmer, 1984). These observations have provoked interest in the fate of the glands in the second half of pregnancy. However, glands can be clearly identified in normal third trimester placental bed biopsies with epithelial markers, although they are often attenuated or compressed (Bulmer et al, 1986).

The leukocytic infiltrate adjacent to the glands contains class II MHC-bearing macrophages, often surrounding the gland structure, and aggregates of CD2-positive granulated lymphocytes (Bulmer and Johnson, 1985b). Scanty CD1-positive and Trf receptor-bearing cells are apparent immediately beneath the epithelium (Bulmer and Sunderland, 1984; Johnson and Bulmer, 1984). Intraepithelial lymphocytes, some of which are granulated, can be identified within the epithelium itself, although their phenotype is not known (Bulmer, unpublished data).

Epithelial cells separated from non-pregnant secretory phase endometrium have been shown to suppress one-way mixed lymphocyte reactions (Johnson et al, 1987). No studies are available for early pregnancy tissues but it is possible that decidual suppression noted in many studies is due to epithelial cells which are a common contaminant in decidual lymphocyte fractions prepared over Ficoll (Ritson and Bulmer, unpublished data), their number depending on the separation technique employed (Ritson and Bulmer, 1987b). Epithelial cells are extremely difficult to separate from other cells in decidual suspensions by morphological criteria alone. It may, therefore, be worthwhile reconsidering the role of endometrial glands in normal pregnancy and embarking on their investigation in pathological conditions.

Decidual spiral arteries

Defective trophoblastic invasion and ensuing physiological changes in spiral arteries has been implicated in the pathogenesis of pre-eclampsia and several immunohistological studies have sought evidence of immune-mediated damage. C3 deposition was reported in spiral arteries of patients with diabetes, hypertension and pre-eclampsia (Kitzmiller and Benirschke, 1973; Kitzmiller et al, 1981), but others have detected C3 deposition in utero-placental arteries in normal pregnancy (Weir, 1981; Hustin et al, 1983; Wells et al, 1987).

Lichtig et al (1985) reported heavy C3 deposition in 14.6% of 110 first trimester placental bed specimens in primiparae. Spiral arteries with the morphological features of acute atherosis had previously been noted in first trimester pregnancies (Lichtig et al, 1984) and the association of acute atherosis, C3 deposition and first pregnancy predominance of pre-eclampsia raised speculation that these may be early pre-eclamptic lesions (Lichtig et al, 1985).

Thus, there is ample evidence for C3 deposition in spiral arteries in normal pregnancy, though the mechanism is disputed. It is debatable whether complement deposition in abnormal pregnancy is a true manifestation of immunopathology.

ABNORMAL PREGNANCY

The concept that various pregnancy disorders are due to failure of the placental allograft causing immune-mediated damage is attractive.

However, concrete evidence of placental immunopathology is surprisingly lacking, partly because the findings in normal pregnancy are often disputed. Furthermore, pathology may arise long before tissues are available for examination: for example, the deficient trophoblast invasion of spiral arteries in pre-eclampsia arises many months before the pregnancy is finally interrupted. All these factors combine to create incomplete and confusing data.

Spontaneous abortion

Of all pregnancy abnormalities, spontaneous abortion most closely resembles graft rejection. Immunological mechanisms for pregnancy failure have gained new importance following reports of successful immunotherapy of women who have suffered three or more consecutive early pregnancy losses (Taylor and Faulk, 1981; Mowbray et al, 1985; Beer et al, 1987; Johnson et al, 1986). These women form a well-defined clinical group under close medical supervision, but there have been few attempts to study their utero-placental tissues. Specimens may be difficult to obtain: pregnancies may be aborted at home and tissue lost, or fetal death may occur several days before evacuation so that decidua and placenta become inflamed. Recent studies have been based on in vitro fertilization (IVF) embryos failing within 30 days of transfer: these form another clearly defined clinical group.

Histopathological and functional studies of utero-placental tissues in spontaneous abortion suggest that immunohistological investigations may be worthwhile. Khong et al (1987) suggested that defective haemochorial placentation may be a cause of recurrent and sporadic miscarriage: 2/7 first trimester and 5/5 second trimester abortions showed no evidence of vascular trophoblast. Khong et al (1987) proposed that spontaneous abortion, pre-eclampsia and small-for-gestational age (SGA) infants represent a continuum of pregnancy failure, sharing a form of defective placentation with specific morphological features but not necessarily indicating a common pathogenesis.

Defective trophoblastic vascular invasion could be an inherent property of trophoblast or may be due to a local abnormality within decidua. The numerous trophoblast antigens defined by mAbs has not so far been investigated in spontaneous abortion tissues, nor have there been any reports relating to trophoblast MHC antigen expression. The 40–41 kD class I MHC antigen on extravillous trophoblast may be involved in local immuno-suppression (Stern et al, 1986a). Defective regulation of MHC antigen expression by villous or extravillous trophoblast could conceivably lead to a maternal anti-fetal rejection response: such a possibility may be clarified by elucidation of MHC regulatory mechanisms in normal pregnancy. Nevertheless, investigation of MHC antigen expression by trophoblast in spontaneous abortions may be worth pursuing.

Decidual leukocyte populations have also been neglected: difficulties arise if tissues are inflamed and it may be impossible to separate inflammatory cells from possible mediators of immune attack. Nebel et al (1986) studied early clinical abortions occurring 22–30 days following embryo transfer (ET) on an IVF–ET programme. Dense infiltrates of lymphocytes were observed in deep decidua and around blood vessels, but the cells were not phenotyped. Functional assays were not possible because of the small tissue samples available. In a study of pregnancies aborting between 8 and 21 weeks' gestational age, Clark et al (1987) reported deficiency of mononuclear cells with large cytoplasmic granules (present in normal pregnancy controls) together with the additional presence of large granular lymphocytes with small cytoplasmic granules. Unfortunately, no criteria were given for distinguishing these two types of granulated cell, nor were there any data regarding their phenotype or function.

Immunopathological studies of spontaneous abortion are at an early developmental stage. Patients suffering spontaneous abortion represent a heterogeneous group with numerous possible causes, including mechanical, hormonal and genetic factors as well as immunological. Investigations may be more worthwhile if confined to well-defined clinical subgroups, such as recurrent (three or more) spontaneous aborters or early pregnancy losses in an IVF–ET programme. As yet, however, there is no conclusive evidence from utero-placental tissues that spontaneous abortion results from immune rejection.

Pre-eclampsia

Several observations support the concept that pre-eclampsia is due to a disturbed materno-fetal immunological interrelationship (see Chapter 5). The placenta is of central importance: pre-eclampsia occurs only when trophoblast is present, does not require a fetus as evidenced by hydatidiform mole and is cured by placental removal. Incidence correlates with placental mass being high in twin pregnancy, molar pregnancy and hydrops fetalis (Fox, 1978). Furthermore, the quantity of trophoblast deposited into uterine veins is increased in pre-eclampsia (Jaameri et al, 1965).

Pathological studies have focused on both placenta and placental bed. The spiral arteries show 'acute atherosis' characterized by fibrinoid necrosis and lipophage infiltration of the vessel wall as well as a perivascular mononuclear cell infiltrate (Robertson et al, 1986). These changes are seen most clearly in decidua parietalis, where vasculopathy is devoid of trophoblast-induced changes. They have been considered to be virtually pathognomonic of albuminuric hypertension in pregnancy (Robertson et al, 1986), but similar lesions have been reported in decidua in intrauterine growth retardation with mild or no hypertension (Sheppard and Bonnar, 1981). Placental changes in pre-eclampsia, namely cytotrophoblast proliferation, syncytial budding and placental infarction (Fox, 1978), are indicative of hypoxia due to these spiral artery lesions.

Acute atherosis resembles vascular changes in rejecting renal and cardiac allografts (Robertson et al, 1967; Hess et al, 1983): an immune pathogenesis has been proposed and supported by detection of complement (C3), IgG and fibrin in placental bed vessels in pre-eclampsia (Kitzmiller and Benirschke, 1973). More recently, C3 and IgM were detected in fibrinoid necrosis and atherosis in decidual vessels in pre-eclampsia, stable chronic hypertension and normotensive diabetes, leading to the suggestion that immunoprotein deposition is related to local intravascular coagulation and fibrinogenesis rather than to an immune reaction (Kitzmiller et al, 1981). Hustin et al (1983), however, reported C3 and IgG deposition in decidual parts of utero-placental arteries in pre-eclampsia, C3 only being found in association with conspicuous IgG deposition. Weir (1981) and Wells et al (1987) have reported fibrin and C3 in spiral arteries in normal pregnancy and, in the latter study, C1q, C4, C6 and C9 were also detected, hence providing support for an immune basis for complement deposition. Reports of complement deposition in normal pregnancy, however, raise doubt regarding the significance in pre-eclampsia. Lichtig et al (1984, 1985) have reported morphological changes of acute atherosis, C3 and occasional IgG deposition in spiral arteries in first trimester terminations. The incidence was significantly higher in primaparae and it was suggested that these may be early pre-eclamptic lesions which may or may not fully develop into the full-blown clinical syndrome. This interesting possibility requires more study.

Various immunopathological observations have been made concerning chorionic villi in pre-eclampsia, but all studies have been performed on third trimester delivered placentae and abnormalities are probably secondary effects. Complement components are normally present in immature and mature placenta (Faulk et al, 1980) but are increased in quantity in pre-eclampsia, particularly in severe disease, possibly reflecting an immune process within villi (Sinha et al, 1984). Pre-eclamptic placentae have been reported to contain connective tissue proteins not present in normal placentae (Vardi and Halbrecht, 1974) and relative concentrations of laminin and type IV collagen in chorionic villi are altered in pre-eclampsia (Risteli et al, 1984). Histologically, villi have been reported to show premature maturation, an observation which may be reflected immunophenotypically: premature expression of the Ca1 antigen, normally only present in third trimester pregnancies, has recently been reported in pre-eclampsia (Bishop et al, 1988). Other trophoblast antigens and MHC antigens have not been studied in detail.

Conversion of uterine spiral arteries into utero-placental arteries is effected by endovascular and perivascular trophoblast and appears to occur in two phases: decidual segments are converted by a wave of endovascular trophoblast migration in the first trimester, and myometrial segments by a subsequent wave in the second trimester (Robertson, 1976; Pijnenborg et al, 1980; Robertson et al, 1986). In pre-eclampsia and in some pregnancies with small-for-gestational age infants (SGA), physiological pregnancy changes are restricted to the decidual segments, myometrial segments retaining their musculoelastic architecture and responding to vasomotor influences (Robertson, 1976; Robertson et al, 1986). Defective physiological change has been attributed to failure of the second wave of trophoblast migration (Robertson, 1976). Khong et al (1986) have recently demonstrated absence of physiologic vascular changes throughout the entire length of the spiral arteries in a proportion of pregnancies complicated by pre-eclampsia or SGA, an abnormality easily detected by examination of the basal plate from the maternal-facing surface of the placenta. Furthermore, intraluminal endovascular trophoblast was demonstrated in third trimester pre-eclamptic tissues, whereas in normal pregnancy arteries re-endothelialize after the second trimester (Khong et al, 1986).

Thus, the maternal vascular response to placentation appears to be inadequate in pre-eclampsia, raising the possibility of abnormal interactions between maternal and fetal cell populations in the placental bed. In an attempt to clarify local materno-fetal relationships, Khong (1987) compared decidual leukocytes in normal and pre-eclamptic pregnancies and noted no difference in either quantity or type of infiltrate. All studies have necessarily been based on third trimester utero-placental tissues, whilst the defect causing pre-eclampsia may arise in the second trimester or even earlier. Pregnancies which will develop pre-eclampsia cannot be predicted and hence it is not feasible to examine tissues at a more appropriate gestational age. Reports that lesions of acute atherosis may be present in early pregnancies before pre-eclampsia is clinically apparent merit further investigation. An interesting application of flow cytometric detection of trophoblast in maternal blood with trophoblast-specific mAbs (Covone et al, 1984) would be to quantitate deported trophoblast elements, which may be 15–20 times more numerous per ml of blood in pre-eclampsia (Jaameri et al, 1965).

Intrauterine growth retardation (IUGR)/small-for-gestational age (SGA)

Well-established causes of small-for-gestational age (SGA) infants include fetal infection, congenital malformations and maternal cigarette smoking. Most cases are unexplained and probably form a heterogeneous group. An immunological aetiology has been proposed based on detection of acute atherosis in placental bed vessels and of chronic villitis of unknown aetiology (VUE). Lesions resembling acute atherosis have been reported in placental bed in association with SGA infants independent of the level of blood pressure (Sheppard and Bonnar, 1976, 1981; DeWolf et al, 1980; Althabe et al, 1985; Labarrere et al, 1985), although it is disputed whether changes are confined to decidua basalis (Robertson et al, 1986) or whether they extend to intramyometrial segments as in pre-eclampsia (Sheppard and Bonnar, 1976, 1981; DeWolf et al, 1980). Immunohistochemical studies have revealed deposition of C3, C1q and IgM in acute atherosis lesions in SGA associated with normotension, hypertension and SLE (Labarrere et al, 1985). In another study, only minute IgG and C3 deposits were noted in placental bed vessels in normotensive SGA but those cases did not show acute atherosis (Hustin et al, 1983). Acute atherosis cannot be considered as specific and has been reported in SGA with and without hypertension, pre-eclampsia with normal birthweight and SGA, sustained chronic hypertension irrespective of superimposed pre-eclampsia, normotensive diabetes and SLE (Labarrere et al, 1985).

A further change in SGA, which is also associated with pre-eclampsia, is lack of physiological changes in spiral arteries. Deficiency of migratory vascular trophoblast in myometrial vessels has been noted in normotensive SGA (Brosens et al, 1977; DeWolf et al, 1980; Gerretson et al, 1981; Khong et al, 1986) and in some cases physiological changes were absent throughout the length of the artery (DeWolf et al, 1980; Althabe et al, 1985; Khong et al, 1986). However, restriction of physiological changes in spiral arteries cannot adequately explain SGA: utero-placental arteries in pre-eclampsia without SGA show changes comparable with those additionally complicated by SGA (Khong et al, 1986).

Chronic VUE has also been associated with SGA: VUE has been reported in 24% cases of SGA (Altshuler et al, 1975). Labarrere et al (1982) noted chronic focal villitis in 26% control placentas and 86% SGA, but lesions were less severe in controls affecting only 1–2% of villi compared with 10% in SGA. Russell (1980) detected VUE in 7–8% of all pregnancies, and also noted correlation between severity of VUE and degree of growth retardation. The cause of VUE is obscure: there is no evidence of haematogenous infection and no infective agent has been found. Infection from uterine sources has been suggested (Russell, 1980) but others have reported a comparable lymphocytic infiltrate in anchoring villi in controls and SGA and have favoured an alternative view, namely that VUE is an immunological disorder resulting from maternal immune attack against fetal tissues (Labarrere et al, 1982). Histologically, an inflammatory infiltrate composed of histiocytes, lymphocytes, fibroblasts, polymorphs, plasma cells and multinucleate giant cells appears to disrupt villous stroma. Inflammatory lesions may also be apparent in intervillous spaces with histiocytes situated on both maternal and fetal sides of the trophoblast (Russell, 1980). It is not known whether inflammatory cells are of maternal or fetal origin, a factor of major importance in consideration of the possibility that VUE represents a maternal immune attack directed against the placental semi-allograft.

Chronic VUE has also been reported as a cause of recurrent SGA (Labarrere and Althabe, 1987) and of recurrent pregnancy failure (Russell et al, 1980). Lesions of chronic VUE have also been noted in association with the typical placental bed vascular lesions in sustained chronic hypertension and pre-eclampsia with normally grown infants (Labarrere and Althabe, 1985).

Systemic lupus erythematosis

Systemic lupus erythematosis (SLE) is associated with a high incidence of spontaneous abortion, prematurity and perinatal death. Poor fetal outcome has been attributed to trophoblast injury but, in the few morphological studies of SLE placentas, there has been no convincing evidence of trophoblast damage (Haustein, 1973; Fox, 1978). Immune complex deposition has been proposed as a cause of trophoblast injury (Theofilopolous et al, 1981): placentae from SLE patients showed granular deposition of C3, IgG and fibrinogen on trophoblast basement membrane, and anti-nuclear and anti-DNA antibodies were eluted in some cases (Grennan et al, 1978). However, C3, IgG and fibrinogen have been detected on trophoblast basement membrane in normal full term placentae (Faulk and Johnson, 1977) and the distinctions in SLE tissues are not clear. Retrovirus particles have been reported in placentae of SLE patients but are also seen in normal human placentae and their significance is uncertain (Imamura et al, 1976; Dirksen and Levy, 1977).

Extensive placental infarcts may also be a feature of SLE and have been attributed to a necrotizing decidual vasculopathy (Abramowsky et al, 1980). Fibrinoid necrosis and a mono- or polymorphonuclear leukocytic infiltrate may occur in spiral arteries in decidua basalis, and acute atherosis akin to that in pre-eclampsia and SGA may be present (Abramowsky et al, 1980; Labarrere et al, 1986). Deposition of IgM, C3, C1q and fibrin in association with acute atherosis has been reported (Abramowsky et al, 1980; Labarrere et al, 1986). Labarrere et al (1986) commented on absence of arterial physiological changes in SLE and also noted chronic VUE in most cases. Other autoimmune diseases showed maternal vascular lesions and chronic VUE but placental vascular damage was more prominent in SLE and IgM deposition in particular appeared related to poor fetal outcome (Labarrere et al, 1986).

Diabetes mellitus

Morphological placental abnormalities are well documented in diabetes mellitus and include cytotrophoblast hyperplasia, focal syncytial necrosis and thickening of trophoblast basement membrane (Fox, 1978; Fox and Jones, 1983). Cytotrophoblast hyperplasia is a response to trophoblast damage but the pathogenesis is not clear: the changes do not suggest hypoxia and electron microscopy does not reveal immune complex deposition which would support immune-mediated damage (Fox and Jones, 1983). Trophoblast damage has been attributed to exposure to abnormal metabolic milieu but factors contributing to trophoblast injury must be partly independent of hyperglycaemia. Similar features occur in both well-controlled gestational diabetes and overt diabetes, although they are more consistent and more prominent in the latter group (Fox and Jones, 1983). Furthermore, placental abnormalities were not modified in patients treated with continuous subcutaneous insulin infusion ensuring near normoglycaemia (Laurini et al, 1987).

In most cases of diabetes mellitus, placentation proceeds normally (Robertson, 1979). Nevertheless, although placental bed vascular lesions were notably absent in some reports (Pinkerton, 1963; Fox, 1978), lesions of fibrinoid necrosis and/or acute atherosis have been detected in spiral arteries in normotensive diabetes (Kitzmiller et al, 1981). Arterial lesions, some of which were occlusive, were noted in both decidua basalis and decidua parietalis in one third of 41 normotensive diabetic patients and were often associated with deposition of IgM and C3. Thus, vascular lesions noted in pre-eclampsia, SGA, SLE and diabetes mellitus show similar morphological and immunopathological features but may arise through different pathogenetic mechanisms (Kitzmiller et al, 1981).

Ectopic pregnancy

Ectopic pregnancy is relatively common, occurring in approximately 1 in 200 conceptions. In 96% of cases, implantation is in the fallopian tube. Placental development proceeds until haemorrhage, tubal distension or rupture necessitates surgical removal. In most cases, tubal pregnancy is considered to be due to tubal abnormalities resulting in a delay in the passage of the fertilized ovum along the fallopian tube, but increased tubal receptivity or factors deriving from the conceptus may play a part in the pathogenesis (Bigelow, 1982). Ectopic pregnancy may follow in vitro fertilization and embryo replacement (Hewitt et al, 1985).

Immunohistochemical investigation of trophoblast and MHC antigen expression by villous and extravillous trophoblast have revealed no major discrepancies between ectopic tubal pregnancy and first trimester intrauterine pregnancy (Earl et al, 1985b, 1986). Granular extracellular NDOG1-reactivity seen around cytotrophoblast shell in normal pregnancy, is notable at the implantation site in ectopic pregnancy even in the ovary or uterine cornua (Figure 3) (Bulmer, 1985; Earl et al, 1985a, 1986). Immuno-localization of hCG, hPL and SP1 is also comparable in early intrauterine pregnancy and extrauterine gestation (Chemnitz et al, 1984; Earl et al, 1986). However, pregnancy-associated plasma protein A (PAPP-A) was reported to be absent in villous syncytiotrophoblast in ectopic tubal pregnancy but present at this site in early intrauterine pregnancy (Chemnitz et al, 1984). Low serum levels of PAPP-A in ectopic pregnancy (Sinosich et al, 1983) and in imminent spontaneous abortion (Westergaard et al, 1983) suggest that synthesis of PAPP-A may be severely compromised, an observation which could be of diagnostic value (Chemnitz et al, 1984).

Decidualization of the tubal mucosa often occurs in ectopic pregnancy but is usually focal and patchy (Pauerstein et al, 1986; Bulmer et al, 1987c; Earl et al, 1987b). Endometrial stromal granulocytes are detectable in ectopic tubal pregnancy only in areas of decidualization and may be entirely absent (Bulmer et al, 1987c). The majority of leukocytes at the tubal implantation site are macrophages. A small number of mature T cells can be identified, but the large population of CD2+ CD7+ granulated lymphocytes identified in decidua in intrauterine pregnancy cannot be detected in the absence of decidualization (Bulmer et al, 1987c; Earl et al, 1987b). Uterine endometrium undergoes decidualization in ectopic pregnancy and shows similar leukocyte populations to those in early intrauterine pregnancy with large populations of macrophages and CD2+ CD7+ granulated lymphocytes (Bulmer et al, 1987c). Thus, macrophages predominate at the ectopic implantation site, whilst granulated lymphocytes are present in intrauterine decidua. Any essential role for granulated lymphocytes in control of tropho-blast invasion or regulation of maternal anti-fetal responses would thus require secretion of a soluble factor capable of exerting its effect at a distant site.

In normal pregnancy, uterine glands lack expression of class I MHC antigens. In tubal pregnancy, however, the epithelium retains class I MHC antigen expression and also shows uniform intense reactivity for class II MHC antigens. HLA-DR,-DP and -DQ antigens could be upregulated by local interferons released as a result of inflammation, but fallopian tube epithelium in early intrauterine pregnancy also expresses class II MHC antigens, suggesting hormonal regulatory mechanisms (Bulmer and Earl, 1987).

Ectopic pregnancy has provided a useful model of early implantation for immunohistological studies and examination of tubal pregnancy may cast light on the functions of maternal leukocytes in normal implantation and placentation. No major abnormalities of trophoblast have been detected, however, and the observations support a mechanical explanation for pathogenesis.

Placenta accreta

Placenta accreta includes all conditions in which chorionic villi adhere to (accreta), invade into (increta) or penetrate through (percreta) the myometrium. The histopathological diagnosis is made when villi oppose directly on the myometrium with no intervening decidua basalis. Placental tissue may be separated from myometrium by a layer of fibrin, and myometrium immediately deep to the villi often appears hyalinized and shows an interstitial chronic inflammatory cell infiltrate (Fox, 1972; Hutton et al, 1983). Placental adherence is often focal and partial with similar focal absence of decidua and the degree of myometrial penetration may not be uniform (Fox, 1972).

Placenta accreta is uncommon and its pathogenesis is uncertain. Several series have noted a high incidence of previous uterine curettage or caesarian section implicating surgical manipulation as an aetiological factor (Hutton et al, 1983). However, Khong and Robertson (1987) have proposed that failure of normal materno-fetal interactions underlies placenta accreta. They highlighted cases in which normal decidua basalis was identified adjacent to focal accreta sites; decidua parietalis was also not diminished in quantity. Extravillous trophoblast accumulated at the villous–decidual junction, was binucleate or mononuclear and multinucleate trophoblast giant cells normally observed in late pregnancy were absent. Some vessels failed to show physiological changes, whilst in others physiological changes extended much more deeply than normal reaching the arcuate system in some cases. Abnormalities of extravillous trophoblast, hyalinization of myometrium and presence of a mononuclear inflammatory cell infiltrate were interpreted as representing decidual destruction of varying degree. Defective interactions between decidua and migratory trophoblast in early pregnancy would thus lead to undue placental adherence and uterine penetration.

No differences in trophoblast phenotype have been detected between normal pregnancy and placenta accreta (Earl et al, 1987a), but immuno-histological studies are limited by the lack of fresh tissues for examination. Furthermore, since tissues cannot be examined until clinical presentation postpartum the hypothesis of defective materno-fetal interactions in early pregnancy is difficult to test. There are reports of placenta accreta in early pregnancy (Hutton et al, 1983) and immunohistochemical studies of such tissues would be worthwhile. Elucidation of the aetiology would be greatly facilitated if it were possible to pinpoint and examine placenta accreta early in gestation. Since this is not feasible, an alternative approach is examination of maternal decidua, decidual leukocytes and extravillous trophoblast in fresh tissues obtained postpartum. Examination of trophoblast oncogene and MHC antigen expression may prove fruitful areas for future study.

Maternal infections

Infections can spread to the placenta via blood or from endometrium and usually take the form of a villitis, villous stroma bearing the brunt of the inflammation. Infections in which inflammation appears limited to tropho-blast are early rubella and herpes virus infection (see Fox and Jones, 1983). Maternal *Plasmodium falciparum* malaria is associated with a high incidence of SGA infants, although congenital malaria is uncommon. Trophoblast damage has been reported and appears to be caused by intratrophoblastic malarial pigment accumulation and pigment-laden macrophages in inter-villous spaces, rather than by the parasite itself (Galbraith et al, 1980b). C1q, C3d, C4, C9, fibrinogen and plasminogen are deposited in increased amounts in the placenta in malaria, although immunoprotein distribution corresponds with that reported for normal placentae (Galbraith et al, 1980b). Trophoblast damage may account for the high incidence of SGA in maternal *P. falciparum* infection. Infective villitis due to other causes is often associated with low birth weight, but this is probably due to trans-placental infection since villitis is rarely sufficient to decrease trophoblast function dramatically (Fox and Jones, 1983).

Trophoblast tumours

The syndromes of hydatidiform mole and choriocarcinoma have been discussed elsewhere (Chapter 6). In Caucasian populations, approximately equal numbers of cases of choriocarcinoma follow normal term delivery, molar pregnancy and non-molar abortion, although the proportion follow-ing hydatidiform mole is higher in Japan. Complete hydatidiform moles are androgenetic in origin and fully allogeneic with the maternal host, as are a proportion of choriocarcinomas.

The distribution of trophoblast antigens is similar to that described for normal pregnancy of matched gestational age (Bulmer et al, 1988b). PLAP is detectable on a minority of hydatidiform moles, reflecting the early gestational age at evacuation (Berkowitz et al, 1986; Bulmer et al, 1988b). Persistent villous stromal labelling with NDOG1 in molar pregnancy may reflect failure of villous development (Sunderland et al, 1985a; Bulmer et al, 1988b). Choriocarcinomas also show heterogeneity of trophoblast antigen expression and most trophoblast phenotypes recognized in normal preg-nancy are present in choriocarcinomas, including a small population of HMFG1-positive cells (Bulmer et al, 1988b). NDOG1 reactivity at the advancing edge of the tumour could reflect the role of hyaluronic acid in disrupting cellular matrices and facilitating trophoblast invasion. PLAP is generally not detected in choriocarcinoma, even in syncytial cells. A pro-portion of choriocarcinomas follow term delivery and may derive from the villous placenta (Brewer and Mazur, 1981). Hence, trophoblast in chorio-carcinoma may revert to a less mature form expressing hCG but not PLAP, as described for normal first trimester villous trophoblast (Kurman et al, 1984a; Bulmer and Johnson, 1985a). It would be worthwhile to compare trophoblast antigen expression in choriocarcinoma following molar pregnancy, non-molar abortion or term delivery.

TLX antigens detected by H316 and polyclonal antisera are expressed by all molar and choriocarcinoma trophoblast and may contribute to the well-established immunogenicity of trophoblast tumours (Berkowitz et al, 1986; Bulmer et al, 1988b). Low molecular weight cytokeratins also appear to be expressed on all trophoblast populations in trophoblast tumours (Sasagawa et al, 1986; Bulmer et al, 1988b): these reagents may aid identification of trophoblast in routinely fixed and embedded sections, particularly for the rare placental site trophoblastic tumour (PSTT) which may cause diagnostic problems.

Placental hormonal products have also been localized in trophoblastic tumours and may be detected in serum (Horne et al, 1984; Kurman et al, 1984a,b). Localization of trophoblast hormones and antigens may identify the cell of origin of tumours: PSTT shows a high hPL content and is unreactive with NDOG1, reflecting its proposed origin from the extravillous ('intermediate') trophoblast (Kurman et al, 1984b; Bulmer et al, 1988b). Examination of mRNA in tissue sections led to the conclusion that hPL gene expression is associated with a higher degree of differentiation and is almost absent in choriocarcinoma (Hoshina et al, 1983).

Phenotypic differences between trophoblast in choriocarcinoma and hydatidiform mole have been of limited value. In immunohistological studies, α_2-macroglobulin and pregnancy protein-5 (PP5) are protease inhibitors which may play a role in trophoblast invasiveness: both were detected in normal placenta and hydatidiform mole, but were absent in invasive mole and choriocarcinoma (Seppala et al, 1979; Saksela et al, 1981). Berkowitz et al (1985a,b) have also reported differential reactivity of choriocarcinomas and hydatidiform moles for sperm- and stage-specific embryonic antigens.

Trophoblast expression of MHC antigens in molar pregnancy is essentially similar to that in normal pregnancy (Berkowitz et al, 1983; Fisher and Lawler, 1984; Sunderland et al, 1985a; Bulmer et al, 1988b). The chorionic villous stroma is class I MHC-positive and probably represents the site of sensitization to paternal MHC antigens (Lawler and Fisher, 1987). Molar extravillous trophoblast proliferating from the villi and in the placental bed expresses a class I MHC antigen comparable with that on extravillous trophoblast in normal pregnancy (Figure 5) (Sunderland et al, 1985a). No differences in HLA expression have been noted between villous and extravillous trophoblast in partial, complete and invasive moles, nor between invasive and non-invasive villi in invasive moles (Sasagawa et al, 1987; Bulmer et al, 1988b).

Choriocarcinoma also shows broadly similar expression of MHC antigens to that in normal pregnancy (Figure 6). Syncytial elements are MHC-negative and certain choriocarcinoma lines lack mRNA for β_2-microglobulin (Tanaka et al, 1981). However, a substantial though variable proportion of cytotrophoblast does express class I HLA antigens (Sunderland et al,

1985c; Bulmer et al, 1988b) and a 40 kD W6/32-reactive, β_2-microglobulin-associated antigen has been identified on the BeWo choriocarcinoma cell line (Ellis et al, 1986; Stern et al, 1986c). Choriocarcinoma is thought to arise from villous trophoblast: the W6/32-reactive cytotrophoblast may be extravillous in origin or could differentiate to an extravillous phenotype following malignant transformation. Class II MHC antigens are absent on normal trophoblast and have not been detected on molar trophoblast or chorio-carcinoma by immunohistology (Sunderland et al, 1985a,c; Bulmer et al, 1988b). Recent studies suggest, however, that the GCH-1 choriocarcinoma line transcribes both α and β class II MHC genes (Takahashi et al, 1987).

There have been few studies of growth factors and their receptors in trophoblast tumours. EGF receptors appear to be decreased in number in

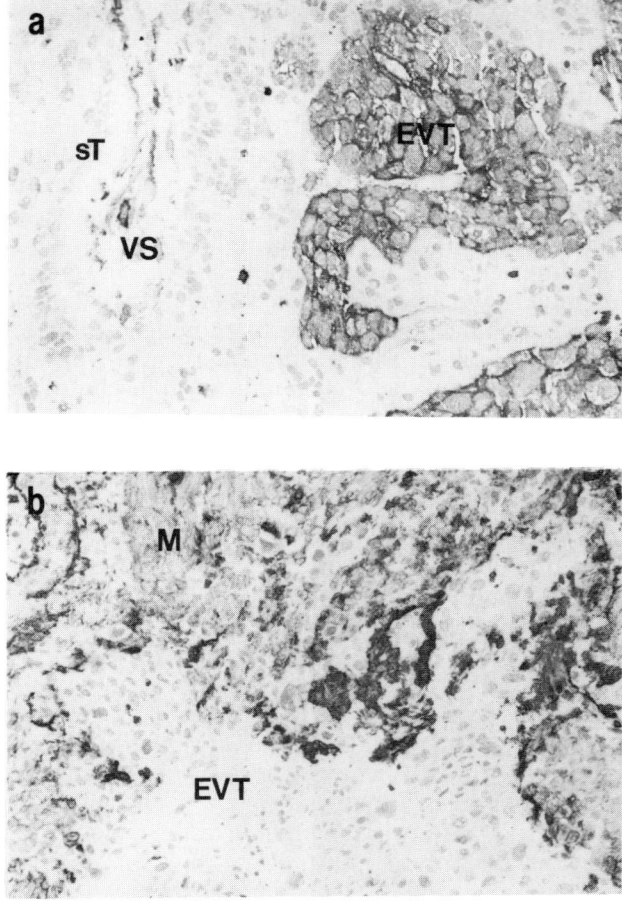

Figure 5. Cryostat sections of invasive mole labelled with (a) W6/32 (class I MHC), and (b) 61.D2 (class I MHC). Note lack of reactivity of W6/32 with villous syncytiotrophoblast (sT) but staining of villous stroma (VS) and extravillous trophoblast (EVT). 61.D2 labels maternal uterine tissues (M), but W6/32-positive extravillous trophoblast is negative. × 105.

molar pregnancy compared with normal tissue of similar gestational age (Carson et al, 1983). Both c-*myc* and c-*ras* have been localized in villous cytotrophoblast in molar pregnancy and in BeWo cells (Sarkar et al, 1986) which also expresses c-*fos* (Muller et al, 1983). Oncogenes may play a role in trophoblast proliferation, but further studies are required to determine whether a specific pattern of oncogene expression is characteristic of invasive trophoblastic neoplasia and could predict malignant potential.

Studies of local maternal host reactions to molar pregnancy and choriocarcinoma have been scarce. C3 and immunoglobulin were not detected at the implantation site in ten complete molar pregnancies (Berkowitz et al, 1982). Studies of cellular immunity suggest a fourfold increase in CD3-positive T lymphocytes with predominance of CD4-positive over CD8-positive T cells (Kabawat et al, 1985b). CD2-positive CD3-negative lymphocytes have also been detected in areas of decidualization and correspond to endometrial stromal granulocytes in molar pregnancy decidua (Bulmer et al, 1988b). Macrophages (class II MHC-positive, CD14-positive, often CD11b-negative) also form a major proportion of leukocytes at the molar implantation site and can be closely associated with extravillous trophoblast (Figure 4; Bulmer et al, 1988b). Macrophages and CD3-positive T cells form the predominant leukocytes associated with choriocarcinoma.

Trophoblast tumours offer enormous scope for immunopathological investigation: studies are limited by both the rarity of the condition in the

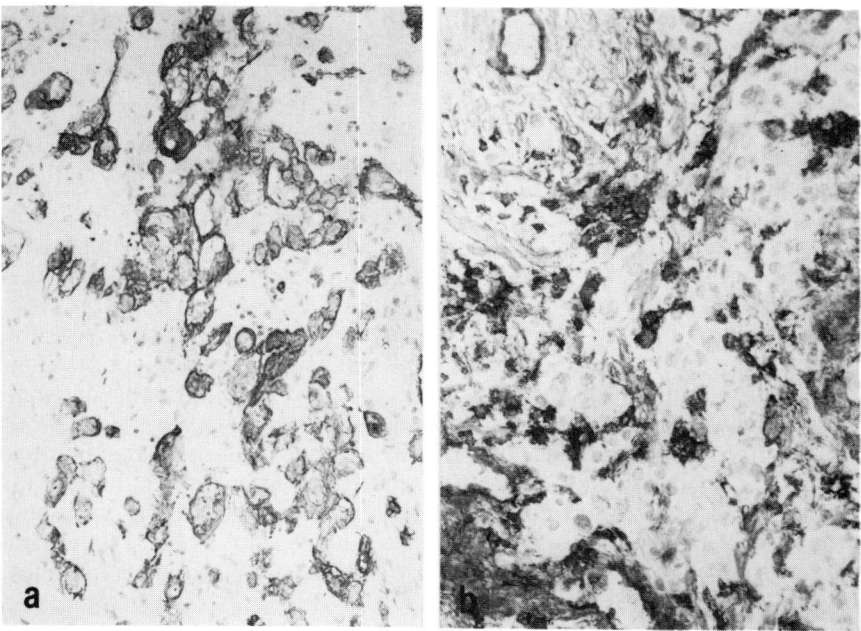

Figure 6. Cryostat sections of choriocarcinoma labelled with (a) CAM 5.2 (low MW cytokeratin), and (b) 61.D2 (class I MHC). Note lack of reactivity of 61.D2 with cytokeratin-positive choriocarcinoma cells. × 160.

West and difficulty in obtaining fresh tissues for detailed immunohistology, in situ hybridization and functional studies which together may help to elucidate materno-fetal interactions in trophoblast tumours.

Pemphigoid gestationis

Pemphigoid gestationis, also termed herpes gestationis, is a rare complication of pregnancy and shows clinical, histological and immunological similarities to bullous pemphigoid. It presents clinically as a pruritic rash around the umbilicus, spreading over the trunk and extremities. Urticated erythematous patches present in the early stages soon develop into papules, vesicles and bullae. Initial onset is in the second or third trimester and the rash persists until parturition. Pemphigoid gestationis invariably recurs in subsequent pregnancies, often presenting earlier and increasing in severity. Fetal prognosis is disputed but the frequency of SGA infants appears to be increased (Holmes et al, 1984).

The histopathology resembles that of bullous pemphigoid with epidermal spongiosis and formation of subepidermal bullae, often containing eosinophils (Holmes et al, 1983). Immunofluorescence shows complement deposition in the basement membrane zone in lesional, perilesional and apparently normal skin. Patients also have a circulating IgG complement-binding auto-antibody (herpes gestationis factor) with specificity for skin basement membrane zone and, in a minority of cases, IgG deposition may be detected at this site. Herpes gestationis factor levels do not correlate with disease severity.

The clinical and immunological similarities between pemphigoid gestationis and bullous pemphigoid suggest that the autoantibodies which cause the former may be induced by placental antigens which cross-react with skin basement membrane zone. Recent studies of placentae from four cases of pemphigoid gestationis have shown increased numbers of class II MHC-bearing leukocytes in chorionic villous stroma compared with normal placentae (Borthwick et al, 1985). Furthermore, using both complement-fixing immunofluorescence and immunoelectron microscopy, Ortonne et al (1987) demonstrated binding of herpes gestationis factor to the basement membrane zone of amnion and chorion laeve, but not to villous syncytio-trophoblast. A further 'pregnancy factor' in pemphigoid gestationis sera, distinct from herpes gestationis factor, was able to fix complement to villous syncytiotrophoblast. Ortonne et al (1987) emphasized the antigenic similarities between amniotic and skin basement membrane zones. Amniotic basement membrane zone is not normally exposed to the maternal immune system and hence the mechanism of sensitisation for maternal autoantibody is not clear. Amniotic antigens have, however, been identified in uterine spiral arteries in pregnancy (Bulmer et al, 1987d) and it is thus possible that extra-villous cytotrophoblast may play a role in evoking maternal autoantibodies.

SUMMARY

Immunological factors have been considered to play a role in the pathogenesis of several pregnancy disorders, but concrete evidence of placental immunopathology is surprisingly deficient. Recent advances in elucidation of materno-fetal relationships in utero-placental tissues in normal pregnancy may provide a more rational basis for investigation of placental immunopathology. This article has reviewed data which have recently accrued from immunohistochemical studies of utero-placental tissues in normal pregnancy. It focused particularly on the heterogeneous villous and extravillous fetal trophoblast populations, describing their expression of MHC antigens, trophoblast antigens, receptor structures, cytokines, oncogenes and hormones. Knowledge of cell types in maternal decidua was also reviewed and the two major decidual leukocyte populations, granulated lymphocytes and macrophages, discussed. The possibility that pregnancy abnormalities may arise from disordered materno-fetal relationships in the placental bed is discussed in relation to the limited data available. Immunopathological findings in pre-eclampsia, intrauterine growth retardation, maternal autoimmune disease, spontaneous abortion, ectopic pregnancy and placenta accreta are described and, wherever possible, related to our knowledge of normal pregnancy. Finally, trophoblast antigens and uterine leukocyte populations in trophoblast tumours are considered.

REFERENCES

Abramowsky CR, Vegas ME, Swinehart G & Gyves MT (1980) Decidual vasculopathy of the placenta in lupus erythematosus. *New England Journal of Medicine* **303:** 668–672.
Adamson ED (1987) Expression of proto-oncogenes in the placenta. *Placenta* **8:** 449–466.
Alberti S & Herzenberg LA (1986) Transfection of DNA from choriocarcinoma cell lines and sperm cells: DNA methylation prevents the expression of genes for the major histocompatibility complex (HLA) class I and the T cell differentiation antigen, Leu 2. In Clark DA & Croy BA (eds) *Reproductive Immunology 1986*, pp 60–66. Amsterdam: Elsevier Science Publishers.
Althabe O, Labarrere C & Telenta M (1985) Maternal vascular lesions in placentae of small-for-gestational-age infants. *Placenta* **6:** 265–276.
Altshuler G, Russell P & Ermocilla R (1975) The placental pathology of small-for-gestational age infants. *American Journal of Obstetrics and Gynecology* **121:** 351–359.
Anderson DJ & Berkowitz RS (1985) γ-Interferon enhances expression of class I MHC antigens in the weakly HLA + human choriocarcinoma cell line BeWo, but does not induce MHC expression in the HLA-choriocarcinoma cell line Jar. *Journal of Immunology* **135:** 2498–2501.
Anderson DJ, Johnson PM, Alexander NJ, Jones WR & Griffin PD (1987) Monoclonal antibodies to human trophoblast and sperm antigens: Report of two WHO-sponsored workshops, 30 June 1986, Toronto. *Journal of Reproductive Immunology* **10:** 231–257.
Beer AE, Shekar SS, Quebbeman JF & Zhu X (1987) Paternal and nonpaternal leukocyte immunization in women with recurrent spontaneous abortions: immune responses and subsequent pregnancy outcome. In Chaouat G (ed.) *Reproductive Immunology: Materno-Fetal Relationship*, pp 161–178. Paris: Inserm.
Berkowitz RS, Mostoufi-Zadeh M, Kabawat SE, Goldstein DP & Driscoll SG (1982) Immunopathologic study of the implantation site in molar pregnancy. *American Journal of Obstetrics and Gynecology* **144:** 925–930.
Berkowitz RS, Anderson DJ, Hunter NJ & Goldstein DP (1983) Distribution of major histocompatibility (HLA) antigens in chorionic villi of molar pregnancy. *American Journal of Obstetrics and Gynecology* **146:** 221–222.

Berkowitz RS, Alberti O, Hunter NJ, Goldstein DP & Anderson DJ (1985a) Localization of stage-specific embryonic antigens in hydatidiform mole, normal placenta and gestational choriocarcinoma. *Gynecologic Oncology* **20:** 71–77.

Berkowitz RS, Alexander NJ, Goldstein DP & Anderson DJ (1985b) Reactivity of anti-human sperm monoclonal antibodies with normal placenta, hydatidiform mole and gestational choriocarcinoma. *Gynecologic Oncology* **22:** 334–340.

Berkowitz RS, Umpierre SA, Johnson PM, McIntyre JA & Anderson DJ (1986) Expression of trophoblast-leukocyte common antigens and placental-type alkaline phosphatase in complete molar pregnancy. *American Journal of Obstetrics and Gynecology* **155:** 443–446.

Bigelow B (1982) Abnormalities and disease of the placenta, membranes and umbilical cord. In Blaustein A (ed.) *Pathology of the Female Genital Tract*, pp 760–783. New York: Springer Verlag.

Bishop PW, Fox H, Morris JA & Malam J (1988) The expression of CA (Oxford) antigen by placental trophoblast in pre-eclampsia and hypertension. *Journal of Pathology* **154:** 103A–104A.

Bohn H, Dati F & Lüben G (1983) Human trophoblast specific products other than hormones. In Loke YW & Whyte A (eds) *Biology of Trophoblast*, pp 317–352. Amsterdam: Elsevier Science Publishers.

Borthwick G, Lawlor F, Holmes RC, Black MM & Stirrat GM (1985) Evidence for an immunological attack on the placenta in pemphigoid gestationis. *British Journal of Dermatology* **113 (supplement 29):** 41–42.

Boyd JD & Hamilton WJ (1970) *The Human Placenta*. Cambridge: W. Heffer.

Braunhut SJ, Blanc WA, Ramanarayanan M, Marboe C & Mesa-Tejada R (1984) Immuno-cytochemical localization of lysozyme and alpha-1-antichymotrypsin in the term human placenta: an attempt to characterize the Hofbauer cell. *Journal of Histochemistry and Cytochemistry* **32:** 1204–1210.

Brewer JI & Mazur MT (1981) Gestational choriocarcinoma. Its origin in the placenta during seemingly normal pregnancy. *American Journal of Surgical Pathology* **5:** 267–277.

Brosens I, Dixon HG & Robertson WB (1977) Fetal growth retardation and the arteries of the placental bed. *British Journal of Obstetrics and Gynaecology* **84:** 656–663.

Bulmer JN (1985) Studies on the immunology of the human placenta in normal and pathological pregnancy. PhD Thesis, University of Bristol.

Bulmer JN & Earl U (1987) The expression of class II MHC gene products by fallopian tube epithelium in pregnancy and throughout the menstrual cycle. *Immunology* **61:** 207–213.

Bulmer JN & Johnson PM (1984) Macrophage populations in the human placenta and amnio-chorion. *Clinical and Experimental Immunology* **57:** 393–403.

Bulmer JN & Johnson PM (1985a) Antigen expression by trophoblast populations in the human placenta and their possible immunobiological relevance. *Placenta* **6:** 127–140.

Bulmer JN & Johnson PM (1985b) Immunohistological characterization of the decidual leuco-cytic infiltrate related to endometrial glands in early human pregnancy. *Immunology* **55:** 35–44.

Bulmer JN & Johnson PM (1986) The T-lymphocyte population in first-trimester human decidua does not express the interleukin-2 receptor. *Immunology* **58:** 685–687.

Bulmer JN & Sunderland CA (1983) Bone marrow origin of endometrial granulocytes in the early human placental bed. *Journal of Reproductive Immunology* **5:** 383–387.

Bulmer JN & Sunderland CA (1984) Immunohistological characterisation of lymphoid cell populations in the early human placental bed. *Immunology* **52:** 349–357.

Bulmer JN, Billington WD & Johnson PM (1984) Immunohistologic identification of tropho-blast populations in early human pregnancy with the use of monoclonal antibodies. *American Journal of Obstetrics and Gynecology* **148:** 19–26.

Bulmer JN, Wells M, Bhabra K & Johnson PM (1986) Immunohistological characterization of endometrial gland epithelium and extravillous fetal trophoblast in third trimester human placental bed tissues. *British Journal of Obstetrics and Gynaecology* **93:** 823–832.

Bulmer JN, Hollings D & Ritson A (1987a) Immunocytochemical evidence that endometrial stromal granulocytes are granulated lymphocytes. *Journal of Pathology* **153:** 281–287.

Bulmer JN, Johnson PM & Bulmer D (1987b) Leukocyte populations in human decidua and endometrium. In Gill TJ III & Wegmann TF (eds) *Immunoregulation and Fetal Survival*, pp 111–134. New York: Oxford University Press.

Bulmer JN, Ritson A, Earl U & Hollings D (1987c) Immunocompetent cells in human decidua.

In Chaouat G (ed.) *Reproductive Immunology: materno-fetal relationship*, pp 89–100. Paris: Inserm.

Bulmer JN, Wells M, Yeh C-JG & Hsi B-L (1987d) Investigation of the expression of amnion antigens by spiral arteries in human uteroplacental tissues. *American Journal of Reproductive Immunology and Microbiology* **14**: 79–83.

Bulmer JN, Smith JC & Morrison L (1988a) Expression of class II MHC gene products by macrophages in human uteroplacental tissues. *Immunology* **63**: 707–714.

Bulmer JN, Johnson PM, Sasagawa M & Takeuchi S (1988b) Immunohistochemical studies of fetal trophoblast and maternal decidua in hydatidiform mole and choriocarcinoma. *Placenta* **9**: 183–200.

Bulmer JN, Smith J, Morrison L & Wells M (1988c) Maternal and fetal cellular relationships in the human placental basal plate. *Placenta* **9**: 237–246.

Carson SA, Chase R, Ulep E, Scommegna A & Benveniste R (1983) Ontogenesis and characteristics of epidermal growth factor receptors in human placenta. *American Journal of Obstetrics and Gynecology* **147**: 932–939.

Chard T, Craig PH, Menabawey M & Lee C (1986) Alpha interferon in human pregnancy. *British Journal of Obstetrics and Gynaecology* **93**: 1145–1149.

Chemnitz J, Tornehave D, Teisner B, Poulsen HK & Westergaard JG (1984) The localization of pregnancy proteins (hPL, SP_1 and PAPP-A) in intra- and extrauterine pregnancies. *Placenta* **5**: 489–494.

Clark DA, Slapsys R, Chaput A et al (1986) Immunoregulatory molecules of trophoblast and decidual suppressor cell origin at the materno-fetal interface. *American Journal of Reproductive Immunology and Microbiology* **10**: 100–104.

Clark DA, Mowbray J, Underwood J & Lidell H (1987) Histopathologic alterations in the decidua in human spontaneous abortion: loss of cells with large cytoplasmic granules. *American Journal of Reproductive Immunology and Microbiology* **13**: 19–22.

Comper WD & Laurent TC (1978) Physiological function of connective tissue polysaccharides. *Physiology Reviews* **58**: 255–315.

Contractor SF (1983) Metabolic and enzymatic activity of human trophoblast. In Loke YW & Whyte A (eds) *Biology of Trophoblast*, pp 236–316. Amsterdam: Elsevier Science Publishers.

Covone AE, Mutton D, Johnson PM & Adinolfi M (1984) Trophoblast cells in peripheral blood from pregnant women. *Lancet* **ii**: 841–843.

Croy BA, Gambel P, Rossant J & Wegmann TG (1985) Characterization of murine decidual natural killer cells and their relevance to the success of pregnancy. *Cellular Immunology* **93**: 315–326.

Dallenbach-Hellweg G (1981) The normal histology of the endometrium. In Histopathology of the Endometrium, pp 22–88. Berlin: Springer-Verlag.

Daya S, Clark DA, Devlin C, Jarrell J & Chaput A (1985) Preliminary characterization of two types of suppressor cells in the human uterus. *Fertility and Sterility* **44**: 778–785.

DeWolf F, Brosens I & Renaer M (1980) Fetal growth retardation and the maternal arterial supply of the human placenta in the absence of sustained hypertension. *British Journal of Obstetrics and Gynaecology* **87**: 678–685.

Dirksen ER & Levy JA (1977) Virus-like particles in placentae from normal individuals and patients with systemic lupus erythematosus. *Journal of the National Cancer Institute* **59**: 1187–1189.

Doellgast GJ & Benirschke K (1979) Placental alkaline phosphatase in hominidae. *Nature* **280**: 601–602.

Doerfler W (1983) DNA methylation and gene activity. *Annual Reviews in Biochemistry* **52**: 93–124.

Drake BL, King NJC, Maxwell LE & Rodger JC (1987) Class I major histocompatibility complex antigen expression on early murine trophoblast and its induction by lymphokines in vitro. *Journal of Reproductive Immunology* **10**: 319–328.

Duc-Goiran P, Lebon P & Chang C (1986) Measurement of interferon in human amniotic fluid and placental blood extract. *Methods in Enzymology* **119**: 541–551.

Earl UM, Bulmer JN & Wells M (1985a) Immunohistological characterization of antigen expression by trophoblast populations in ectopic cornual implantation. Case report. *British Journal of Obstetrics and Gynaecology* **92**: 843–846.

Earl U, Wells M & Bulmer JN (1985b) The expression of major histocompatibility complex

728   J. N. BULMER

antigens by trophoblast in ectopic tubal pregnancy. *Journal of Reproductive Immunology*
8: 13–24.

Earl U, Wells M & Bulmer JN (1986) Immunohistochemical characterisation of trophoblast
antigens and secretory products in ectopic tubal pregnancy. *International Journal of
Gynaecological Pathology* **5:** 132–142.

Earl U, Bulmer JN & Briones A (1987a) Placenta accreta: an immunohistological study of
trophoblast populations. *Placenta* **8:** 273–282.

Earl U, Lunny DP & Bulmer JN (1987b) Leucocyte populations in ectopic tubal pregnancy.
Journal of Clinical Pathology **40:** 901–905.

Ellis SA, Sargent IL, Redman CWG & McMichael AJ (1986) Evidence for a novel HLA
antigen found on human extravillous trophoblast and a human choriocarcinoma cell line.
Immunology **59:** 595–601.

Epenetos AA, Travers PJ, Gatter KC, Oliver RDT, Mason DY & Bodmer WF (1984) An
immunohistological study of testicular germ cell tumours using two different monoclonal
antibodies against placental alkaline phosphatase. *British Journal of Cancer* **49:** 11–15.

Faulk WP & Johnson PM (1977) Immunological studies of human placentae: identification and
distribution of proteins in mature chorionic villi. *Clinical and Experimental Immunology*
27: 365–375.

Faulk WP & McIntyre JA (1981) Trophoblast survival. *Transplantation* **32:** 1–5.

Faulk WP, Temple A, Lovins RE & Smith N (1978) Antigens of human trophoblasts: a working
hypothesis for their role in normal and abnormal pregnancies. *Proceedings of the National
Academy of Sciences USA* **75:** 1947–1951.

Faulk WP, Jarret R, Keane M, Johnson PM & Boackle RJ (1980) Immunological studies of
human placentae: complement components in immature and mature chorionic villi.
Clinical and Experimental Immunology **40:** 299–305.

Fisher RA & Lawler SD (1984) The expression of major histocompatibility antigens in
chorionic villi of molar placentae. *Placenta* **5:** 237–242.

Flynn A (1984) Stimulation of interleukin-1 production from placental monocytes. *Lymphokine Research* **3:** 1–5.

Fox H (1972) Placenta accreta, 1945–1969. *Obstetrical and Gynaecological Survey* **27:** 475–490.

Fox H (1978) *Pathology of the Placenta*. London, Philadelphia and Toronto: WB Saunders.

Fox H & Kharkongor NF (1969) Enzyme histochemistry of the Hofbauer cells of the human
placenta. *Journal of Obstetrics and Gynaecology of the British Commonwealth* **76:** 918–
921.

Fox H & Jones CJP (1983) Pathology of trophoblast. In Loke YW & Whyte A (eds) *Biology of
Trophoblast*, pp 137–185. Amsterdam: Elsevier Science Publishers.

Galbraith GMP, Galbraith RM & Faulk WP (1980a) Immunological studies of transferrin and
transferrin receptors on human placental trophoblast. *Placenta* **1:** 33–46.

Galbraith RM, Fox H, Hsi B et al (1980b) The human materno-foetal relationship in malaria.
II. Histological, ultrastructural and immunopathological studies of the placenta. *Transactions of the Royal Society of Tropical Medicine and Hygiene* **74:** 61–72.

Galbraith RM, Kantor RRS, Ferrara GB, Ades EW & Galbraith GMP (1981) Differential
anatomical expression of transplantation antigens within the normal human placental
chorionic villus. *American Journal of Reproductive Immunology* **1:** 331–335.

Gazit E, Gothelf Y, Gil R et al (1984) Alloantibodies to PHA-activated lymphocytes detect
human Qa-like antigens. *Journal of Immunology* **132:** 165–169.

Gerretsen G, Huisjes HJ & Elema JD (1981) Morphological changes of the spiral arteries in the
placental bed in relation to pre-eclampsia and fetal growth retardation. *British Journal of
Obstetrics and Gynaecology* **88:** 876–881.

Gosseye S & Fox H (1984) An immunohistological comparison of the secretory capacity of
villous and extravillous trophoblast in the human placenta. *Placenta* **5:** 329–348.

Goustin AS, Betsholtz C, Pfeifer-Ohlsson S et al (1985) Coexpression of the *sis* and *myc*
proto-oncogenes in developing human placenta suggests autocrine control of trophoblast
growth. *Cell* **41:** 301–312.

Grennan DM, McCormick JN, Wojtacha D, Carty M & Behan W (1978) Immunological
studies of the placenta in systemic lupus erythematosus. *Annals of the Rheumatic Diseases*
37: 129–134.

Halloran PF, Wadgymar A & Autenried P (1986) The regulation of expression of major
histocompatibility complex products. *Transplantation* **41:** 413–420.

Haustein UF (1973) Elektronmikroscopische Untersuchungen der Plazenta bei Lupus erythematodes visceralis. *Zentralblatt für Gynäkologie* **95:** 1818–1823.

Head JR, Drake BL & Zuckermann FA (1987) Major histocompatibility antigens on trophoblast and their regulation: implications in the maternal–fetal relationship. *American Journal of Reproductive Immunology and Microbiology* **15:** 12–18.

Hess ML, Hastillo A, Mohanakumar T et al (1983) Accelerated atherosclerosis in cardiac transplantation: Role of cytotoxic B-cell antibodies and hyperlipidemia. *Circulation* **68**(supplement II): II94–II101.

Hewitt J, Martin R, Steptoe PC, Rowland GF & Webster J (1985) Bilateral tubal ectopic pregnancy following in vitro fertilisation and embryo replacement. *British Journal of Obstetrics and Gynaecology* **92:** 850–852.

Holmes RC & N Black MM (1984) The fetal prognosis of pemphigoid gestationis (herpes gestationis). *British Journal of Dermatology* **110:** 67–72.

Holmes R, Black MM, Jurecka W et al (1983) Clues to the aetiology and pathogenesis of herpes gestationis. *British Journal of Dermatology* **109:** 131–139.

Horne CHW, Rankin R & Bremner RD (1984) Pregnancy-specific proteins as markers for gestational trophoblastic disease. *International Journal of Gynecological Pathology* **3:** 27–40.

Hoshina M, Hussa R, Pattillo R & Boime I (1983) Cytological distribution of chorionic gonadotrophin subunit and placental lactogen messenger RNA in neoplasms derived from human placenta. *Journal of Cell Biology* **97:** 1200–1206.

Howatson AG, Farquharson M, Meager A, Foulis AK & McNicol AM (1988) Localisation of apparently constitutive alpha-interferon in the human feto-placental unit. *Journal of Pathology* **154:** 103A.

Hoyes AD (1975) Structure and function of the amnion. *Obstetrics and Gynecology Annual* **4:** 1–38.

Hsi B-L, Yeh C-JG & Faulk WP (1984) Class I antigens of the major histocompatibility complex on cytotrophoblast of human chorion laeve. *Immunology* **52:** 621–629.

Hunt JS, King CR Jr & Wood GW (1984) Evaluation of human chorionic trophoblast cells and placental macrophages as stimulators of maternal lymphocyte proliferation in vitro. *Journal of Reproductive Immunology* **6:** 377–391.

Hunt JS, Andrews GK & Wood GW (1987) Normal trophoblast resist induction of class I HLA. *Journal of Immunology* **138:** 2481–2487.

Hustin J, Foidart JM, Lambotte R (1983) Maternal vascular lesions in pre-eclampsia and intrauterine growth retardation: light microscopy and immunofluorescence. *Placenta* **4:** 489–498.

Hutton L, Yang SS & Bernstein J (1983) Placenta accreta: a 26-year clinicopathologic review (1956–1981). *New York State Journal of Medicine* **6:** 857–866.

Imamura M, Phillips PE & Mellors RC (1976) The occurrence and frequency of type C virus-like particles in placentas from patients with systemic lupus erythematosus and from normal subjects. *American Journal of Pathology* **83:** 383–394.

Jaameri KEU, Koivuniemi AP & Carpen EO (1965) Occurrence of trophoblasts in the blood of toxaemic patients. *Gynaecologia* **160:** 315–320.

Jenkins DM, O'Neill M & Johnson PM (1983) HLA-DR positive cells in the human amniochorion. *Immunology Letters* **6:** 65–67.

Johnson PM (1984) Immunobiology of the human trophoblast. In Crighton DB (ed.) *Immunological Aspects of Reproduction in Mammals*, pp 109–131. London: Butterworths Press.

Johnson PM & Bulmer JN (1984) Uterine gland epithelium in human pregnancy often lacks detectable maternal MHC antigens but does express fetal trophoblast antigens. *Journal of Immunology* **132:** 1608–1610.

Johnson PM & Molloy CM (1983) Localization in human term placental bed and amniochorion of cells bearing trophoblast antigens identified by monoclonal antibodies. *American Journal of Reproductive Immunology* **4:** 33–37.

Johnson PM, Chia KV & Risk JM (1986) Immunological question marks in recurrent spontaneous abortion. In Clark DA & Croy BA (eds) *Reproductive Immunology 1986*, pp 239–245. Amsterdam: Elsevier Science Publishers.

Johnson PM, Cheng HM, Molloy CM, Stern CMM & Slade MB (1981) Human trophoblast-specific surface antigens identified using monoclonal antibodies. *American Journal of Reproductive Immunology* **1:** 246–254.

Johnson PM, Arnaud P, Werner P & Galbraith RM (1985) Native α_2-macroglobulin binds to a surface component of human placental trophoblast. *Placenta* **6:** 323–328.

Johnson PM, Risk JM, Bulmer JN, Niewola Z & Kimber I (1987) Antigen expression at human maternofetal interfaces. In Gill TJ III & Wegmann TG (eds) *Immunoregulation and Fetal Survival*, pp 181–196. New York: Oxford University Press.

Jones CJP & Fox H (1976) An ultrahistochemical study of the distribution of acid and alkaline phosphatases in placentae from normal and complicated pregnancies. *Journal of Pathology* **118:** 143–150.

Jordan BR, Caillol D, Damotte T et al (1985) HLA class I genes: from structure to expression, serology and function. *Immunological Reviews* **85:** 73–92.

Kabawat SE, Mostoufi-Zadeh M, Berkowitz RS, Driscoll SG & Bhan AK (1985a) Implantation site in normal pregnancy. A study with monoclonal antibodies. *American Journal of Pathology* **118:** 76–84.

Kabawat SE, Mostoufi-Zadeh M, Berkowitz RS et al (1985b) Implantation site in complete molar pregnancy: a study of immunologically competent cells with monoclonal antibodies. *American Journal of Obstetrics and Gynecology* **152:** 97–99.

Kawata M, Parnes JR & Herzenberg LA (1984) Transcriptional control of HLA-A, B, C antigen in human placental cytotrophoblast isolated using trophoblast and HLA-specific monoclonal antibodies and the fluorescence-activated cell sorter. *Journal of Experimental Medicine* **160:** 633–651.

Khong TY (1987) Immunohistologic study of the leukocytic infiltrate in maternal uterine tissues in normal and pre-eclamptic pregnancies at term. *American Journal of Reproductive Immunology and Microbiology* **15:** 1–8.

Khong TY & Robertson WB (1987) Placenta creta and placenta praevia creta. *Placenta* **8:** 399–409.

Khong TY, DeWolf F, Robertson WB & Brosens I (1986) Inadequate maternal vascular response to placentation in pregnancies complicated by pre-eclampsia and by small-for-gestational age infants. *British Journal of Obstetrics and Gynaecology* **93:** 1049–1059.

Khong TY, Liddell HS & Robertson WB (1987) Defective haemochorial placentation as a cause of miscarriage: a preliminary study. *British Journal of Obstetrics and Gynaecology* **94:** 649–655.

Kitzmiller JL & Benirschke K (1973) Immunofluorescent study of placental bed vessels in pre-eclampsia of pregnancy. *American Journal of Obstetrics and Gynecology* **115:** 248–251.

Kitzmiller JL, Watt N & Benirschke K (1981) Decidual arteriopathy in hypertension and diabetes in pregnancy: immunofluorescent studies. *American Journal of Obstetrics and Gynecology* **141:** 773–779.

Kurman RJ, Main CS & Chen H-C (1984a) Intermediate trophoblast: a distinctive form of trophoblast with specific morphological, biochemical and functional features. *Placenta* **5:** 349–370.

Kurman RJ, Young RH, Norris HJ et al (1984b) Immunocytochemical localization of placental lactogen and chorionic gonadotrophin in the normal placenta and trophoblastic tumors, with emphasis on intermediate trophoblast and the placental site trophoblastic tumor. *International Journal of Gynecological Pathology* **3:** 101–121.

Labarrere C & Althabe O (1985) Chronic villitis of unknown etiology and maternal arterial lesions in pre-eclamptic pregnancies. *European Journal of Obstetrics, Gynecology and Reproductive Biology* **20:** 1–11.

Labarrere C & Althabe O (1987) Chronic villitis of unknown aetiology in recurrent intrauterine fetal growth retardation. *Placenta* **8:** 167–173.

Labarrere C, Althabe O & Telenta M (1982) Chronic villitis of unknown aetiology in placentae of idiopathic small for gestational age infants. *Placenta* **3:** 309–318.

Labarrere C, Alonso J, Manni J, Domenichini E & Althabe O (1985) Immunohistochemical findings in acute atherosis associated with intrauterine growth retardation. *American Journal of Reproductive Immunology and Microbiology* **7:** 149–155.

Labarrere CA, Catoggio LJ, Mullen EG & Althabe OH (1986) Placental lesions in maternal autoimmune diseases. *American Journal of Reproductive Immunology and Microbiology* **12:** 78–86.

Lala PK, Parhar RS, Kearns M, Johnson S & Scodras JM (1986) Immunological aspects of the decidual response. In Clark DA & Croy BA (eds) *Reproductive Immunology 1986*, pp 190–198. Amsterdam: Elsevier Science Publishers.

Lalani E-NMA, Bulmer JN & Wells M (1987) Peroxidase-labelled lectin binding of human extravillous trophoblast. *Placenta* **8**: 15–26.

Lanier LL, Le AM, Civin CI, Loken MR & Phillips JH (1986) The relationship of CD16 (leu 11) and leu 19 (NKH1) antigen expression on human peripheral blood NK cells and cytotoxic T lymphocytes. *Journal of Immunology* **136**: 4480–4486.

Laurini RN, Visser GHA, Van Ballegooie E & Schoots CJF (1987) Morphological findings in placentae of insulin-dependent diabetic patients treated with continuous subcutaneous insulin infusion (CSII). *Placenta* **8**: 153–165.

Lawler SD & Fisher RA (1987) Immunogenicity of hydatidiform mole. *Placenta* **8**: 195–199.

Lew AM, Lillehoj EP, Cowan EP, Maloy WL, Van Schravendijk MR & Coligan JE (1986) Class I genes and molecules: an update. *Immunology* **57**: 3–18.

Lichtig C, Deutch M & Brandes J (1984) Vascular changes of endometrium in early pregnancy. *American Journal of Clinical Pathology* **81**: 702–707.

Lichtig C, Deutsch M & Brandes J (1985) Immunofluorescent studies of the endometrial arteries in the first trimester of pregnancy. *American Journal of Clinical Pathology* **83**: 633–636.

Lipinski M, Parks DR, Rouse RV & Herzenberg LA (1981) Human trophoblast cell-surface antigens defined by monoclonal antibodies. *Proceedings of the National Academy of Sciences, USA* **78**: 5147–5150.

Loke YW, Eremin P, Ashby J & Day S (1982) Characterization of the phagocytic cells isolated from the human placenta. *Journal of the Reticuloendothelial Society* **31**: 317–324.

Magid M, Nanney LB, Stoscheck CM & King LE Jr (1985) Epidermal growth factor binding and receptor distribution in term human placenta. *Placenta* **6**: 519–526.

McDicken IW, Stamp GH, McLaughlin PJ & Johnson PM (1983) Expression of human placental-type alkaline phosphatase in primary breast cancer. *International Journal of Cancer* **32**: 205–209.

McDicken IW, McLaughlin PJ, Tromans PM, Luesley DM & Johnson PM (1985) Detection of placental-type alkaline phosphatase in ovarian cancer. *British Journal of Cancer* **52**: 59–64.

McIntyre JA & Faulk WP (1979) Antigens of human trophoblasts: effects of heterologous anti-trophoblast sera on lymphocyte responses in vitro. *Journal of Experimental Medicine* **149**: 824–836.

McIntyre JA, Faulk WP, Verhulst SJ & Colliver J (1983) Human trophoblast–lymphocyte cross-reactive (TLX) antigens define a new alloantigen system. *Science* **222**: 1135–1137.

McLaughlin PJ, Cheng HM, Slade MB & Johnson PM (1982) Expression on cultured human tumour cells of placental trophoblast membrane antigens and placental alkaline phosphatase defined by monoclonal antibodies. *International Journal of Cancer* **30**: 21–26.

McLaughlin PJ, Warne PH, Hutchinson GE, Johnson PM & Tucker DF (1987) Placental-type alkaline phosphatase in cervical neoplasia. *British Journal of Cancer* **55**: 197–201.

Mowbray JF, Gibbings C, Liddell H, Reginald PW, Underwood JL & Beard RW (1985) Controlled trial of treatment of recurrent spontaneous abortion by immunisation with paternal cells. *Lancet* **i**: 941–943.

Muller R, Tremblay JM, Adamson ED & Verma IM (1983) Tissue and cell type-specific expression of two human c-*onc* genes. *Nature* **304**: 454–456.

Nebel L, Fein A, Rudak E, Blank M, Mashiach S, Dor J, Lerran D & Goldman B (1986) Structural aspects of embryo failure following in-vitro fertilization and embryo transfer; immune rejection or malimplantation. In Clark DA & Croy BA (eds) *Reproductive Immunology 1986*, pp 227–235. Amsterdam: Elsevier Science Publishers.

Nehemiah JL, Schnitzer JA, Schulman H & Novikoff AB (1981) Human chorionic trophoblasts, decidual cells and macrophages: a histochemical and electron microscopic study. *American Journal of Obstetrics and Gynecology* **140**: 261–268.

Neighbour PA, Huberman HS & Kress Y (1982) Human large granular lymphocytes and natural killing: ultrastructural studies of strontium-induced degranulation. *European Journal of Immunology* **12**: 588–595.

Oksenberg JR, Mor Yosef S, Persitz E et al (1986) Antigen presenting cells in human decidual tissue. *American Journal of Reproductive Immunology and Microbiology* **11**: 82–88.

Ortonne J-P, Hsi B-L, Verrando P et al (1987) Herpes gestationis factor reacts with the amniotic epithelial basement membrane. *British Journal of Dermatology* **117**: 147–154.

Pattillo RA, Hussa RO, Yorde DE & Cole LA (1983) Hormone synthesis by normal and neoplastic human trophoblast. In Loke YW & White A (eds) *Biology of Trophoblast*, pp 283–316. Amsterdam: Elsevier Science Publishers.

Pauerstein CJ, Croxatto HB, Eddy CA, Ramzy I & Walters MD (1986) Anatomy and pathology of tubal pregnancy. *Obstetrics and Gynecology* **67**: 301–308.

Pfeifer-Ohlsson S, Goustin AS, Rydnert J et al (1984) Spatial and temporal pattern of cellular *myc* oncogene expression in developing human placenta: implications for embryonic cell proliferation. *Cell* **38**: 585–596.

Pijnenborg R, Dixon G, Robertson WB & Brosens I (1980) Trophoblast invasion of human decidua from 8–18 weeks of pregnancy. *Placenta* **1**: 3–19.

Pinkerton JHM (1963) The placental bed arterioles in diabetes. *Proceedings of the Royal Society of Medicine* **56**: 1021–1022.

Redman CWG (1983) HLA-DR antigen on human trophoblast: a review. *American Journal of Reproductive Immunology* **3**: 175–177.

Redman CWG, McMichael AJ, Stirrat GM, Sunderland CA & Ting A (1984) Class I major histocompatibility complex antigens on human extravillous trophoblast. *Immunology* **52**: 457–468.

Richards RC, Beardmore JM, Brown PJ, Molloy CM & Johnson PM (1983) Epidermal growth factor receptors on isolated human placental syncytiotrophoblast plasma membrane. *Placenta* **4**: 133–138.

Risteli J, Roidart JM, Risteli L, Boniver J & Goffinet G (1984) The basement membrane proteins laminin and type IV collagen in isolated villi in pre-eclampsia. *Placenta* **5**: 541–550.

Ritson A & Bulmer JN (1987a) Endometrial granulocytes in human decidua react with a natural-killer (NK) cell marker. NKH1. *Immunology* **62**: 329–331.

Ritson A & Bulmer JN (1987b) Extraction of leucocytes from human decidua. A comparison of dispersal techniques. *Journal of Immunological Methods* **104**: 231–236.

Robertson WB (1976) Uteroplacental vasculature. *Journal of Clinical Pathology* **29** (supplement; Royal College of Pathology), **10**: 9–17.

Robertson WB (1979) Uteroplacental bloodflow in maternal diabetes. In Sutherland HW & Stowers JM (eds) *Carbohydrate Metabolism in Pregnancy and the Newborn, 1978*, pp 63–75. Berlin, Heidelberg and New York: Springer-Verlag.

Robertson WB, Brosens I & Dixon HG (1967) The pathological response of the vessels of the placental bed to hypertensive pregnancy. *Journal of Pathology and Bacteriology* **93**: 581–592.

Robertson WB, Khong TY, Brosens I et al (1986) The placental bed biopsy: review from three European centers. *American Journal of Obstetrics and Gynecology* **155**: 401–412.

Russell P (1980) Inflammatory lesions of the human placenta. III: The histopathology of villitis of unknown aetiology. *Placenta* **1**: 227–244.

Russell P, Atkinson K & Krishnan L (1980) Recurrent reproductive failure due to severe placental villitis of unknown etiology. *Journal of Reproductive Medicine* **24**: 93–98.

Saksela O, Wahlstrom T, Lehtovirta P, Seppala M & Vaheri A (1981) Presence of α_2-macroglobulin in normal but not in malignant human syncytiotrophoblast. *Cancer Research* **41**: 2507–2513.

Sarkar S, Kacinski BM, Kohorn EI, Merino MJ, Carter D & Blakemore KJ (1986) Demonstration of myc and ras oncogene expression by hybridisation in situ in hydatidiform mole and in the BeWo choriocarcinoma cell line. *American Journal of Obstetrics and Gynecology* **154**: 390–393.

Sasagawa M, Watanabe S, Ohmomo Y et al (1986) Reactivity of two monoclonal antibodies (Troma 1 and CAM 5.2) on human tissue sections: analysis of their usefulness as a histological trophoblast marker in normal pregnancy and trophoblastic disease. *International Journal of Gynecological Pathology* **5**: 345–356.

Sasagawa M, Ohmomo Y, Kanazawa K & Takeuchi S (1987) HLA expression by trophoblast of invasive moles. *Placenta* **8**: 111–118.

Seppala M, Wahlstrom T & Bohn H (1979) Circulating levels and tissue localization of placental protein 5 (PP5) in pregnancy and trophoblastic disease: absence of PP5 expression in the malignant trophoblast. *International Journal of Cancer* **24**: 6–10.

Sheppard BL & Bonnar J (1976) The ultrastructure of the arterial supply of the human placenta in pregnancy complicated by growth retardation. *British Journal of Obstetrics and Gynaecology* **83**: 948–959.

Sheppard BL & Bonnar J (1981) An ultrastructural study of uteroplacental spiral arteries in hypertensive and normotensive pregnancy and fetal growth retardation. *British Journal of Obstetrics and Gynaecology* **88**: 695–705.

Sinha D, Wells M & Faulk WP (1984) Immunological studies of human placentae: complement components in pre-eclamptic chorionic villi. *Clinical and Experimental Immunology* **56**: 175–184.

Sinosich MJ, Smith DH, Grudzinskas JG et al (1983) The prediction of pregnancy failure by measurement of pregnancy-associated plasma protein A (PAPP-A) following in-vitro fertilization and embryo transfer. *Fertility and Sterility* **40**: 539–541.

Slapsys RM, Richards CD & Clark DA (1986) Active suppression of host-versus-graft reaction in pregnant mice. VIII. The uterine decidua-associated suppressor cell is distinct from decidual NK cells. *Cellular Immunology* **99**: 140–149.

Soubiran P, Zapitelli JP & Schaffar L (1987) IL2-like material is present in human placenta and amnion. *Journal of Reproductive Immunology* **12**: 225–234.

Stern PL, Beresford N, Friedman CI et al (1986a) Class I-like MHC molecules expressed by baboon placental syncytiotrophoblast. *Journal of Immunology* **138**: 1088–1091.

Stern PL, Beresford N, Thompson S et al (1986b) Characterization of the human trophoblast-leukocyte antigenic molecules defined by a monoclonal antibody. *Journal of Immunology* **137**: 1604–1609.

Stern PL, Morris AC, Beresford N, Johnson PM & Hole N (1986c) Molecular characterisation of human teratocarcinoma-trophoblast cell surface antigens. In Clark DA & Croy BA (eds) *Reproductive Immunology 1986*, pp 67–74. Amsterdam: Elsevier Science Publishers.

Stromberg K, Pigott DA, Ranchalis JE & Twardzik DR (1982) Human term placenta contains transforming growth factors. *Biochemical and Biophysical Research Communications* **106**: 354–361.

Sunderland CA, Naiem M, Mason DY, Redman DWG & Stirrat GM (1981a) The expression of major histocompatibility antigens by human chorionic villi. *Journal of Reproductive Immunology* **3**: 323–331.

Sunderland CA, Redman CWG & Stirrat GM (1981b) HLA-A, B, C antigens are expressed on nonvillous trophoblast of the early human placenta. *Journal of Immunology* **127**: 2614–2615.

Sunderland CA, Redman CWG & Stirrat GM (1981c) Monoclonal antibodies to human syncytiotrophoblast. *Immunology* **43**: 541–546.

Sunderland CA, Davies JO & Stirrat GM (1984) Immunohistology of normal and ovarian cancer tissue with a monoclonal antibody to placental alkaline phosphatase. *Cancer Research* **44**: 4496–4502.

Sunderland CA, Redman CWG & Stirrat GM (1985a) Characterization and localization of HLA antigens on hydatidiform mole. *American Journal of Obstetrics and Gynecology* **151**: 130–135.

Sunderland CA, Bulmer JN, Luscombe M, Redman CWG & Stirrat GM (1985b) Immuno-histological and biochemical evidence for a role for hyaluronic acid in the growth and development of the placenta. *Journal of Reproductive Immunology* **8**: 197–212.

Sunderland CA, Sasagawa M, Kanazawa K, Stirrat GM & Takeuchi S (1985c) An immuno-histochemical study of HLA antigen expression by gestational choriocarcinoma. *British Journal of Cancer* **51**: 809–814.

Suni J, Narvanen A, Wahlstrom T, Aho M, Pakkanen R, Vaheri A, Copeland T, Cohen M & Oroszlan S (1984) Human placental syncytiotrophoblastic Mr 75 000 polypeptide defined by antibodies to a synthetic peptide based on a cloned human endogenous retroviral sequence. *Proceedings of the National Academy of Science USA* **81**: 6197–6201.

Sutton L, Mason DY & Redman CWG (1983) HLA-DR positive cells in the human placenta. *Immunology* **49**: 103–113.

Sutton L, Gadd M, Mason DY & Redman CWG (1986) Cells bearing class II MHC antigens in the human placenta and amniochorion. *Immunology* **58**: 23–29.

Takahashi H, Adachi S, Yoshiya N, Suzuki T, Kanazawa K & Takeuchi S (1987) Expression of HLA-DR molecules in human gestational choriocarcinoma cell lines and malignant cell lines. *Placenta* **8**: 293–298.

Tanaka K, Nabeshima Y, Takahashi H, Takeuchi S, Nabeshima Y & Ogata K (1981) Lack of effective messenger RNA for β_2-microglobulin in a gestational human choriocarcinoma cell line (GCH-1). *Cancer Research* **41:** 3639–3641.

Tawfik OW, Hunt JS & Wood GW (1986) Implication of prostaglandin E_2 in soluble factor-mediated immune suppression by murine decidual cells. *American Journal of Reproductive Immunology and Microbiology* **12:** 111–117.

Taylor C & Faulk WP (1981) Prevention of recurrent abortions with leukocyte transfusions. *Lancet* **ii:** 68–70.

Tekelioglu-Uysal M, Edwards RG & Kisnisci HA (1975) Ultrastructural relationships between decidua, trophoblast and lymphocytes at the beginning of human pregnancy. *Journal of Reproduction and Fertility* **42:** 431–438.

Theofilopoulos AN, Gleicher N, Pereira AB & Dixon FJ (1981) The biology of immune complexes and their possible role in pregnancy. *American Journal of Reproductive Immunology and Microbiology* **1:** 92–105.

Toder V, Altaratz H, Shepshelovich J, Fein A & Nebel L (1987) Immunoregulation of cytokines at the placenta. In Chaouat G (ed.) *Reproductive Immunology: Materno-Fetal Relationship*, pp 131–139. Paris: Inserm.

van Leeuwen A, Giphart MJ, de Groot G, Festenstein H & van Rood JJ (1985) Two different T-cell systems in humans, one of which is probably equivalent to Qa or Tla in mice. *Human Immunology* **12:** 235–246.

Vardi I & Halbrecht I (1974) Toxemia of pregnancy: 1. Antigens associated with toxaemia of pregnancy in placental connective tissue. *American Journal of Obstetrics and Gynecology* **118:** 552–558.

Wahlstrom T, Nieminen P, Narvanen A, Suni J, Lehtovirta P, Saksela E & Vaheri A (1984) Monoclonal antibody defining a human syncytiotrophoblastic polypeptide immunologically related to mammalian retrovirus structural protein p30. *Placenta* **5:** 465–474.

Webb PD, Evans PW, Molloy CM & Johnson PM (1985) Biochemical studies of human placental microvillous plasma membrane proteins. *American Journal of Reproductive Immunology and Microbiology* **8:** 113–117.

Weir PE (1981) Immunofluorescent studies of the uteroplacental arteries in normal pregnancy. *British Journal of Obstetrics and Gynaecology* **88:** 301–307.

Wells M, Hsi B-L & Faulk WP (1984) Class I antigens of the major histocompatibility complex on cytotrophoblast of the human placental basal plate. *American Journal of Reproductive Immunology* **6:** 167–174.

Wells M, Bennett J, Bulmer JN, Jackson P & Holgate CS (1987) Complement component deposition in uteroplacental (spiral) arteries in normal human pregnancy. *Journal of Reproductive Immunology* **12:** 125–135.

Westergaard JG, Sinosich MJ, Bugge M et al (1983) Pregnancy-associated plasma protein A in the prediction of early pregnancy failure. *American Journal of Obstetrics and Gynecology* **145:** 67–69.

Whyte A (1983) Biochemistry of the human syncytiotrophoblastic plasma membrane. In Loke YW & Whyte A (eds) *Biology of Trophoblast*, pp 513–533. Amsterdam: Elsevier Science Publishers.

Whyte A, Ragge N, Loke YW & Thiry L (1985) Human syncytiotrophoblast membrane proteins defined using a heterologous antiserum. *Clinical and Experimental Immunology* **59:** 227–234.

Wild AE (1983) Trophoblast cell surface receptors. In Loke YW & Whyte A (eds) *Biology of Trophoblast*, pp 472–512. Amsterdam: Elsevier Science Publishers.

Wislocki GB & Bennett HS (1943) The histology and cytology of the human and monkey placenta, with special reference to the trophoblast. *American Journal of Anatomy* **73:** 335–449.

Wood GW (1980) Mononuclear phagocytes in the human placenta. *Placenta* **1:** 113–123.

Yeh C-JG, Hsi B-L, Samson M et al (1987) Monoclonal antibodies (GB16, GB18, GB19, GB22) raised against human placental microvilli recognize the transferrin receptor. *Placenta* **8:** 627–638.

Zuckerman FA & Head JR (1986) Expression of the MHC antigens on murine trophoblast and their modulation by interferon. *Journal of Immunology* **137:** 846–853.

9

Pregnancy and host resistance

C. A. HART

In mammalian pregnancy, the antigenically foreign fetus and placenta are tolerated by the mother. It has been suggested that maternal immune responsiveness is depressed and this might assist the fetal allograft to implant and survive (Rocklin et al, 1979). Whether this diminished response is entirely limited to the fetal allograft or extends to other facets of the immune system is unclear. This chapter examines the effect of pregnancy on host resistance. If diminished maternal immune responsiveness in pregnancy does depress host resistance (Purtilo et al, 1972), this would manifest itself in at least four areas (Table 1). Infection may occur more frequently in immunocompromised hosts; it may be more severe, it may become disseminated more easily, or latent viruses such as varicella-zoster may reactivate more readily. Administration of vaccines to immunocom-

Table 1. Manifestations of decreased host resistance in pregnancy.

Infection
  Increased incidence
  Localized infection becoming generalized
  More severe infection
  Low grade pathogens producing symptomatic infection
  Recurrence of infection to which individual is immune
  Increased frequency of recurrence of latent infection
  Increased frequency of reactivation of latent viruses
  Diminished immune response to latent viruses
  Increased risk due to mechanical or hormonal factors
  Increased risk due to presence of placenta and fetus

Immunization
  Vaccine take
  Immune response to vaccine
  Effect of live attenuated vaccine

Malignant tumours
  Increased incidence
  Secondary spread

Transplantation
  Graft survival
  Graft vs host

promised patients may result in lack of response, as measured immunologically or as seen by lack of protection, or there may be problems with live attenuated vaccines in producing the disease which they are designed to prevent. Immune surveillance is an important mechanism for preventing or limiting the spread of malignant tumours, and decreased host resistance may become obvious by an increased incidence of malignancies. Finally, the resistance to other tissue allografts might also be diminished in pregnancy.

SUSCEPTIBILITY TO INFECTION

There are tremendous logistical problems in determining whether there is an increased risk of susceptibility to infection in pregnant women and it is necessary to follow large numbers of pregnancies. Perhaps because of this, there is a dearth of information on the incidence and severity of infection in pregnancy. Similarly, there is a paucity of comparative information on non-pregnant women of child-bearing age. Some information is available on specific infections, however, and will be reviewed here. In contrast, there is a wealth of information on transplacental infection of the fetus and its effect on the neonate (Lambert and Wood, 1981); the temptation to concentrate on this aspect will be avoided.

Incidence of infection

There are two major surveys published on infections in pregnancy, both of which concentrate on viral infections. A survey in the United States was carried out over the period 1958 to 1964 involving a total of 30 059 pregnancies (Sever and White, 1968; Catalano and Sever, 1971). Approximately 1600 women (5.2%) experienced definite or presumed viral infection during pregnancy. All viral illnesses were included except for the common cold. A single infective episode was experienced by 4.8% of the women, two episodes by 0.4% and more than two episodes by 0.03%. The majority (58%) of these were 'flu-like' upper respiratory tract infections. Herpes labialis occurred at a rate of 12 per 1000 pregnancies, laryngotracheitis at 3.2 per 1000, gastroenteritis at 1.7 per 1000 and conjunctivitis at 0.4 per 1000 pregnancies. Of the childhood infectious diseases, rates of 1.5 per 1000 pregnancies were complicated by mumps, 1.1 per 1000 by rubella (this rose to 22–30 per 1000 in epidemics), 0.7 per 1000 by chickenpox and 0.4 per 1000 by measles. Viral pneumonia, infectious mononucleosis and hepatitis were reported far less frequently. Serological investigation confirmed 66% of the cases of rubella, 20% of measles (30% of suspected cases proved to be rubella) and 70% of varicella-zoster and mumps. In addition, 2% of the women were found subsequently to have had subclinical viral infections on serological testing.

A British survey revealed that, of 16 994 pregnancies delivered in one week in 1958, 34 (0.2%) were complicated by one of seven infectious diseases (Butler, 1973). Three women had chickenpox, seven had shingles, eleven had rubella, four had mumps, two had measles, five had infectious hepatitis and one had pertussis.

To derive any conclusions from these studies, it is necessary to have control data from age-matched women who were not pregnant, over the same time period, and from the same geographical areas. The latter two points are of some importance since the incidence of infectious diseases varies over time and will now be influenced by immunization programmes. Unfortunately, no such control data are available. The rates of infection quoted in the two surveys, however, do not seem very high. For example, it is estimated that each adult will have at least one episode of gastroenteritis and two to three episodes of upper respiratory tract infection each year.

Localized infection becoming generalized

Examples of pathogens that cause localized infection becoming generalized in the immunocompromised host include herpes simplex virus (labialis or genitalis) or herpes zoster (shingles) in renal transplant recipients or patients on chemotherapy, *Neisseria gonorrhoea* in individuals with defects in the final components of the complement cascade and *Candida albicans* in neonates (Hensey et al, 1984).

There is little evidence to suggest that pregnancy encourages such dissemination. Gonorrhoea does occur in pregnancy, but the major risk is of the neonate acquiring ophthalmia neonatorum during delivery. Vaginal thrush is also a not uncommon problem during pregnancy and there is no evidence of dissemination. A total of 43 cases of zoster occurring in pregnancy have been reported (Brazin et al, 1979; Enders, 1984; Paryani and Arvin, 1986). Only one (2%) of these patients showed evidence of dissemination (ten cutaneous lesions outside the primary dermatome). However, a few extradermatomal lesions can be found in cases of zoster in otherwise healthy individuals (Schauf and Toplin, 1984). In contrast, between 25% and 50% of immunocompromised patients with zoster will show major dissemination of the virus (Schauf and Toplin, 1984). Similarly, of 29 women who acquired genital herpes during pregnancy, none had disseminated disease (Brown et al, 1987). There is one report of primary oral mucocutaneous herpes simplex becoming disseminated in pregnancy leading to infection of the fetus and death (Peacock and Sarubbi, 1983). Pregnancy does seem to increase the risk of dissemination of the fungal pathogen *Coccidiodes immitis* (Purtilo, 1975).

Increased severity of infection

Many micro-organisms produce a much more severe infection in the immunocompromised host. Examples include measles virus which produces giant cell pneumonia only in the immunocompromised host (Mitus et al, 1959), and cytomegalovirus which can produce pneumonitis, enteritis and hepatitis. In pregnant women, severity of infection can be assessed in terms of severity of the disease itself and by the effect of the infection on the continuation of the pregnancy. The latter point will be discussed in a later section.

The evidence available on severity of viral and non-viral infections in pregnancy is summarized in Tables 2 and 3, respectively.

Pregnancy increases the susceptibility of mice to Coxsackie B virus (Dalldorf and Gifford, 1954), and cases of aseptic meningitis, pleurodynia and pericarditis due to Coxsackie B-5 are reported to occur more readily in pregnant women (Plager et al, 1962). Similarly, pregnancy and parturition may be associated with a greater risk of paralysis by poliovirus infection (Siegel and Greenberg, 1955). Early reports indicated that hepatitis had an increased mortality during pregnancy (Snyderman, 1985). However, these were based mostly on clinical diagnosis and could be related more to malnutrition and anaemia rather than immune depression (D'Cruz et al, 1968).

There is no evidence to suggest that infection by rubellavirus, lymphocytic choriomeningitis virus, morbillivirus or mumps virus is associated with a more severe disease, but infection by mumps virus in the immunocompromised host does not differ from that in healthy hosts. Initial reports suggested that Asian 'flu' was associated with a higher mortality in pregnant women (Freeman and Barno, 1959). This was not observed in subsequent surveys (Butler, 1973). There are several reports that infection with the arenavirus that causes Lassa fever is associated with stillbirth and increased mortality (see C. J. Peters, 1984). However, the pathogenesis of Lassa fever involves decomplementation and it is conceivable that the complement cascade is more readily activated in pregnancy. There are no reports of human immune deficiency virus (HIV) being acquired by women during pregnancy but, in one woman who became infected via a blood transfusion immediately after delivery, the natural history of the infection was not abnormal (Ziegler et al, 1985). Several cohorts of pregnant women who were already infected by HIV have been studied and it does not seem that there is an increased risk of development of the acquired immune deficiency syndrome (AIDS) during pregnancy (e.g. Thomas et al, 1987). Being already infected with HIV does not appear to affect the outcome of pregnancy (Johnstone et al, 1988).

The recently described human parvovirus (B19) causes erythema infectiosum. B19 infections occurring in six pregnant women resulted in clinical manifestations in only two (Anand et al, 1987). The two human polyomaviruses, JC and BK, reactivate more frequently in pregnancy but produce no clinical manifestations (Coleman et al, 1980). In contrast, JC virus is known to cause progressive multifocal leucoencephalopathy in the immunocompromised host (Walker, 1978). Much of the evidence for increased severity of hepatitis B virus and non-A non-B hepatitis (due to several viruses, including a retrovirus) comes from the surveys described above (Snyderman, 1985). Subsequent studies have shown that there is no greater risk with hepatitis B virus or non-A non-B hepatitis (Gerety and Schweitzer, 1977), but infections in the last trimester might increase the risk of prematurity (Hieber et al, 1977).

Of the herpes viruses, neither cytomegalovirus (CMV) nor Epstein–Barr virus (EBV) seem to be associated with increased severity in pregnancy. For example, of three women who seroconverted with EBV during pregnancy,

Table 2. Severity of viral infections during pregnancy.

	Increase	No increase
RNA viruses		
Picornaviridae		
Poliovirus	+	−
Coxsackie B	+	−
Hepatitis A (Enterovirus 72)	+	+
Reoviridae		
Rotavirus	−	+
Togaviridae		
Rubellavirus	−	+
Arenaviridae		
Lassa	+	−
Lymphocytic choriomeningitis	−	+
Retroviridae		
HIV	−	+
Myxoviridae		
Influenza	+	+
Measles	−	+
Mumps	−	+
DNA viruses		
Parvoviridae		
B19	−	+
Polyomaviridae		
BK	−	+
JC	−	+
Hepadnaviridae		
Hepatitis B	+	+
Herpetoviridae		
Herpes simplex	(+)	+
Varicella-zoster	+	+
Cytomegalovirus	−	+
Epstein–Barr virus	−	+
Poxviridae		
Smallpox	+	−
Miscellaneous		
Non-A non-B hepatitis	−	+

Table 3. Severity of non-viral infections in pregnancy.

	Increase	No increase
Bacteria		
Listeria monocytogenes	−	+
Mycobacterium tuberculosis	+	+
Chlamydia psittaci	+	−
Treponema pallidum	−	+
Protozoa		
Plasmodium falciparum	+	−
Toxoplasma gondii	−	+

all had unremarkable disease (Fleisher and Bolognese, 1984). Apart from the case alluded to earlier (Peacock and Sarubbi, 1983), infection with herpes simplex virus in pregnancy appears no more likely to be severe than in other healthy individuals. It does appear that varicella pneumonia occurs more readily in pregnant women with chickenpox (Harris and Rhoades, 1965; Enders, 1984; Paryani and Arvin, 1986). Moreover, of 21 reported cases of varicella pneumonia in pregnancy, 8 (38%) proved fatal (Harris and Rhoades, 1965; Paryani and Arvin, 1986) whereas the mortality in 173 non-pregnant adults was 17% (quoted in Harris and Rhoades, 1965). The increased risk of varicella pneumonia has been attributed to decreased maternal respiratory activity, presumably due to pressure from the conceptus (Pickard, 1968). If this were so, cases of varicella pneumonia should occur more commonly in the second half of pregnancy; it is noteworthy that seventeen of twenty (85%) cases where gestational age was given occurred at six months or later (Harris and Rhoades, 1965; Paryani and Arvin, 1986). Shingles is no more severe in pregnancy than at other times.

Smallpox infection used to occur in pregnant women and such infections were reported to be more frequently fatal. In unvaccinated pregnant women in Madras, 61% who contracted smallpox died compared with an overall mortality of 35%, and 27% of vaccinated women who became infected in pregnancy died compared with a mortality of 6% in all cases (Rao, 1972). In addition, 50% of the cases of haemorrhagic smallpox seen in Madras had occurred in pregnant women (Rao, 1972). This might bear some relationship to the increased mortality in pregnant women observed with the haemorrhagic fever, Lassa fever (C. J. Peters, 1984). Apart from a few exceptions, there is little specific information on severity of non-viral infections in pregnancy. This would suggest that such infections are unlikely to be problematical. The Gram-positive bacillus *Listeria monocytogenes* is known to damage the developing fetus and neonate. It can produce a spectrum of disease in the immunocompetent host ranging from fatal meningitis and septicaemia to a 'flu-like' illness. Examination of outbreaks reveals that the pattern of infection in pregnant women does not differ significantly from the normal spectrum (e.g. Lennon et al, 1984).

Although there were suggestions of development of anergy to tuberculin in pregnancy, there is no clinical evidence of relapse of tuberculosis (De March, 1975).

The Ewe Abortion Agent (*Chlamydia psittaci*), as its name implies, is a cause of abortion and stillbirth in sheep. Infection of pregnant women (generally farmers' wives) by this agent has been described and is severe, being accompanied by disseminated intravascular coagulation and septic shock (Johnson et al, 1985). However, infection occurring in non-pregnant individuals has not been described and hence it is difficult to ascertain whether infection is more severe in pregnancy.

The protozoon *Toxoplasma gondii* can produce both symptomatic and inapparent infection. Although toxoplasma can cross the placenta to infect the fetus, with dire consequences, the spectrum of maternal infection does not differ from that in other adults. For example, of 746 cases of maternal toxoplasmosis, 40% had signs of infection which were usually mild and associated with persistent occipital or submaxillary adenitis (Daffos et al, 1988).

Finally, malaria (especially if due to *Plasmodium falciparum*) appears to be more hazardous during pregnancy (Bruce-Chwatt, 1983). In areas where malaria is highly endemic and adults may have some immunity, the prevalence of clinical malaria is higher and the disease more severe in pregnant women than in other adults especially if it occurs in the final trimester (Bray and Anderson, 1979). The mechanism is unclear, but it has been suggested that there is a suppression of both specific antibody formation and cell-mediated immunity (Weidanz, 1982).

Low grade pathogen producing symptomatic disease

This section overlaps to a large extent with the previous one. Infections with cytomegalovirus largely go unnoticed, although occasionally the syndrome of infectious mononucleosis can occur. There is no evidence that this pattern is altered in pregnancy. Pregnancy does not increase the risk of acquiring CMV infection and several surveys have demonstrated that primary CMV infections in pregnancy are asymptomatic (see Stagno and Whitley, 1985). Infection with rubella virus is inapparent in about 50% of all cases (Green et al, 1965) and approximately 67% of cases occurring in pregnancy are also subclinical (Sever et al, 1965).

Recurrence of infection to which the individual is imune

There are anecdotal reports of second or even third attacks of childhood infectious disease occurring in previously infected individuals, including rubella and measles (Watson, 1965) and chickenpox. There is no evidence that this happens in pregnancy, despite undoubtedly high frequency of exposure.

LATENT AND PERSISTENT INFECTION

Many pathogens remain in close association with their host for long periods after the initial infection. These may be divided broadly into latent and persistent infections, although there is some overlap between the two. The majority of such infections are viral.

Latent infections follow an acute or primary infection. The virus remains dormant within the tissues and is usually not detectable antigenically. Viral genome can be detected and can be reactivated, generally using organ culture. The virus may be reactivated in vivo, when it can be detected immunologically or by simple culture. If the virus produces a lesion following reactivation, this is termed recrudescence (Wildy et al, 1982). With persistent infection, virus is present continuously and can be detected either antigenically or by simple culture. Persistent infection may be either asymptomatic, as is the case with cytomegalovirus, or can occasionally produce disease as is the case with hepatitis B virus and glomerulonephritis.

In general, virus does not replicate during latency and is present either integrated into the host cell chromosomes or as an episome. With persistent infection, the virus is continually replicating. Examples of latent and persistent infections, together with sites of infection, are given in Table 4.

Table 4. Latent and persistent viral infection.

Virus	Site of latency
Latent	
Human immune deficiency virus	$CD4^+$ lymphocytes, brain cells
Herpes simplex	Trigeminal or sacral ganglia
Varicella-zoster	Dorsal root ganglia
JC and BK viruses	Kidney
Human papillomavirus	Squamous epithelium
Persistent	
Measles	Brain (in subacute sclerosing panencephalitis)
Hepatitis B virus	Hepatocytes
Cytomegalovirus	Mononuclear leukocytes, ?cervical and oral mucosae
Epstein–Barr virus	B lymphocytes, pharyngeal mucosa
Adenovirus	Lymphoid tissue

Latent infection

Herpes simplex virus is an α-herpesvirus and causes a mild or inapparent primary infection in childhood during which virus is transported intra-axonally to the trigeminal (herpes labialis) or sacral (herpes genitalis) ganglia, depending upon the site of primary infection. During latency, viral DNA, but not RNA, can be detected. The whole genome except for the terminal repeats is present, suggesting that virus is integrated into the chromosome or present as concatemers (Puga et al, 1984). HSV reactivates relatively frequently and passes again intra-axonally to the mucosa. The mechanism of reactivation is unknown but DNA demethylation might be involved (Whitby et al, 1987). Virus may be shed asymptomatically (the more frequent event), or produce the characteristic vesicles of herpes labialis ('cold sore') or herpes genitalis (Spruance, 1984). The development of lesions or recrudescence depends upon many factors, including the presence of prostaglandins (Harbour et al, 1978). The role of the immune system in preventing reactivation is unclear. Virus is transported from the ganglion intracellularly to the body surface and virus-specific antigens do not seem to be present on the neuronal cell surface (Wildy and Gell, 1985). Recrudescence is under immunological control and immune deficiency leads to a higher incidence of recrudescence, to longer periods of virus shedding and to prolongation of symptoms (Corey and Spear, 1986). There are no large longitudinal studies of serological response, asymptomatic viral shedding or recrudescence of HSV1 or HSV2 during pregnancy, but there is little evidence to suggest an increase. In a longitudinal survey of nine women who acquired primary genital herpes before 30 weeks gestation and of 13 women with established genital herpes, 56% and 69% respectively, showed at least one recrudescence during the pregnancy and rates of recrudescence were 0.23 and 0.31 per month (Brown et al, 1987). Asymptomatic excretion was more common after a primary infection (10.6% of patients per week) than in those patients with recrudescence (0.5% of patients per week). These figures are not significantly different from those for non-pregnant women (Corey and Spear, 1986). The frequency of shedding does not fluctuate during gestation (Horger et al, 1983).

The primary infection with varicella-zoster virus (VZV; chickenpox) is followed by intra-axonal transport to the dorsal root ganglia (generally thoracic). The virus remains in firm latency (unlike HSV) and does not reactivate spontaneously. When immunity wanes, recrudescence occurs with the classical features of shingles. Again, shingles occurs frequently in immunocompromised patients. Little is known about the frequency of occurrence of zoster in pregnancy (Enders, 1984). However, in a recent survey, one of 43 women who developed varicella in pregnancy developed zoster during the same pregnancy (Paryani and Arvin, 1986). Antibody response to VZV in pregnancy does not differ from that in the non-pregnant woman (Enders, 1984).

The polyoma viruses BK and JC both reactivate more frequently in pregnancy than in non-pregnant women. Serological evidence indicates that reactivation occurs in 5–10% of pregnant women compared with less than 5% in adults (Hogan et al, 1984). It is suggested that increased reactivation is due to immunological alterations in pregnancy, since excretion of virus ceases after birth (Coleman et al, 1980).

Human papillomaviruses are DNA viruses that cause genital and other warts. An association between human papillomaviruses 16 and 33 and cervical intraepithelial neoplasia has been described (McCance et al, 1983; Campion et al, 1986; Beaudenon et al, 1986). This virus has not been cultured and detection of antigen is difficult. Viral DNA can, however, often be found integrated in the host cell chromosome. Carcinoma of the cervix is thought to be more invasive in pregnancy.

Persistent infection

Following primary infection with the γ-herpesvirus, Epstein–Barr virus (EBV), a persistent infection is set up in the pharyngeal epithelium and B lymphocytes can be shown to contain EBV genome (Rickinson et al, 1985). At any one time between 10 and 25% of those infected can be shown to be excreting EBV. It appears that there are two populations, 'high-virus shedders' from whom large numbers of virus particles are excreted on each occasion tested, and 'low-virus shedders' from whom low numbers of EBV are detected infrequently. Renal allograft recipients become 'high-shedders' on immunosuppression and over 90% of such patients are EBV excretors. This occurs in the presence of high antibody titres to antigens expressed by replicating virus. EBV appears to be reactivated more readily during pregnancy. Persistently infected pregnant women (55%) are more likely to have antibody to early antigen (marker for replication) than non-pregnant women (25%), and are more likely to be pharyngeal virus excreters (29% versus 18%) (Stagno and Whitley, 1985). Such reactivations do not seem to harm the fetus (Fleisher and Bolognese, 1984).

Apart from rubellavirus, the β-herpesvirus cytomegalovirus (CMV) is probably the best studied virus in pregnancy. Unlike rubellavirus, there is no vaccine for CMV. Primary infection with CMV is inapparent in the vast majority of cases, but exceptions include the mononucleosis syndrome which is most commonly due to transfusion of infected blood. The site of virus persistence is certain. Virus can be recovered from peripheral blood mononuclear cells and is excreted in urine, saliva and cervical secretions (Griffiths, 1987). Excretion rates vary and, as is the case for EBV, there appear to be both high and low virus shedders. Approximately 10% of pregnant and non-pregnant women excrete CMV from one or more sites, but excretion drops after the age of 30. Early reports indicated that CMV excretion rose as pregnancy progressed. When longitudinal studies on a cohort of women were carried out, it became apparent that CMV excretion was suppressed in early pregnancy and rose to 'normal' levels as pregnancy progressed (Stagno et al, 1975). The mechanism of suppression is unclear, although a hormonal link was suggested by the finding that certain human chorionic gonadotrophin (hCG) preparations inhibited CMV replication. Unfortunately, pure hCG had no effect.

Excretion of CMV occurs in the presence of high titres of specific antibody and titres do not fluctuate unduly in pregnancy (Gehrz et al, 1981). Information on cell-mediated immunity (CMI) to CMV is conflicting. Several studies have demonstrated depressed CMI to CMV in mothers and their congenitally infected offspring. A longitudinal study of CMI (as measured by lymphocyte transformation) to CMV in seropositive pregnant women revealed that responses to CMV antigen became markedly depressed by the third trimester. This depression was specific for CMV, since response to phytohaemagglutinin did not alter, but none of the subjects excreted CMV during the study (Gehrz et al, 1981). Brunham and colleagues (1983) found that lymphocyte transformation responses to phytohaemagglutinin (and to *Chlamydia trachomatis*, *Candida albicans*, streptokinase–streptodornose, tetanus toxoid and mumps virus) were depressed in pregnancy compared both with the same individuals post partum and with a group of non-pregnant women. Clearly, there is much still to learn about specific CMI responses to CMV and other microbes in pregnancy.

Similar assays were carried out on 14 women acquiring primary CMV infection during pregnancy (H. Stern et al, 1986). Eight of the women showed a brisk response and there was no correlation between response and period of gestation; all of these women delivered uninfected babies. Four of the remaining six who had a negative response delivered congenitally infected babies. One of the six, who had an initially negative response, became positive at 35 weeks. Again the depressed response was specific for CMV. CMV excretion occurred in both responders and non-responders. More information on CMI in pregnancy to both latent and persistent infections is needed.

Mechanical, social and hormonal factors

Factors other than those involved in the classic specific immune system may also be important in alterations in host resistance during pregnancy. At a simple level, holding large antenatal clinics may increase the risk to patients of acquiring upper respiratory tract infections or other infectious diseases, especially if the mothers also bring their other children.

During pregnancy, the ureter gradually dilates above the pelvic brim. After delivery, the dilatation recedes but there may be some residual defect. This dilatation is probably a result of hormonally induced relaxation of smooth muscle and physical obstruction by the enlarging uterus. Bacteriuria occurring in pregnancy can be asymptomatic or present as overt urinary tract infection. Overt infection will develop in 11–40% of those with asymptomatic bacteriuria, and in 1–3% of those who do not. The prevalence of bacteriuria is not increased in pregnancy (2–10%) compared with that in infertile women or those who have never been pregnant (McFadyen, 1986; Campbell-Brown et al, 1987). Asymptomatic bacteriuria is more likely to become symptomatic in pregnant women than others. This is due to a mixture of slowing of urine flow and the composition of the urine, which contains large quantities of nutrients for bacterial growth. There is a greater risk to the fetus if the mother develops bacteriuria, with a greater chance of mid-trimester abortion and a perinatal mortality rate twice that of those who were not infected (McFadyean, 1986).

INFECTION OF THE FETUS AND PLACENTA

Host resistance might be decreased in pregnancy because of the presence of the placenta and fetus, either because the new cells are more susceptible to infection than maternal tissues or because the fetus is immunologically incompetent. The fetus and placenta can be infected either via the haematogenous route or by micro-organisms ascending from the vagina. Nevertheless, the fetus is well protected and intrauterine infection is rare. The membranes and amniotic fluid which contains antibacterial glycopeptides (C. M. M. Stern, 1981) protect the fetus against ascending infection. The placenta may also protect the fetus from blood-borne infection. Infection in pregnancy may result in early pregnancy loss, in stillbirth, in congenital infection or in congenital malformation.

Early pregnancy loss

Anecdotal reports suggest that any severe infection can lead to abortion. More systematic information is needed to confirm this. Fetal loss has been associated with a wide variety of micro-organisms, many of which have also been recovered from the products of conception (Overall and Glasgow, 1970; Peckham and Marshall, 1979).

A prospective study has demonstrated that there is an association between gestational mumps and spontaneous abortion; 27% of 33 women who suffered mumps in the first trimester lost the fetus (Siegal et al, 1966).

Mumps virus has been isolated from the fetus in such cases (Kurtz et al, 1982). Similar findings have also implicated a variety of pathogens, including smallpox virus, vaccinia virus, poliovirus, rubella virus, *Treponema pallidum*, *Chlamydia psittaci*, *Escherichia coli*, *Mycoplasma lominis* and *Ureoplasma urealyticum*.

The role of CMV in spontaneous abortion provides an intriguing puzzle. CMV can certainly cross the placenta to infect the fetus and can produce congenital malformation. There is some evidence that CMV might cause early abortion. CMV or CMV-like organisms were obtained from 14 of 59 instances of pregnancy wastage (Kriel et al, 1970), but there was no correlation between isolation of CMV and maternal complement-fixing anti-CMV antibodies. Later studies have shown that women suffering imminent abortion were more likely to have IgM antibody against CMV late antigen than those with a normal pregnancy (14.7% vs 6.0%) (Gartner et al, 1982), and that women with spontaneous abortion (5.35%), especially those with loss in the second trimester (18.75%), were more likely to have IgM anti-CMV antibodies than control pregnant women (0%) (Luerti et al, 1983). The data on virus culture must be interpreted with care, since the aborted material will have come through a cervix already excreting CMV. Searching for virus particles in the tissue by electron microscopy, looking for viral inclusions by light microscopy, or detection of virally-encoded RNA transcripts would help to differentiate between the infection and virus acquired in transit.

In contrast, we have recently demonstrated that women suffering unexplained recurrent spontaneous abortions were less likely to have anti-CMV antibody (measured by complement fixation and ELISA) than non-pregnant women; this was not the case for anti-HSV antibodies. Furthermore, CMV-seropositive women with recurrent spontaneous abortion had a decreased lymphoproliferation response to CMV antigen than controls (Radcliffe et al, 1986). Clearly, more information on the interaction between the placenta, the fetus, mothers and CMV is needed.

Congenital infection and congenital malformation

The micro-organisms that are known to cross the placenta to infect the fetus and to cause congenital damage are shown in Table 5. That congenital infection has occurred is determined by both isolation of the pathogen from the neonate and by demonstrating a raised IgM antibody to the pathogen in cord blood. The manifestations of congenital damage may be present at birth (e.g. hydrancephaly, hepatosplenomegaly, microcephaly or chorioretinitis) or may take years to become apparent (e.g. mental retardation, deafness or carcinoma).

Rubellavirus is the prototype of a transplacental pathogen. If acquired in the first trimester, spontaneous abortion occurs in 20% of cases and the risk of major malformation is between 10 and 52% of cases. Between 22 and 33% of infants whose mothers acquired rubella between the 16th and 20th week of pregnancy showed evidence of infection. Those infants who became infected in the first trimester continue to excrete rubellavirus for long

Table 5. Transplacental infection and congenital damage.

	Congenital infection	Congenital damage
Well established agents		
Cytomegalovirus	+	+
Herpes simplex virus	+	±
Varicella-zoster virus	+	±
Rubellavirus	+	+
Human parvovirus	+	+
Smallpox virus	+	−
Treponema pallidum	+	+
Listeria monocytogenes	+	+
Less well established agents		
Influenza virus	+	(+)
Mumps virus	+	(+)
Measles virus	+	−
Lymphocytic choriomeningitis virus	+	(+)
Enteroviruses	+	(+)
Human immune deficiency virus	(+)	−
Hepatitis B virus	+	−
Vaccinia virus	+	−
Epstein–Barr virus	+	−
Mycobacterium tuberculosis	+	−
Borrelia burgdorferi	+	+
Plasmodium	(+)	−
Filaria	(+)	−

periods after birth, indicating some form of immune tolerance (see Best and Banatvala, 1987).

Both herpes simplex and varicella zoster viruses cross the placenta to infect the fetus, but only rarely produce congenital damage. Varicella zoster virus infection poses the greatest risk to the fetus if maternal infection occurs less than five days before delivery. It produces fatal fulminant chickenpox in the neonate. If infection occurs earlier, then the virus becomes latent in the neonate but can reactivate at 4–6 months after delivery, presumably as maternally derived antibody levels fall (Brunell, 1981). Three cases of congenital malformation following zoster have been described (Webster and Smith, 1977).

With the advent of safe and effective rubella vaccines, CMV has become the most important cause of congenital infection and damage. Congenital CMV infection occurs in between 0.2 to 2.2% of pregnancies and is more common in higher income groups. Approximately 10% of those who are congenitally infected will have congenital damage ranging from gross cerebral damage to learning difficulties (Stagno and Whitley, 1985). CMV tends to be excreted for long periods by congenitally infected infants despite a brisk immune response (Griffiths, 1987). Congenital infection does not occur only in a primary infection, and recurrent (either reactivation or infection with a new strain of virus) infections do produce infection but are less likely to produce damage (Huang et al, 1980; Stagno et al, 1982).

Human parvovirus B19 infects erythroid precursor cells and can produce aplastic crises in individuals with a rapid marrow turnover (e.g. in hereditary spherocytosis). Transplacental infection has been observed and can result in abortion and hydrops fetalis, presumably by infecting fetal erythroid cells (Anand et al, 1987).

There is some evidence that other micro-organisms can infect the fetus in utero and produce damage but it is less well-established (Table 5). It is more likely that HIV and hepatitis B virus are transmitted to the neonate during delivery, than across the placenta, but at present it is difficult to detect neonatal IgM anti-HIV which would prove the latter possibility. Suggestions that EBV is acquired transplacentally have not been proven in the studies carried out (Fleisher and Bolognese, 1984).

Viral infections during pregnancy have also been linked to increased risk of perinatal death (Butler, 1973) and a higher risk of subsequent development of cancers (Butler, 1973; Fine et al, 1985). For example, higher than expected rates of perinatal death were observed following infective hepatitis and possibly glandular fever and poliomyelitis (Butler, 1973), and an excess of cancers (16 vs 7) were clustered among those exposed to CMV or VZV in utero (Fine et al, 1985). However, virological confirmation in the former group was not obtained and the figures are based on clinical diagnoses, thus subclinical cases would not have been considered.

Premature delivery and stillbirth

Many of the pathogens causing congenital infection are said to be responsible for premature delivery and stillbirth. Again, conclusive evidence is lacking. Anecdotal evidence links *Campylobacter fetus* (Editorial, 1984) and *Chlamydia psittaci* with such occurrences; both of these agents cause abortion in animals. The spirochaete *Borrelia burgdorferi* that causes Lyme disease is also able to cross the placenta to infect the fetus causing stillbirth and cardiac defects (MacDonald et al, 1987).

The genital mycoplasmas *Mycoplasma hominis* and *Ureaplasma urealyticum* have been associated with premature delivery and perinatal death when they infect the placenta (Kundsin et al, 1984). These agents probably infect the placenta by ascending from the genital tract.

The placenta as a site for infection

Placental tissue does support the growth of many viruses. Human amnion cells are used in many diagnostic virology laboratories to grow, for example, CMV, VZV, HSV, enteroviruses and measles virus. In vivo, the placenta may be infected by exogenous and endogenous agents. Evidence for endogenous retroviruses in human placentae has been obtained from both serological and electron microscopic studies as well as by detection of reverse transcriptase (Nelson et al, 1978; Suni et al, 1984). C-type retroviruses have been described in human and primate placentae, but their role is still unclear. Exogenous infections for the most part are derived from maternal blood. In most cases, the infection is not confined to the placenta alone but *Chlamydia psittaci* does appear to have a tropism for the placenta. Rubellavirus infects the placenta and induces higher levels of interferon in placentally derived cells than does Sendai virus (Banatvala et al, 1973). This apparently does not protect the fetus. The evidence for infection by other viruses is variable and has been reviewed by Kalter (1983).

Perhaps of greater interest is the role of the immune system in limiting infection of the placenta. Syncytiotrophoblast does not express classical transplantation antigens and virus-specific cytotoxic T-cells depend upon the expression of both major histocompatibility antigens and viral proteins on the infected cell surface in order to kill effectively (Zinkernagel and Doherty, 1979). The presence of specific antibodies bound to Fcγ receptors on the trophoblast membrane might facilitate adherence of bacteria and viruses to the trophoblast. Viruses that could not normally infect trophoblast because their receptor was not expressed might thus be able to infect via an antibody bridge. Finally, the ability of viruses to infect the placenta and fetus could be restricted by the stage of differentiation of the host. Thus, CMV was unable to infect human embryonal carcinoma cells but did replicate in their differentiated progeny (Gonczol et al, 1985).

IMMUNIZATION

Maternal antibody responses to micro-organisms causing infection during pregnancy do not appear to differ from those occurring outside pregnancy. Indeed, these form the basis for diagnosis of infections occurring during pregnancy. Far less is known of cell-mediated immune responses to specific pathogens in pregnancy. Some surveys have demonstrated a diminution of lymphoproliferative response to a mycobacterial antigen (PPD), to tetanus toxoid and to streptokinase–streptodornase (Covelli and Wilson, 1978; Lopatin et al, 1980) towards the later stages of pregnancy. However, it seems that this does not affect generalized systemic immunity, otherwise the rubella vaccination campaign would not have been successful in preventing congenital rubella.

Vaccine take

Because most vaccines are used to prevent the commonly occurring childhood infectious diseases, they are administered early in life and it is not often that pregnant women are immunized. Administration of vaccinia was generally contraindicated in pregnancy, except for immediate contacts of a smallpox case. When this has been done, there is little evidence that take of vaccine is diminished (Rahjvajn et al, 1973). Similarly there is no evidence that administration of the 17D Yellow Fever vaccine or of live attenuated polio (Sabin) vaccine during pregnancy gives lesser protection (Smith et al, 1958).

Immune response to vaccine

Most of the information on the serological response to vaccine given in pregnancy comes from the trials to prevent neonatal tetanus (MacLennan et al, 1965). Immunization produces high titre antibody that crosses the placenta and protects the neonate from the effects of infection by *Clostridium tetani*. Indeed, it has been shown that the fetus can also mount an antibody response to tetanus toxoid administered during pregnancy (Gill et al, 1983).

Live attenuated vaccines

Live attenuated vaccines should not be given to immunocompromised patients. If immunity to infection were depressed in pregnancy it might be expected that the vaccine strains would be more likely to produce infection either in the mother or the fetus. The live attenuated vaccines available for use include rubella, polio, vaccinia, yellow fever, measles, mumps, varicella zoster and BCG. It is unlikely that measles, mumps or varicella zoster vaccines would be given, but mumps virus vaccine has been found to be transmitted to the placenta (Yamauchi et al, 1974). In order to assess this finding, we need to know how frequently viraemia follows administration of mumps vaccine.

Vaccinia

Vaccinia virus can infect the fetus and placenta (Levine et al, 1974) but is apparently no more dangerous for the pregnant than the non-pregnant woman. In a large survey of vaccination in pregnancy, no case of fetal vaccinia was seen but there was some evidence of excess fetal wastage, especially if administered in the first trimester (MacArthur, 1952). Although vaccinia is no longer used to protect against smallpox, it may be administered in the future as a polyvalent vaccine.

Rubella

Rubella vaccine virus does infect the fetus and can cause congenital malformation (Modlin et al, 1976), although the risk is low (5.5% of those immunized). The vaccine does not cause a more severe infection in pregnancy.

BCG, polio and yellow fever

There is no evidence of fetal infection nor of increased risk of infection in the pregnant woman. Despite this, the use of live attenuated vaccines in pregnancy is to be avoided unless there are strong indications for their use.

MALIGNANT TUMOURS

There are numerous anecdotal reports of increased severity of malignancy in pregnancy, including ovarian, colonic and uterine cervical carcinoma. Immune suppression would be expected to be associated with an increased incidence and severity of malignancy. In practice, the malignancies most often associated with immune-depressed patients are lymphomata. However, if pregnancy were associated with decreased host resistance to cancer, tumours might occur more frequently, might metastasize more readily, and the growth of existing tumours might be enhanced or previously treated tumours might recur.

Carcinomas of the breast occurring during pregnancy is the malignancy that has received the greatest attention (Anderson, 1979). Approximately 3% of breast cancers occur during a pregnancy and about 1 in 3000 pregnancies is complicated by breast cancer. Although this occurrence was previously regarded with great pessimism, there is little evidence to support this view. Overall, the 5-year survival is the same for pregnant and non-pregnant women. For example, in a survey of 63 cases at the Mayo Clinic, the 5-year survival was 80% for patients with localized malignancy (King et al, 1985). Previous surveys had found that the incidence of nodal metastases was greater in pregnant (76%) than non-pregnant women (see Anderson, 1979). This may, however, be related to delay in treatment rather than increased spread. In one series, only 7% of 150 patients received treatment within one month of detection.

Survival is said to be less good in pregnant women with nodal metastases but, when patients are matched for age and stage of tumour, the difference is insignificant (Anderson, 1979). Patients under 30 have a poorer outlook and in one series the 5-year survival for patients treated in the second half of pregnancy was 11% compared with 48% for those treated in the first half (M. V. Peters, 1968). It has been proposed that malignant growth is accelerated in pregnancy because of increased stimulation by sex hormones, prolactin and corticosteroids. For these reasons, therapeutic abortion and oophorectomy have been advocated. No significant difference in 5-year survival has been observed between patients who underwent mastectomy and termination (43%) and those who only had mastectomy (59%) (King et al, 1985). This group found that pregnancy increased the risk of nodal metastasis and scirrhous changes on histopathology. Survival of those who become pregnant after treatment for breast cancer appears to be greater than for the non-pregnant (M. V. Peters, 1968), especially if pregnant within two years of treatment. The survival of those acquiring breast cancer during lactation is no different from other groups (M. V. Peters, 1968).

TRANSPLANTATION AND PREGNANCY

Pregnancy may interact with transplantation in several ways. Firstly, and numerically the most likely, a transplantee may become pregnant when immune suppression is low, secondly there may be rejection episodes during pregnancy, and thirdly a transplant might be carried out on a pregnant woman. The majority of data on transplantation and pregnancy concerns renal or hepatic transplants.

There is one case report of a renal transplant being inadvertently performed in pregnancy (Burleson et al, 1983). Renal allotransplantation took place during the second trimester, with standard immune suppression using azothioprine and prednisolone. One rejection episode occurred (pregnancy did not decrease host resistance to the allograft) which was managed with methylprednisolone. The pregnancy was delivered at 35 weeks gestation. The neonate had no gross abnormalities, but was subsequently found to have an atrial septal defect and linginal thyroid. At 2.5 years, she was on the 20th centile for weight and the 8th centile for height. Postpartum, the maternal renal function remained stable.

There are two large surveys of pregnancy occurring after transplantation, of 59 pregnancies in 40 renal or hepatic transplant recipients (Penn et al, 1980) and of 440 pregnancies in renal recipients (Rudolph et al, 1979). In the former, gestation occurred at a mean of 50 months post-renal transplant and there were eight abortions (one spontaneous, the rest at the patient's request). Pre-eclampsia occurred in 27%, but two thirds of these had pre-existing problems. Of 56 pregnancies, there was one stillbirth due to carbon monoxide poisoning and 47 live births including one set of twins. In the latter study, 52% of renal transplant recipients who became pregnant had term infants with no serious complications. A further 12% had pre-term deliveries, 5% spontaneous abortion and 25% therapeutic abortion. Rejection episodes occurred in 9% of patients, and in four patients pregnancy appeared to trigger the episode. Unfortunately, comparative data of rejection episodes in a non-pregnant group of age-matched women were not available.

From the above, it can be seen that pregnancy is not greatly affected by having been a clinical tissue allograft recipient, but nor does pregnancy greatly lower host resistance to allow improved survival of the renal allograft since rejection episodes do occur.

SUMMARY

Apart from a few exceptions, the hypothesis that pregnancy lowers host resistance to infection, to cancer, to transplantation and in immunization appears unproven. Certainly, the consequences of smallpox and Lassa fever infection are more likely to be fatal in pregnant women, but this could be due to a lability of the complement and clotting cascades rather than to depression of specific immunity. That varicella pneumonia and risks of bacteriuria are greater in pregnancy might be attributable to mechanical factors rather than defects in immunity. The observation that pregnancy increases excretion of CMV has now been shown to be a return from suppression of excretion back to normal levels, although there is some evidence that EBV is excreted in higher amounts and more frequently in pregnancy.

The humoral immune responses to pathogens or immunogens in pregnancy seems to be no different from that in the non-pregnant woman. Immunity does not appear to wane with the onset of pregnancy or this would render the rubella immunization programme ineffective. There is conflicting data on cell-mediated immune responses to specific pathogens in pregnancy, and this would warrant much more study. Caution must be exercised in interpreting such studies, which should always be compared with age and sex matched controls in longitudinal studies. The use of live vaccines in pregnancy is contraindicated but more because of theoretical or proven risks to the fetus than of risks of dissemination in the mother. The placenta and fetus do, however, appear to have a decreased host resistance. The developing fetus and the placenta contain cell populations with differing susceptibilities to infection by different pathogens. In addition, the fetal immune system is evolving and may be tolerant to some pathogens (e.g. with rubella and CMV) if infection occurs early enough. Immunity of the placenta to infection might also be diminished by virtue of the absence of major histocompatibility antigens and binding of immunoglobulin to the trophoblast surface via Fcγ receptors.

Breast cancer appears to have no worse a prognosis in pregnancy, providing that diagnosis is early and it occurs in the first half of pregnancy. Diminished host resistance in pregnancy does not appear to favour survival of the transplanted kidney since rejection episodes still occur.

It seems that a pregnant woman *does* bloom with health.

REFERENCES

Anand A, Gray ES, Brown T et al (1987) Human parvovirus infection in pregnancy and hydrops fetalis. *New England Journal of Medicine* **316:** 183–186.

Anderson JM (1979) Mammary cancers and pregnancy. *British Medical Journal* **i:** 1124–1127.

Banatvala JE, Potter JE & Webster MJ (1973) Foetal interferon responses induced by rubella virus. In Ciba Foundation Symposium 10. *Intrauterine Infections*, pp 77–99. Amsterdam: Elsevier.

Beaudenon S, Kremsdorf D & Croissant O et al (1986) A novel type of human papillomavirus associated with genital neoplasias. *Nature* **321:** 246–249.

Best JM & Banatvala JE (1987) Rubella. In Zuckerman AJ, Banatvala JE & Pattison JR (eds) *Principles and Practice of Clinical Virology*, pp 315–353. London: John Wiley & Sons.

Bray RS & Anderson MJ (1979) Falciparum malaria and pregnancy. *Transactions of the Royal Society of Tropical Medicine and Hygiene* **73:** 427–431.

Brazin SA, Simkowich JW & Johnson T (1979) Herpes zoster during pregnancy. *Obstetrics and Gynecology* **53:** 175–181.

Brown ZA, Vontver LA, Benedetti J et al (1987) Effects on infants of a first episode of genital herpes during pregnancy. *New England Journal of Medicine* **317:** 1246–1251.

Bruce-Chwatt LJ (1983) Malaria and pregnancy. *British Medical Journal* **286:** 1457–1458.

Brunell PA (1981) Epidemiology of varicella-zoster virus infections. In Nahmias AJ, Dowdle WR & Schinazi RF (eds) *The Human Herpesviruses*, pp 153–158. New York: Elsevier.

Brunham RC, Martin DH, Hubbart TW et al (1983) Depression of the lymphocyte transformation response to microbial antigens and phytohemagglutinin during pregnancy. *Journal of Clinical Investigation* **72:** 1629–1638.

Burleson RL, Sunderji SG, Aubry RH et al (1983) Renal allotransplantation during pregnancy: successful outcome for mother, child and kidney. *Transplantation* **36:** 334–335.

Butler NR (1973) Epidemiological approach to intrauterine infections. In Ciba Foundation Symposium 10. *Intrauterine Infections*, pp 151–163. Amsterdam: Elsevier.

Campbell-Brown M, McFadyean IR, Seal DV & Stephenson ML (1987) Is screening for bacteriuria in pregnancy worth while? *British Medical Journal* **294:** 1579–1582.

Campion MJ, McCance DJ, Cuzick J & Singer A (1986) Progressive potential of mild cervical atypia: prospective cytological, colposcopic and virological study. *Lancet* **ii:** 237–240.

Catalano LW & Sever JL (1971) The role of viruses as causes of congenital defects. *Annual Review of Microbiology* **25:** 255–282.

Coleman DV, Wolfendale MR, Daniel RA et al (1980) A prospective study of human polyomavirus infection in pregnancy. *Journal of Infectious Diseases* **142:** 1–8.

Corey L & Spear PG (1986) Infection with herpes simplex viruses. *New England Journal of Medicine* **314:** 686–691; 749–757.

Covelli HD & Wilson RT (1978) Immunologic and medical considerations in tuberculin sensitized pregnant patients. *American Journal of Obstetrics and Gynecology* **132:** 256–262.

Daffos F, Forestier F, Capello-Pavlovsky M et al (1988) Perinatal management of 746 pregnancies at risk for congenital toxoplasmosis. *New England Journal of Medicine* **318:** 271–275.

Dalldorf G & Gifford R (1954) Susceptibility of gravid mice to coxsackie virus infection. *Journal of Experimental Medicine* **99:** 21–27.

D'Cruz IA, Balini SG & Lyer LS (1968) Infectious hepatitis and pregnancy. *Obstetrics and Gynecology* **31:** 449–454.

De March (1975) Tuberculosis and pregnancy. *Chest* **68:** 800–804.

Editorial (1984) Premature labor and neonatal sepsis caused by *Campylobacter fetus subsp. fetus*—Ontario. *Morbidity and Mortality Weekly Report* **33:** 483–489.

Enders G (1984) Varicella-zoster virus infection in pregnancy. *Progress in Medical Virology* **29:** 166–196.

Fine PE, Adelstein AM, Snowman J, Clarkson JA & Evans SM (1985) Long term effects of exposure to viral infections in utero. *British Medical Journal* **i:** 509–511.

Fleisher G & Bolognese R (1984) Epstein–Barr virus infections in pregnancy: A prospective study. *Journal of Pediatrics* **104:** 374–379.

Freeman DW & Barno A (1959) Death from Asian influenza associated with pregnancy. *American Journal of Obstetrics and Gynecology* **78:** 1172–1175.

Gartner VL, Stranz G & Herrman C (1982) Occurrence of IgM antibodies against cytomegalovirus-induced late antigen in women with imminent abortion as compared to women with normal course of pregnancy. *Zentralblatt fur Gynakologie* **104:** 1005–1008.

Gehrz RC, Christianson WR, Linner KM et al (1981) Cytomegalovirus-specific humoral and cellular responses in human pregnancy. *Journal of Infectious Diseases* **143:** 391–395.

Gerety RJ & Schweitzer IL (1977) Viral hepatitis type B during pregnancy, the neonatal period and infancy. *Journal of Pediatrics* **90:** 368–374.

Gill TJ, Repetti CF, Metlay LA et al (1983) Transplacental immunization of the human fetus to tetanus by immunization of the mother. *Journal of Clinical Investigation* **72:** 987–996.

Gonczol E, Andrews PW & Plotkin SA (1985) Cytomegalovirus infection of human teratocarcinoma cells in culture. *Journal of General Virology* **66:** 509–515.

Green RH, Balsamo MR, Giles JP et al (1965) Studies of the natural history and prevention of rubella. *American Journal of Diseases of Children* **110:** 348–365.

Griffiths PW (1987) Cytomegalovirus. In Zuckerman AJ, Banatvala JE & Pattison JR (eds) *Principles and Practice of Clinical Virology*, pp 75–109. London: John Wiley & Sons.

Harbour DA, Blyth WA & Hill TJ (1978) Prostaglandin enhanced spread of herpes simplex virus in cell cultures. *Journal of General Virology* **41:** 87–95.

Harris RE & Rhoades ER (1965) Varicella pneumonia complicating pregnancy. *Obstetrics and Gynecology* **25:** 734–740.

Hensey OJ, Hart CA & Cooke RWI (1984) *Candida albicans* skin abscesses. *Archives of Diseases of Childhood* **59:** 479–480.

Hieber JP, Dalton D, Shorey J & Combes B (1977) Hepatitis and pregnancy. *Journal of Pediatrics* **91:** 545–549.

Hogan TF, Padgett BL & Walker DL (1984) Human polyomaviruses. In Belshe RB (ed.) *Textbook of Human Virology*, pp 969–995. Massachusetts: PSG Publishing Co.

Horger JH, Pazin GJ, Armstrong JA, Breinig MC & Ho M (1983) Characteristics and management of pregnancy in women with genital herpes simplex infection. *American Journal of Obstetrics and Gynecology* **145:** 784–791.

Huang E-S, Alford CA, Reynolds DW, Stagmo S & Pass RF (1980) Molecular epidemiology of cytomegalovirus infections in women and their infants. *New England Journal of Medicine* **303:** 958–962.

Johnson FWA, Matheson BA, Williams H et al (1985) Abortion due to infection with *Chlamydia psittaci* in a sheep farmer's wife. *British Medical Journal* **290:** 592–594.

Johnstone FD, MacCallum L, Brettle R et al (1988) Does infection with HIV affect the outcome of pregnancy? *British Medical Journal* **296:** 467.

Kalter SS (1983) Viral expression in trophoblast. In Loke YW & Whyte A (eds) *Biology of Trophoblast*, pp 627–662 Amsterdam: Elsevier.

King RM, Welch JS, Martin JK & Coulam CB (1985) Carcinoma of the breast associated with pregnancy. *Surgery, Gynecology and Obstetrics* **160**: 228–232.

Kriel RL, Gates GA, Wulff H et al (1970) Cytomegalovirus isolations associated with pregnancy wastage. *American Journal of Obstetrics and Gynecology* **106**: 885–892.

Kundsin RB, Driscoll SG, Monson RR et al (1984) Association of *Ureaplasma urealyticum* in the placenta with perinatal morbidity and mortality. *New England Journal of Medicine* **310**: 941–945.

Kurtz JB, Tomlinson AH & Pearson J (1982) Mumps virus isolated from a fetus. *British Medical Journal* **284**: 471.

Lambert HP & Wood CBS (1981) *Immunological Aspects of Infection in the Fetus and New-born*. London: Academic Press.

Lennon D, Lewis B, Mantell C et al (1984) Epidemic perinatal listeriosis. *Pediatric Infectious Disease* **3**: 30–34.

Levine MM, Edsall G & Bruce-Chwatt LJ (1974) Live vaccine in pregnancy—risks and recommendations. *Lancet* **ii**: 34–38.

Lopatin DE, Kornman KS & Loesche WJ (1980) Modulation of immunoreactivity to periodontal disease associated micro-organisms during pregnancy. *Infection and Immunity* **28**: 713–718.

Luerti M, Santini A, Bernini O, Costigliani M & Ragni MC (1983) ELISA antibodies to cytomegalovirus in pregnant patients: Prevalence in and correlation with spontaneous abortion. *Biological Research in Pregnancy* **4**: 181–183.

MacArthur P (1952) Congenital vaccinia and Vaccinia gravidarum. *Lancet* **ii**: 1104–1106.

McCance DJ, Walker PG, Dyson JL, Coleman DV & Singer A (1983) Presence of human papillomavirus DNA sequences in cervical intraepithelial neoplasia. *British Medical Journal* **286**: 784–788.

MacDonald AB, Benach JL & Burgdorfer W (1987) Stillbirth following maternal Lyme disease. *New York State Journal of Medicine* **87**: 615–616.

McFadyen IR (1986) Urinary tract infection in pregnancy. In Andreucci VE (ed.) *The Kidney in Pregnancy*, pp 205–229. Amsterdam: Martinus Nijhoff.

MacLennan R, Schofield FD, Pittman M, Hardegree MC & Barlie MF (1965) Immunization against neonatal tetanus in New Guinea: Antitoxin response of pregnant women to adjuvant and plain toxoid. *Bulletin of the WHO* **32**: 683–697.

Mitus A, Enders JF, Craig JM et al (1959) Persistence of measles virus and depression of antibody formation in patients with giant cell pneumonia after measles. *New England Journal of Medicine* **261**: 882–889.

Modlin JF, Herrman K, Brandling-Bennett B, Eddins DL & Hayden G (1976) Risk of congenital abnormality after inadvertent rubella vaccination of pregnant women. *New England Journal of Medicine* **294**: 272–274.

Nelson J, Leong J-A & Levy JA (1978) Normal human placentas contains RNA directed DNA polymerase activity like that in viruses. *Proceedings of the National Academy of Sciences USA* **75**: 6263–6267.

Overall JC & Glasgow LA (1970) Virus infections of the fetus and newborn infant. *Fetal and Neonatal Medicine* **77**: 315–333.

Paryani SG & Arvin AM (1986) Intrauterine infection with varicella-zoster virus after maternal varicella. *New England Journal of Medicine* **314**: 1542–1546.

Peacock JE & Sarubbui FA (1983) Disseminated herpes simplex virus infection during pregnancy. *Obstetrics and Gynecology* **61** (supplement 3): 8–13.

Peckham C & Marshall WC (1979) Rubella and other virus infections in pregnancy. *Journal of Antimicrobial Chemotherapy* **5** (supplement A): 71–80.

Penn I, Makowski EL & Harrris P (1980) Parenthood following renal and hepatic transplantation. *Transplantation* **30**: 397–400.

Peters CJ (1984) Arenaviruses. In Belshe RB (ed.) *Textbook of Human Virology*, pp 513–545. Massachusetts: PSG Publishing Co.

Peters MV (1968) The effect of pregnancy in breast cancer. In Forrest APM & Kunkler PB (eds) *Prognostic factors in breast cancer*, pp 65–80. Edinburgh: ES Livingstone Ltd.

Pickard RF (1968) Varicella pneumonia in pregnancy. *American Journal of Obstetrics and Gynecology* **101**: 504–506.

Plager H, Beebe R & Miller JK (1962) Coxsackie B-5 pericarditis in pregnancy. *Archives of Internal Medicine* **110:** 737–738.

Puga A, Cantin EM, Wohlenberg C et al (1984) Different sizes of restriction endonuclease fragments from the terminal repetitions of the herpes simplex virus type 1 genome latent in trigeminal ganglia of mice. *Journal of General Virology* **65:** 437–444.

Purtilo DT (1975) Opportunistic mycotic infections in pregnant women. *American Journal of Obstetrics and Gynecology* **122:** 607–612.

Purtilo DT, Hallgren HM & Yunis EJ (1972) Depressed maternal lymphocyte response to phytohaemagglutinin in human pregnancy. *Lancet* **i:** 769–771.

Radcliffe JJ, Hart CA, Francis WJA & Johnson PM (1986) Cytomegalovirus in women with unexplained recurrent spontaneous abortion. *American Journal of Reproductive Immunology and Microbiology* **12:** 103–105.

Rahjvajn B, Krznar B, Stiljkovic C, Orescanin M & Smerdel S (1973) Vaccination against smallpox in early pregnancy. *Acta Medica Jugoslavica* **27:** 351–357.

Rao AR (1972) *Smallpox*. Bombay: Kothari Book Depot.

Rickinson AB, Yao Y & Wallace LE (1985) Epstein–Barr virus as a model of virus–host interactions. *British Medical Bulletin* **41:** 75–79.

Rocklin RE, Kitzmiller JL & Kaye MD (1979) Immunobiology of the maternal–fetal relationship. *Annual Review of Medicine* **30:** 375–396.

Rudolph JE, Schweitzer RT & Bartus SA (1979) Pregnancy in renal transplant recipients. *Transplantation* **27:** 26–29.

Schauf V & Toplin M (1984) Varicella-zoster virus. In Belshe RB (ed.) *Textbook of Human Virology*, pp 829–851. Massachusetts: PSG Publishing Co.

Sever JL & White LR (1968) Intrauterine viral infections. *Annual Review of Medicine* **19:** 471–486.

Sever JL, Nelson KB & Gilkeson MR (1965) Rubella epidemic, 1964: Effect on 6000 pregnancies. *American Journal of Diseases of Children* **110:** 395–401.

Siegel M & Greenberg M (1955) Incidence of poliomyelitis in pregnancy: Its relation to maternal age, parity and gestational period. *New England Journal of Medicine* **253:** 841–845.

Siegel M, Fuerst HT & Peress NG (1966) Comparative fetal mortality in maternal virus disease. *New England Journal of Medicine* **274:** 768–771.

Smith HH, Penna HA & Paoliello A (1958) Yellow fever vaccination with cultured virus (17D) without immune serum. *American Journal of Tropical Medicine* **18:** 437–463.

Snyderman D (1985) Hepatitis in pregnancy. *New England Journal of Medicine* **313:** 1398–1401.

Spruance SL (1984) Pathogenesis of herpes simplex labialis: excretion of virus in the oral cavity. *Journal of Clinical Microbiology* **19:** 675–679.

Stagno S & Whitley RC (1985) Herpesvirus infections of pregnancy: 1 cytomegalovirus and Epstein–Barr virus infections. *New England Journal of Medicine* **313:** 1270–1274.

Stagno S, Reynolds D, Tsiantos A et al (1975) Cervical cytomegalovirus excretion in pregnant and non-pregnant women: suppression in early gestation. *Journal of Infectious Diseases* **131:** 522–527.

Stagno S, Pass RF, Dworsky ME (1982) Congenital cytomegalovirus infection. *New England Journal of Medicine* **306:** 945–949.

Stern CMM (1981) Bactericidal glycopeptide in human amniotic fluid. *Journal of Antimicrobial Chemotherapy* **8:** 3–4.

Stern H, Hannington G, Booth J & Moncrieff D (1986) An early marker of fetal infection after primary cytomegalovirus infection in pregnancy. *British Medical Journal* **292:** 718–720.

Suni J, Närvänen A, Wahlström T et al (1984) Human placental syncytiotrophoblastic Mr 75,000 polypeptide defined by antibodies to a synthetic peptide based on a cloned human endogenous retroviral DNA sequence. *Proceedings of the National Academy of Sciences USA* **81:** 6197–6201.

Thomas PA, Lubin K, Milberg J et al (1987) Cohort comparison study of children whose mothers have acquired immune deficiency syndrome and children of well inner city mothers. *Pediatric Infectious Diseases* **6:** 247–251.

Walker DL (1978) Progressive multifocal leukoencephalopathy: An opportunistic viral infection of the central nervous system. In Vinken PJ & Bruyn GW (eds) *Handbook of Clinical Neurology*, vol. 34, pp 307–329. Amsterdam: North Holland Publishing Co.

Watson GI (1965) Serological studies on second attacks of measles and rubella. *Lancet* **i**: 80–81.

Webster MH & Smith CS (1977) Congenital abnormalities and maternal herpes zoster. *British Medical Journal* **2**: 1193.

Weidanz WP (1982) Malaria and alterations in immune reactivity. *British Medical Bulletin* **38**: 167–172.

Whitby AJ, Blyth WA, Hill TJ (1987) The effect of DNA hypomethylating agents on the reactivation of herpes simplex virus from latently infected mouse ganglia in vitro. *Archives of Virology* **97**: 137–144.

Wildy PW & Gell PG (1985) The host response to herpes simplex virus. *British Medical Bulletin* **41**: 86–91.

Wildy PW, Field HJ & Nash AA (1982) Classical herpes latency revisited. In Mahy BWJ, Minson AC & Darby GK (eds) *Virus Persistence: Society for General Microbiology Symposium 33*, pp 133–167. Cambridge: Cambridge University Press.

Yamauchi T, Wilson C & St Geme JW (1974) Transmission of live attenuated mumps virus to the human placenta. *New England Journal of Medicine* **290**: 710–712.

Ziegler JB, Cooper DA, Johnson RD & Gold J (1985) Postnatal transmission of AIDS-associated retrovirus from mother to infant. *Lancet* **i**: 896–897.

Zinkernagel RM & Doherty PC (1979) MHC restricted cytotoxic T cells: studies on the biological role of polymorphic major transplantation antigens determining T-cell restriction-specificity, function and responsiveness. *Advances in Immunology* **27**: 51–177.

10

Birth control vaccines

A. BASTEN

The world population continues to increase despite the provision of family planning services to many of the countries on our planet. According to World Health Organization (WHO) estimates, there are over 300 million couples of reproductive age in developing countries, 80% of whom do not use adequate means of birth control (Ada et al, 1985). Among the reasons for this is the lack of an effective, safe, cheap and easy to administer form of contraception. A fertility-regulating vaccine offers one viable solution to the problem for several reasons: firstly, immunization as a prophylactic measure enjoys widespread acceptance in all countries; secondly, recent advances in our knowledge of reproduction and materno-placental interactions in early pregnancy have provided a sound scientific base hitherto unavailable for such an approach; thirdly, the application of recombinant DNA and immunological techniques means that vaccines which need to be directed at highly specific target molecules and to be free of unwanted cross-reactions are now a realistic goal.

THE IDEAL VACCINE

In theory, vaccine protocols can be based on the principle of either active or passive immunization. Passive immunization with antibodies, however, is of too short a duration to be a practical proposition in fertility control, which needs to be sustained for years rather than weeks. Furthermore, it is impractical to produce sufficient quantities of purified antibody even by means of hybridoma technology for this purpose. Thus, effective fertility-regulating vaccines depend on the identification of immunogenic moieties capable of stimulating an active immune response which will interfere with conception.

For active immunization, any antigen to be used as a candidate for a fertility-regulating vaccine should conform to the following criteria:

1. It should be present transiently and in relatively low amounts compared to the predicted immune (antibody) response. This criterion applies even if the antigen is sequestered.
2. It should be specific, that is restricted to the vaccine target, and should

not carry cross-reactive epitopes shared with other tissues or related molecules (e.g. hormones).

3. Its precise structure should be known and should preferably be a protein rather than a carbohydrate to facilitate manufacture by modern methods of recombinant DNA technology, which can be scaled up for mass production.
4. Its expression should be confined to gametes and/or early products of the fertilization process. In this context, complete functional characterization is preferable, although not absolutely essential.

To be acceptable, the vaccine itself should have the following characteristics:

1. A minimum efficacy rate of 90%.
2. A highly reproducible immune response of sufficient magnitude, desired type (antibody versus cell-mediated) and duration irrespective of genetic (for example, Ir gene) and nutritional status. Ir gene effects become of particular importance in the case of peptide vaccines expressing a very restricted number of immunogenic determinants.
3. An anti-fertility effect which is potentially reversible spontaneously or by relatively simple manipulation.
4. Free of significant side-effects, including unwanted immune reactions (for example, autoimmunity, allergy and pathogenic immune complexes).
5. Pharmacologically inert according to standard criteria laid down by regulatory authorities.
6. Suitable for widespread usage in developing countries, i.e. it should require relatively few injections and be acceptable to the social mores of the target population.

An appropriate homologous animal model is most desirable for assessment of safety, teratogenicity, clinical efficacy, reversibility and the mechanism(s) of the anti-fertility effect induced. This is particularly important for fertility-regulating vaccines since a pregnancy could occur post-immunization and certain potential targets are oncofetal antigens the response to which could have unpredictable consequences including the risk of development of neoplasia (Tung, 1986).

POTENTIAL VACCINE CANDIDATES

In principle it is possible to use immunological methods to interfere with fertility in both the male and female. Thus, immunization of male and female experimental animals has resulted in production of antibodies and reduced fertility (reviewed in Jones, 1982). In practice, however, the antigens currently being seriously considered as vaccine candidates in humans are restricted to those capable of fertility control in women.

There are four potential stages in the female reproductive process during which fertility-regulating vaccines may act: ovulation; sperm transport and/or fertilization; implantation; blastocyst development. At each stage the vaccine target (examples of which are listed in Table 1) differs. Discussion will be restricted to human chorionic gonadotrophin (hCG), sperm, zona pellucida and trophoblast, since studies on them comprise the bulk of relevant work in the field.

Table 1. Examples of antigens of relevance to fertility control in women.

Stage of reproduction	Target	References
Ovum/ovulation	Zona pellucida	Dunbar, 1983
		Sacco, 1981
	LH–RH	Jones, 1982
	Relaxin	Kemp and Niall, 1984
Sperm transport and/or fertilization	Sperm	Alexander and Anderson, 1987
Implantation	hCG (β-subunit)	Stevens, 1981b
		Griffin, 1986
	Trophoblast	Johnson and Stern, 1986
Blastocyst development	hCG (β-subunit)	Stevens, 1981b

HORMONE-BASED VACCINE CANDIDATES

Human chorionic gonadotrophin

Among the potential targets for fertility-regulating vaccines, hCG (particularly its β-subunit) best fulfils the criteria for an ideal vaccine. A glycoprotein with an approximate molecular weight of 38 kD (Bahl, 1977), hCG has a known structure and amino acid sequence (Morgan et al, 1973). The α-subunit is identical in primary structure to those of hormones such as luteinizing hormone (hLH), follicle stimulating hormone (hFSH) and thyroid stimulating hormone (hTSH); the β-subunit, which includes the determinants responsible for its unique biological activity, differs significantly from the corresponding parts of hFSH and hTSH and to a lesser extent hLH. As expected, antibodies directed towards the intact hCG molecule show extensive cross-reactions with those other hormones, particularly hLH. Furthermore, some degree of cross-reactivity with hLH, albeit much reduced, still occurs when β-hCG is used as the immunogen (Jones, 1982). However, β-hCG has a total of 145 amino acid residues compared with 115 in the case of β-hLH. Thus, with the exception of one position between residues 111 and 115, the 35 amino acid sequence of the carboxy-terminus of β-hCG has no counterpart in hLH (Jones, 1982). Based on this observation, a series of peptides of differing length were derived from the carboxy-terminus of the β-subunit and checked for specificity and hCG neutralizing activity. The results indicated that the optimal peptides for immunization consisted of the 111–145 and 109–145 regions since they elicited high affinity antibodies which were specific for hCG and lacked any cross-reactivity with hLH (Stevens, 1981a,b). Of these two peptides, the 109–145 peptide has the added advantage of containing a cysteine residue at position 10, which is particularly useful as a site for conjugation to protein carrier molecules, such as diphtheria toxoid.

The potential value of hCG as a vaccine candidate is further enhanced by its biological properties. Thus, it is only secreted at physiological levels in pregnancy, i.e. hCG is a pregnancy-specific hormone (Jones, 1982). From the immunological point of view, this means that in the non-pregnant state: (i) autoreactive B cells are likely to be present rather than being deleted; and (ii) any antibodies generated would not be expected to interfere with normal ovarian function or the menstrual cycle. Indeed, both these predictions have now been verified (see below, and section on Clinical trials).

Human chorionic gonadotrophin is first detected at the time of implantation between days seven and eight of pregnancy (Hearn, 1980). It is thought to be produced initially by the pre-implantation blastocyst (Saxena et al, 1974) and subsequently by the early trophoblast (Hearn, 1980). From this stage onwards, hCG plays an important role in the maintenance of pregnancy. Interference with its biological activity by pre-existing antibodies, or possibly activated lymphocytes, has the potential therefore to disrupt pregnancy at a very early stage before implantation is complete (Figure 1).

Developmental work with β-hCG and its 109–145 C-terminal peptide (CTP) has been facilitated by studies in other primates, including Rhesus monkeys (Talwar, 1980), marmosets (Hearn, 1980) and baboons (Stevens,

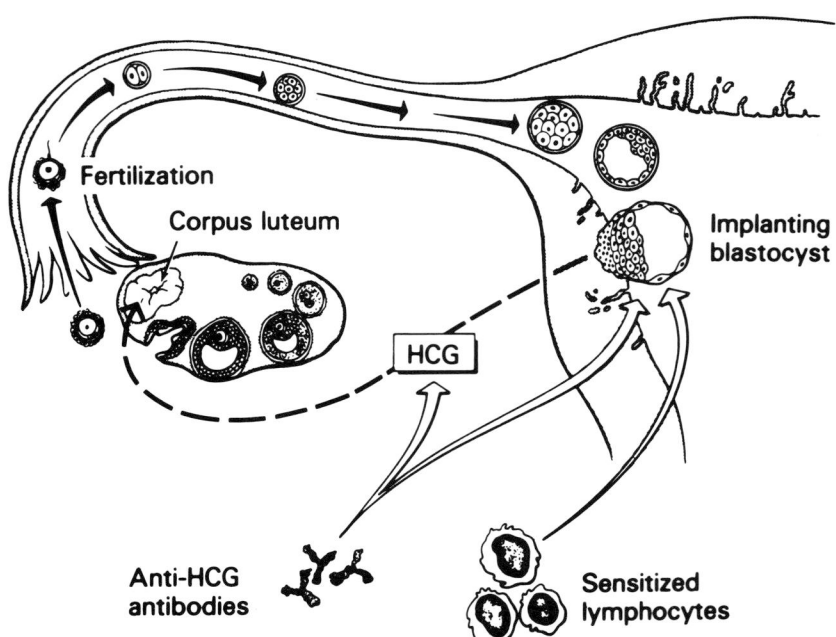

Figure 1. *Possible modes of action of anti-hCG vaccine.* Antibodies capable of neutralizing hCG may inhibit its luteotrophic action on the corpus luteum. Cytotoxic anti-hCG antibodies or sensitized lymphocytes may disrupt the early peri-implantation blastocyst. From Jones WR, 1982.)

1976), all of which, like humans, secrete chorionic gonadotrophins throughout the major part of pregnancy. Antisera raised in rabbits and baboons to intact hCG and its β-subunit have been shown by Stevens (1976) to cross-react with baboon CG (bCG), the degree of cross-reactivity being sufficient to mediate anti-fertility effects in these animals following immunization with hCG or its β-subunit. Consequently, it was possible to use fertile baboons as a model for testing the safety and efficacy of a vaccine based on the 109–145 CTP of the hCG β-subunit (Stevens, 1981a). For this purpose, the peptide was conjugated to diphtheria toxoid and administered in a squalene–arlacel–water emulsion together with MDP-1 as adjuvant (Stevens et al, 1981). Controls received unconjugated toxoid, MDP and emulsion vehicle. Successful pregnancies occurred in 70% of the control animals compared with only 4.6% of the group given complete vaccine. These results were most encouraging since the antibodies raised to the vaccine cross-reacted significantly with intact hCG but to a much lesser extent (3–15%) with bCG. In other words, close to 100% protection could be predicted in a homologous (human) system where a higher level of cross-reactivity would be expected. Equally encouraging was the fact that the anti-fertility effect was reversible and no significant toxicity was demonstrated either in these baboons or in rodents and rabbits immunized with this particular vaccine preparation (Griffin, 1986).

The next logical step was to develop a fully homologous model for fertility-regulation in baboons. This required the cloning and sequencing of the genes for bCG expressed during early pregnancy with the aim of identifying a unique peptide corresponding to the human 109–145 CTP. Such a peptide was found although it differed significantly from the corresponding human β-subunit sequence with 10 of the 37 carboxy-terminal residues changed (Crawford et al, 1986). Despite repeated attempts, antibodies raised to the baboon peptide have failed to react with the native bCG molecule, whereas antibodies to the same region in hCG do so (Stevens, personal communication). The reasons for this enigma remain unclear and currently preclude the use of the baboon as a fully homologous system.

Other hCG-based approaches

The majority of the work on the CTP from the β-subunit of hCG has been carried out under the auspices of the WHO Task Force on Vaccines for Fertility Regulation. At the same time, research supported by the Population Council, New York, has been directed towards development of alternative vaccine candidates based on the β-subunit, of which two are of particular interest since they are now undergoing clinical trials in parallel with the CTP peptide. The first is α-ovine LH-β-hCG conjugated to the two carriers tetanus toxoid (TT) and cholera toxin chain B (CHB) (Talwar and Gur, 1986). The rationale for annealing α-oLH to β-hCG was based on evidence in Bonnet monkeys that this manoeuvre enhanced the immunogenicity of β-hCG apparently without leading to production of anti-hLH antibodies (Sharma et al, 1986a). The use of two, rather than a single, carrier was designed to generate a more consistent antibody response by minimizing the chance of obtaining variable antibody titres due to Ir gene effects in recipients (Sharma et al, 1986b).

The second preparation consists of a mixture of β-oLH and β-hCG, each linked to the carriers tetanus toxoid and cholera toxin chain B. The combination of conjugates was shown to be eight- to thirteenfold more immunogenic in monkeys and rodents than β-hCG conjugated to tetanus toxoid on its own (Talwar et al, 1986). As expected, this preparation led to partial neutralization of LH in monkeys and a shortened luteal phase, but was claimed not to interfere with ovulation (Thau et al, 1979). The potential advantage of such a vaccine is that it can exert a dual anti-fertility effect, while the obvious disadvantage is the extent (largely unpredictable) to which it could interfere with hLH activity when used in humans over long periods of time. Beta-oLH has been given repeatedly to Rhesus monkeys without evidence of pituitary or renal pathology or other unwanted side-effects (Thau et al, 1986).

NON-HORMONAL VACCINE CANDIDATES

In contrast to hCG, these vaccine candidates (sperm, trophoblast and zona pellucida) are all complex structures with multiple components most of which have yet to be fully characterized, biologically or chemically. Thus, although anti-fertility effects have been demonstrated with crude preparations (Jones, 1982), there are no antigen preparations sufficiently well defined to warrant testing in clinical trials at this stage. Nevertheless, it is clear that non-cross-reactive antigens do exist within these structures and further research is justified, particularly if a vaccine can be produced which will inhibit fertilization rather than preventing implantation as occurs with β-hCG based vaccines.

Owing to the complexity of the antigens, a combination of recombinant DNA and immunological techniques is required. cDNA libraries are already available for the human testis and placenta. These libraries can then be screened with monoclonal antibodies, polyclonal antisera and/or oligonucleotide probes in order to isolate clones expressing the required immunogen(s). Once a promising antigen has been identified, the next step is to carry out extensive immunolocalization and specificity studies followed by in vitro and in vivo assessment of its capacity to elicit a fertility-regulating response. The ultimate goal of generating large quantities of material at reasonable cost for vaccination means that research must focus on proteins, the genes for which can be expressed in appropriate over-production systems.

Sperm antigens

Of the non-hormone vaccine candidates, sperm antigens may be the most attractive option on the basis of current knowledge. There are several reasons for this:

1. The immunogenicity and anti-fertility effects of sperm have been well established by experiments in animals and the finding of anti-sperm antibodies in infertile men or post-vasectomy (Anderson and Alexander, 1983; Alexander et al, 1986). In addition, the anti-fertility effect is reversible, at least following immunization with LDH-C4 in baboons.
2. No serious consequences have been reported in humans with anti-sperm antibodies. In particular, the incidence of coronary artery disease is not increased in vasectomized males despite the presence of circulating immune complexes as well as anti-sperm antibodies in these subjects (Alexander and Anderson, 1987) and the increased severity of diet-induced atherosclerosis in vasectomized primates (Alexander and Clarkson, 1978).
3. Sperm are present only transiently in the female reproductive system and are normally sequestered in the male.
4. The fact that there are a number of sperm-reactive antibodies (poly-clonal and monoclonal) which can block sperm function in vitro points to the existence of antigenic targets, an immune response to which has the potential to interfere with the normal physiological activity of sperm (Anderson et al, 1987).
5. A number of sperm antigens (e.g. LDH-C4, RSA-1 and FA-1) are highly conserved molecules, which means that animal models for testing safety and efficacy are readily available.
6. Certain sperm antigens are also expressed on the surface of the embryo, thereby offering an opportunity for fertility regulation both before and after fertilization.

The major drawback of a sperm-based vaccine is the need for induction of adequate levels of antibody of the appropriate class (e.g. IgA) in the reproductive tract. Nevertheless, precedents do exist for generation of mucosal immune responses. For example, oral administration of antigen (possibly incorporated into a salmonella vector) following primary systemic immunization has been shown to elicit significant local antibody responses (McCaughan and Basten, 1983).

Numerous human sperm antigens have now been described (Table 2;

Table 2. Examples of human sperm antigens (After Alexander and Anderson, 1987).

Antigen	Nature
LDH-C4	12 kD isoenzyme of LDH
Acrosin	Sperm acrosomal antigen
Hyaluronidase	Sperm acrosomal antigen
RSA-1, MA-29, FA-1	Antigens identified by polyclonal antisera
SO3, S37, S61	Antigens identified by monoclonal antibodies
HT	Expressed on sperm surface ?
ABO antigens	Adherent to sperm surface

Alexander and Anderson, 1987). Of these, LDH-C4, an isoenzyme of LDH confined to male germ cells, is the best characterized: its amino acid sequence and crystallographic structure are known (Goldberg, 1971; Goldberg et al, 1981). Immunization of female baboons, both systemically and locally, has resulted in reduced fertility without evidence of interference with the ovulatory cycle or other side-effects. However, neither LDH-C4 nor synthetic peptides derived from it appear to be sufficiently immunogenic to achieve the desired anti-fertility level of 90% or greater (Goldberg et al, 1981). The search for alternative vaccine candidates has therefore continued. For example, antibodies have been raised to the two acrosomal enzymes, acrosin and hyaluronidase, but neither appear to be sufficiently immunogenic for vaccine purposes, presumably because of their location within the acrosome. More recently, three monoclonal antibodies (S20, S37 and S61) were identified from a panel presented at a WHO-sponsored workshop (Anderson et al, 1987) which recognize sperm-specific targets, and work is now proceeding to characterize these antigens by molecular and immunochemical techniques. It is hoped that one of them will meet the criteria required of an effective fertility-regulating vaccine.

Trophoblast antigens

The early trophoblast, although even more complex in structure than sperm, does have the dual advantage of being expressed at a single anatomical site post-fertilization and being in intimate contact with the maternal blood supply from a very early stage in pregnancy, perhaps within ten days of ovulation in the human. Thus, systemic immunization with trophoblast-specific antigens is a feasible option as the basis for a fertility-regulating vaccine (Johnson and Stern, 1986).

In immunological terms, the function of the trophoblast is to 'protect' the embryo from destruction by the maternal immune system. Not surprisingly, it therefore lacks classical class I and class II MHC antigens due to down-regulation of the genes concerned (Bulmer and Johnson, 1985). Nevertheless, it does appear that the maternal immune system can recognize other antigens on trophoblast, the immune response to which is inhibitory in nature and designed to preserve the fetal allograft (Hunziker and Wegmann, 1986; Johnson and Stern, 1986). Further evidence in support of this concept comes from studies on women with recurrent idiopathic abortions, in whom normal regulatory responses are absent (Beer et al, 1985; MacIntyre et al, 1986) or overridden by the presence of anti-paternal antibodies (Hole et al, 1987).

Several trophoblast antigens have now been identified by means of monoclonal antibodies. Among the most interesting is a novel 41 kD class I-like MHC glycoprotein linked to β-2 microglobulin and expressed on extra-villous cytotrophoblast cells (Redman et al, 1984; Bulmer and Johnson, 1985). These molecules may be an analogue of the murine Qa-Tla antigens (Van Leeuwen et al, 1985) and could well play a role in protection of the fetus from attack by maternal cytotoxicity mechanisms (Johnson and Stern, 1986). Given its limited tissue distribution, the 41 kD glycoprotein could be one possible candidate for an anti-fertility vaccine.

Theoretically, the plasma membrane of the syncytiotrophoblast could also provide a potential vaccine target. Thus, in addition to bearing growth factor and hormone receptors, it expresses two polymorphic cell surface antigen systems which have now been characterized in some detail. The first is the heat-stable isoenzyme placental alkaline phosphatase (PLAP). PLAP is a dimeric 130 kD sialoglycoprotein (Bulmer and Johnson, 1985) and has been identified in both syncytiotrophoblast and some extravillous cyto-trophoblast cells as well as some human tumours (Stigbrand and Fishman, 1984). However, it does not appear until after the first trimester of pregnancy, and hence is not a suitable vaccine candidate. The second antigen is the trophoblast–leukocyte common (TLX) antigen. It was originally identified by rabbit antisera (Faulk and MacIntyre, 1983), but more recently a monoclonal antibody (H316) has been raised against a monomorphic epitope on the molecule (McLaughlin et al, 1982). As its name implies, the expression of this antigen is not restricted to trophoblast and it is, in fact, found on blood leukocytes and epithelial cells from endometrial glands. Although TLX may well play a role in materno-fetal interactions, its widespread distribution precludes it from being a potential vaccine candidate.

The difficulty in identifying suitable vaccine candidate molecules was confirmed at the 1987 WHO-Sponsored Workshop on Monoclonal Antibodies to Human Trophoblast and Sperm Antigens (Anderson et al, 1987), at which only two antibodies were identified that recognized trophoblast-restricted antigens. In addition to characterizing these antigens, what is now required includes development of a suitable homologous animal, extensive use of the recently available placental cDNA libraries and improvements in in vitro systems for culturing human trophoblast cells (Loke et al, 1986).

Zona pellucida

The zona pellucida (ZP) is the complex extracellular glycoprotein matrix which surrounds the oocyte. Antibodies to crude heterologous ZP preparations have been shown to reduce fertility in a number of animal species (Dunbar, 1983). These antibodies interfere with the sperm–ZP interaction in vitro by inhibiting binding and penetration of sperm (Sacco, 1981). Active immunization with ZP, however, leads to disruption of follicular development and alterations in normal ovarian function (Dunbar, 1983; Skinner et al, 1984), which are unacceptable side-effects for a fertility-regulating vaccine.

Zonae have been isolated from ova of several animal species, including the pig, mouse and rabbit. Of these, porcine ZP has attracted the most interest, since it possesses cross-reactive antigens shared with ZP from humans and other primates. On two-dimensional gels, four major families of glycoproteins have been identified with apparent molecular weights of 90 kD, 65 kD, 55 kD and 21 kD (Hedrick and Wardrip, 1981; Sacco et al, 1981). The 55 kD antigen complex comprises 60% of the porcine zona and has been isolated in relatively pure form (Yurewicz et al, 1985), although it appears to be much less immunogenic than the original crude ZP extract. At the same time, parallel studies of murine ZP have led to identification of three proteins designated ZP-1 (200 kD), ZP-2 (140 kD) and ZP-3 (83 kD). ZP-3 is the sperm receptor on murine ZP, and a monoclonal antibody to it has been successfully used to prevent fertilization in vivo (Zona Pellucida Workshop, 1986). A cDNA clone has now been isolated which encodes the epitope recognized by this antibody and cross-hybridizes with human DNA. It should therefore be possible to isolate the human ZP-3 gene, thereby providing the basis for the study of the sperm receptor in man as a possible vaccine candidate testable in vitro and in vivo. Further work, particularly involving recombinant DNA techniques, clearly has comparable potential for identifying ZP vaccine targets as it does for trophoblast antigens.

ASSESSMENT OF VACCINE CANDIDATES

Irrespective of the source of a vaccine, all candidate antigens must be subjected to the same stringent tests of safety and efficacy outlined in the Report of the Task Force on Immunological Methods for Fertility Regulation (1978) before they can be considered for clinical trials in humans. Such an evaluation includes the following:

1. Description and quality control of vaccine components including carrier molecules and adjuvants.
2. Acute toxicity testing in at least two rodent species and one non-rodent species.
3. Long-term toxicity testing in at least two species, one of which should preferably be a non-human primate (Mitchison, 1974);
4. Immunosafety testing, preferably in a homologous model. This involves:
   (a) monitoring the cell-mediated and humoral response to the vaccine preparation;
   (b) stringent assays for cross-reactivity of antibodies produced;
   (c) recording of allergic, autoantibody and immune complex-mediated reactions.
   Immunosafety testing is particularly important in the case of fertility-regulating vaccines since many potential candidates are isoimmunogens which will only elicit an adequate response when coupled to foreign carriers and in the presence of potent adjuvants.
5. Assessment of anti-fertility efficacy in an adequate number of non-human primates and influence on both ovulation and hormone levels in the case of hormone-based vaccines.
6. Identification of any teratogenic effects in offspring born to female animals which have conceived post-immunization (Stevens, 1986):

CLINICAL TRIALS

First generation vaccines

To date the only fertility-regulating vaccines which have been deemed to meet the safety and efficacy requirements outlined above are those based on hCG and its β-subunit. The first Phase I clinical trial was carried out some years ago by Talwar and his colleagues (Nash et al, 1980; Shahani et al, 1982) using the intact β-subunit of hCG coupled to tetanus toxoid. Sixty-three fertile women received four injections (80–160 μg β-hCG per dose) at fortnightly intervals, 61 of whom produced at least some antibody against hCG and tetanus toxoid. Considerable variation in duration and titre of the response was observed but, in high responders (25%), the levels of antibody reached a peak at five months and then declined towards zero at 18 months. Due to the variable responses, ten pregnancies occurred in eight women despite the presumed use of concurrent contraceptive methods (Shahani et al, 1979). Nine were terminated while one proceeded to a term delivery of a normal infant. In none of them did pregnancy (equivalent to a boost with soluble hCG) lead to an increase in antibody levels. No interference with ovulation was recorded. Menstrual cycles were said to remain normal, as did the hormone profile, despite the fact that some sera cross-reacted with hLH in both binding and biological assay systems. Presumably this may have been due to the low affinity of the cross-reactive antibodies for shared determinants on hLH. Finally, the injection regime was well tolerated, there being no evidence for untoward allergic or autoimmune reactions over the four-year period of follow-up. The development of significant but reversible antibody responses in at least some subjects, together with the lack of significant side-effects, pointed to the feasibility of using hCG-based vaccines for fertility control. On the other hand, the limited efficacy and production of hLH cross-reactive antibodies highlighted the need for a better formulation.

During the past two years, a second series of Phase I clinical trials has been initiated using the improved formulations described in the section on hCG Vaccine Candidates. The first three preparations are being tested under the auspices of the Population Council, New York, in India and Scandinavia (Talwar et al, 1987). They include β-hCG–TT, α-oLH–β-hCG coupled to tetanus toxoid and cholera toxin chain B, and the combination of β-oLH–TT/CHB plus β-hCG–TT/CHB given with alum and lipopolysaccharide in the first injection only. Preliminary results with the β-hCG–TT formulation indicate that measurable levels of anti-hCG antibodies were detectable in the first 21 women immunized (Talwar and Gaur, 1986).

The second preparation consists of CTP-β-hCG coupled to diphtheria toxoid injected in a squalene–arlacel–water emulsion together with MDP-1 as adjuvant. This WHO-sponsored trial has now been completed at one centre in Australia and the results published (Jones et al, 1988). In brief, a total of 30 surgically sterilized subjects participated and were divided into five groups. Within each group, four subjects received two injections of the active preparation containing 50, 100, 200, 500 or 1000 μg CTP, and two the vehicle only. The vaccine proved to be immunogenic at all doses tested, although there was some inter-subject variation and the antibody titres had fallen significantly by six months. The question of whether the levels of antibody achieved might have been sufficient to prevent implantation needs to be considered in the context of the predicted hCG concentration post-fertilization. Normally the hCG concentration in the maternal circulation at the time of expected menses (i.e. two weeks after ovulation in a conceptual cycle) is of the order of 100 mIU/ml, i.e. 0.2 nmol/litre or 8 ng/ml. If one assumes the biological neutralizing activity of the antibodies produced in vivo to be about 50% of their in vitro binding capacity, the data obtained shows that even the lower doses of vaccine elicited an antibody response well in excess of that required to neutralize the predicted hCG concentrations in the maternal circulation. The only side-effect of definite significance was the occurrence of myalgia and arthralgia in subjects given the higher doses of vaccines and adjuvant which was shown to be due to emulsion instability and was readily corrected. No allergic or immune complex-mediated reactions were observed. Occasional autoantibodies were detected by immunofluor-escence, including one displaying cross-reactivity with somatostatin-secreting cells in the baboon and rat pancreas, although their occurrence was not associated with abnormalities in blood glucose. The transient appearance of autoantibodies following immunization is not surprising since a potent adjuvant like MDP was being used. Furthermore, if autoantibodies were sought with the same thoroughness after other vaccine procedures, it is very likely that they would be detected in this situation as well. In view of these encouraging results, a second trial is now being planned based on a similar formulation with the aim of determining anti-fertility efficacy in fertile women.

Second generation vaccines

At the same time as alternative vaccine candidates are being sought, a substantial amount of research is now being directed towards development of better formulations. The major goal of these efforts is production of better vaccine delivery systems to overcome the practical difficulties associ-ated with multiple injections and the limited duration of the protective response. This is particularly important in the case of fertility-regulating vaccines for several reasons: firstly, the anti-fertility effect is likely to be of relatively short duration despite the addition of adjuvants, since most antigens will be isoimmunogens; secondly, the vaccines will be used largely in developing countries where the opportunity for follow-up may be limited; and, finally, the stability of current formulations (for example, two–three weeks for the CTP-β-hCG vaccine) is suboptimal.

A number of delivery systems are being examined, including liposomes (Gregoriadis, 1985), iscoms (Morein et al, 1984) and biodegradable micro-spheres (Lewis, 1985), which could have the potential of eliciting sustained anti-fertility effects following a single injection. From preliminary work carried out by Stevens (personal communication) with the CTP vaccine, it would appear that at least for this preparation the microsphere system is the most promising. However, sustained release systems will clearly be of benefit in the case of a wide range of vaccines including those to infectious agents.

The other area of research currently receiving attention is the possible development of a vaccine based on cellular, rather than antibody-dependent responses. The stimulus for this work has come from the demonstration of cell-mediated immune responses in both the male and female reproductive tracts (Anderson and Hill, 1988), coupled with the fact that experimental allergic orchitis can be transferred by activated T-cells (Tung et al, 1987). Furthermore, cytokines have been shown to interfere with sperm function (Hill et al, 1987a), trophoblast immunogenicity and viability (Head et al, 1987) and embryo development (Hill et al, 1987b).

The development of T cell-specific vaccines would require the selection of different epitopes on candidate antigens, since all the present studies involve delineation of antibody-reactive epitopes. However, this is now feasible with the availability of algorithms for predicting T cell epitopes in protein molecules (Berzofsky, 1985). The potential advantage of a T cell-based vaccine is the long duration of T cell memory compared with that of the B cell, although considerable work will be required to determine whether systemic immunization can elicit a local cell-mediated reaction of sufficient specificity to induce a prolonged anti-fertility response free from side-effects.

SUMMARY

Fertility-regulating vaccines offer the most practical way of controlling the birth rate, particularly in developing countries. Ideological and political pressure has limited the scope of research being directed towards the goal. Nevertheless, recent advances in reproductive endocrinology, immunology and molecular biology have made an acceptable anti-fertility vaccine a realistic possibility for the next decade. Among the various vaccine candidates under study, the β-subunit of hCG and its unique C-terminal peptide are the most advanced since extensive work in experimental animals and Phase I clinical trials in humans have demonstrated the safety, potential efficacy and reversibility of this hormone-based vaccine in women. It is now also clear that complex structures such as sperm, trophoblast and zona pellucida express antigens, the distribution of which are largely restricted to reproductive tissues. Furthermore, immune responses to them have been shown to interfere with the processes of fertilization and implantation. More research is required, however, before any of the candidate molecules from these sources can be considered for clinical trials in humans. The first generation vaccines based on the β-subunit of hCG require multiple injections for efficacy and appear to exert their effect through antibody-dependent mechanisms. In the future, better delivery systems (e.g. microspheres) designed to induce sustained fertility control following a single injection, and antigens capable of eliciting T-cell dependent responses, could well become the basis of the second and third generations of vaccines.

REFERENCES

Ada GL, Basten A & Jones WR (1985) Prospects for developing vaccines to control fertility. *Nature* **317**: 288–289.

Alexander NJ & Clarkson TB (1978) Vasectomy increases the severity of diet-induced athero-sclerosis in Macaca fascilularis. *Science* **201:** 538–541.

Alexander NJ & Anderson DJ (1987) Immunology of semen. *Fertility and Sterility* **47:** 192–205.

Alexander NJ, Fulghan DL, Plunkett RR & Witkin SS (1986) Anti-sperm antibodies and circulating immune complexes of vasectomised men with and without coronary events. *American Journal of Reproductive Immunology and Microbiology* **12:** 38–44.

Anderson DJ & Alexander NJ (1983) A new look at anti-fertility vaccines. *Fertility and Sterility* **40:** 557–571.

Anderson DJ & Hill JA (1988) Cell-mediated immunity in infertility. *American Journal of Reproductive Immunology* (in press).

Anderson DJ, Johnson PM, Alexander NJ, Jones WR & Griffin PD (1987) Monoclonal antibodies to human trophoblast and sperm antigens: Report of two WHO-sponsored workshops, 30 June, 1986, Toronto. *Journal of Reproductive Immunology* **10:** 231–257.

Bahl OP (1977) Human chorionic gonadotrophin, its receptor and mechanism of action. *Federation Proceedings* **36:** 2119–2127.

Beer AE, Semprini AE, Xiaoyn Z & Quebberman JP (1986) Pregnancy outcome in human couples with recurrent spontaneous abortion: the role(s) of female serum, mixed lympho-cyte culture blocking factors, potentiating factors and local uterine immunity before and after paternal leucocyte immunisation. *Experimental and Clinical Immunogenetics* **2:** 1–12.

Berzofsky JA (1985) Intrinsic and extrinsic factors in protein antigenic structure. *Science* **229:** 932–940.

Bulmer JN & Johnson PM (1985) Antigen expression by trophoblast populations in the human placenta and their possible immunobiological significance. *Placenta* **6:** 127–140.

Crawford RJ, Tregear GW & Niall HD (1986) The nucleotide sequence of baboon chorionic gonadotrophin. Beta-subunit genes have diverged from the human. *Gene* **46:** 161–169.

Dunbar BS (1983) Antibodies to Zona Pellucida antigens and their role in fertility. In Wegmann T, Gill T, Cumming C & Nisbet-Brown B (eds) *Immunology of Reproduction*, pp 506–534. New York: Oxford University Press.

Faulk WP & McIntyre JA (1983) Immunological studies of human trophoblast: markers, subsets and functions. *Immunological Reviews* **75:** 139–175.

Goldberg E (1971) Immunochemical specificity of lactate dehydrogenase. *Proceedings of the National Academy of Sciences USA* **68:** 349–352.

Goldberg E, Wheat TE, Powell JE & Stevens VC (1981) Reduction of fertility in female baboons immunised with lactate dehydrogenase. *Fertility and Sterility* **35:** 214–217.

Gregoriadis G (1985) Liposomes for drugs and vaccines. *Trends in Biotechnology* **3:** 235–241.

Griffin PD (1986) A fertility regulating vaccine based on the carboxyl-terminal peptide of the beta-subunit of human chorionic gonadotrophin. In Talwar GP (ed.) *Immunological Approaches to Contraception and Fertility*, pp 43–59. New York: Plenum Press.

Head JR, Drake BL & Zuckermann FA (1987) Major histocompatibility antigens on tropho-blast and their regulation: implications in the materno-foetal relationship. *American Journal of Reproductive Immunology* **15:** 12–18.

Hearn JP (1980) The immunology of chorionic gonadotrophin. In Hearn JP (ed.) *Immuno-logical Aspects of Reproduction and Fertility Control*, p 229, Lancaster: MTP Press.

Hedrick JL & Wardrip N (1981) Microheterogeneity in the glycoproteins of the zona pellucida is due to the carbohydrate moiety. *Journal of Cell Biology* **91:** 177a.

Hill JA, Hacmovici F, Politch JA & Anderson DJ (1987a) Effects of soluble products of activated lymphocytes and macrophages (lymphokines and monokines) on human sperm motion parameters. *Fertility and Sterility* **47:** 460–465.

Hill JA, Hacmovici F & Anderson DJ (1987b) Products of activated lymphocytes and macro-phages inhibit mouse embryo development in vitro. *Journal of Immunology* **139:** 2250–2254.

Hole N, Cheng HM & Johnson PM (1987) Antibody reactivity against human trophoblast membrane antigens in the context of normal pregnancy and unexplained recurrent miscarriage. In Chaouat G (ed.) *Inserm Colloque on Materno-Fetal Relations* **154:** 213–224.

Hunziker RD & Wegmann TG (1986) Placental immunoregulation. *CRC Reviews in Immunology* **6:** 245–285.

Johnson PM & Stern PJ (1986) Antigen expression at human maternal–foetal interfaces.

Progress in Immunology VI: 1056–1069. New York: Academic Press.

Jones WR (1982) *Immunological Fertility Regulation.* Oxford: Blackwell Scientific Publications.

Jones WR, Bradley J, Judd SJ et al (1988) Phase 1 clinical trial of a World Health Organisation Birth Control Vaccine. *Lancet* ii: 1295–1298.

Kemp BE & Niall HD (1984) Relaxin. In Aurbach G (ed.) *Vitamins and Hormones* 42: 79–115.

Lewis DH (1985) Overview of controlled release systems for male contraception. In Zatuchni GI, Goldsmith A & Sciarra JJ (eds). Philadelphia: Harper and Row.

Loke YW, Butterworth BH, Margetts JJ & Burland K (1986) Identification of cytotrophoblast colonies in cultures of human placental cells using monoclonal antibodies. *Placenta* 7: 221–231.

McCaughan GW & Basten A (1983) Immune system of the gastrointestinal tract. In Young JA (ed.) *Gastrointestinal Physiology IV* 28: 131–157. Baltimore: University Park Press.

McLaughlin PJ, Cheng HM, Slade MB & Johnson PM (1982) Expression on cultured human tumour cells of placental trophoblast membrane antigens and placental alkaline phosphatase defined by monoclonal antibodies. *International Journal of Cancer* 30: 21–26.

McIntyre JA, Faulk WP, Nichols-Johnson VR & Taylor CG (1986) Immunological testing and immunotherapy in recurrent spontaneous abortion. *Obstetrics and Gynecology* 67: 169–175.

Mitchison NA (1974) Long term hazards in immunological methods of fertility control. In Diczfalusy E (ed.) *Seventh Karolinska Symposium on Research Methods in Reproductive Endocrinology: Immunological Approaches to Fertility Control* (Supplement 194), pp 405–418, *Acta Endocrinologica.*

Morein B, Sundqvist B, Hoglund S, Dalsgaard K & Osterhaus A (1984) Iscom, a novel structure for antigenic presentation from enveloped viruses. *Nature* 308: 457–460.

Morgan JF, Birken S & Canfield RE (1973) Human chorionic gonadotrophin: a proposal for the amino acid sequence. *Molecular and Cellular Biochemistry* 2: 97–99.

Nash HA, Talwar GP, Segal S, Luuckainen T & Johansson EDB (1980) Observations on the antigenicity and clinical effects of a candidate anti-pregnancy vaccine: Beta-subunit of human chorionic gonadotrophin linked to Tetanus Toxoid. *Fertility and Sterility* 34: 328–335.

Redman CWG, McMichael AJ, Sturrat GM, Sunderland CA & Ting A (1984) Class I major histocompatibility complex antigens on human extravillous trophoblast. *Immunology* 52: 457–468.

Sacco AG (1981) Immunocontraception: consideration of the Zona Pellucida as a target antigen. In Wynn RM (ed.) *Obstetrics and Gynecology Annual,* vol. 10, pp 1–26.

Sacco AG, Yurewicz EC, Subramanian MG & De Mayo FJ (1981) Zona Pellucida composition: species cross-reactivity and contraception potential of antiserum to a purified pig zone antigen (PPZA) *Biology of Reproduction* 25: 997–1008.

Saxena BB, Hasan SH, Haour F & Schmidt-Gollwitzer M (1974) Radioreceptor assay of human chorionic gonadotrophin: detection of early pregnancy. *Science* 184: 793–795.

Shahani SM, Kulkarni PP & Patel KL (1979) Evaluation of immunological and safety data in women treated with PR-β-hCG-TT vaccine. In Talwar GP (ed.) *Recent Advances in Reproduction and Regulation of Fertility,* pp 473–476. Amsterdam: Elsevier/North Holland.

Shahani SM, Kulkarni PP, Patel KL, Salahuddin M, Das C & Talwar GP (1982) Clinical and immunological response to Pr-β-hCG-TT vaccine. *Contraception* 25: 421–434.

Sharma NC, Singh O, Gaur A et al (1986a) Improved immunogenic formulations for anti-gonadotrophin response. In Talwar GP (ed.) *Immunological Approaches to Contraception and Fertility,* pp 37–41. New York: Plenum Press.

Sharma NC, Kaul S, Rao LV, Singh O, Gaur A & Talwar GP (1986b) Reduction of individual variability of anti-hCG response by mixed carriers. *Progress in Immunology VI* (Abstract No. 6.23.2.) New York: Academic Press.

Skinner SM, Mills T, Kirchick HJ & Dunbar BS (1984) Immunisation with Zona Pellucida proteins results in abnormal ovarian follicular differentiation and inhibition of gonadotrophin-induced steroid secretion. *Endocrinology* 111: 2418–2432.

Stevens VC (1976) Perspectives of development of a fertility control vaccine from hormonal antigens of the trophoblast. In *Development of Vaccines for Fertility Regulation (WHO Symposium),* pp 93–110. Copenhagen: Scriptor.

Stevens VC (1981a) Preparation and formulation of a hCG anti-fertility vaccine: selection of a peptide immunogen. *American Journal of Reproductive Immunology* **6**: 307–314.

Stevens VC (1981b) Vaccines against pregnancy. In Fen CC, Griffin D & Woolman A (eds) *Symposium on Recent Advances in Fertility Regulation*, pp 211–227. Geneva: Atar, SA.

Stevens VC (1986) Current status of anti-fertility vaccines using gonadotrophin immunogens. *Immunology Today* **7**: 369–374.

Stevens VC, Cinader B, Powell JE, Lee AC & Kohn SW (1981) Preparation and formulation of a hCG anti-fertility vaccine: selection of adjuvant and vehicle. *American Journal of Reproductive Immunology* **6**: 315–321.

Stigbrand T & Fishman WH (1984) *Human Alkaline Phosphatases*. New York: Alan R. Liss.

Talwar GP (1980) *Immunology of Contraception*. London: Edward Arnold.

Talwar GP & Gaur A (1986) Recent developments in immunocontraception. In Ratnam SS & Teoh ES (eds) *Advances in Fertility and Sterility Series*, vol. 6, pp 39–45. Camforth: Parthenon.

Talwar GP, Singh O, Singh V et al (1986) Enhancement of anti-gonadotrophin response to the beta-subunit of ovine luteinising hormone by carrier conjugation and combination with the beta-subunit of human chorionic gonadotrophin. *Fertility and Sterility* **46**: 120–126.

Talwar GP, Gaur A, Gupta SK & Singh SO (1987) Immunological control of fertility. In Thompson RA (ed.) *Recent Advances in Clinical Immunology*, pp 183–200. Edinburgh: Churchill Livingstone.

Task Force on Immunological Methods for Fertility Regulation (1978) Evaluating the safety and efficacy of placental antigen vaccines for fertility regulation. *Clinical and Experimental Immunology* **33**: 360–375.

Thau RB, Sundaram K, Thornton YS & Seidman LS (1979) Effects of immunisation with the beta-subunit of ovine luteinising hormone on corpus luteum function in the rhesus monkey. *Fertility and Sterility* **31**: 200–204.

Thau RB, Bond MG, Witkin SS, Sundaram K & Sawyer JK (1986) Lack of toxicological effects following seven years of active immunisation of rhesus monkeys with the beta-subunit of ovine luteinising hormone. In Talwar GP (ed.) *Immunological Approaches to Contraception and Fertility*, pp 25–33. New York: Plenum Press.

Tung KSK (1986) Immunopathologic aspects of anti-sperm immunity. In Clark DA & Croy BA (eds) *Reproductive Immunology*, pp 143–151. Amsterdam: Elsevier.

Tung KSK, Yule TD, Mahi-Brown CA & Listrom MB (1987) Distribution of histopathology and Ia positive cells in actively induced and passively transferred experimental auto-immune orchitis. *Journal of Immunology* **138**: 752–759.

Van Leeuwen A, Giphart MJ, de Groot G et al (1985) Two different T-cell systems in humans, one of which is probably equivalent to Qa or Tla in mice. *Human Immunology* **12**: 235–246.

Yurewicz EC, Sacco AG & Submanian MG (1985) Isolation and preliminary characterisation of a purified pig zona antigen (PPZA) from porcine oocytes. *Biology of Reproduction* **29**: 511–523.

Zona Pellucida Workshop (1986) *Family Health International*, pp 1–7.

11

Immunological approaches to prenatal diagnosis

M. ADINOLFI

This chapter analyses selected topics involving the use of immunological techniques for the prenatal diagnosis of inherited disorders. Some arguments, such as the detection and prevention of isoimmune haemolytic disease of the newborn, have already been analysed extensively and critically in recent articles (see Acker et al, 1986; Mollison et al, 1987; also Chapter 3). The same applies to the diagnostic value of estimating levels of α-fetoprotein (AFP) in amniotic fluid or maternal sera for the prenatal diagnosis of neural tube defects (NTD) (Norgaard-Pedersen, 1976; Adinolfi, 1979; Cederqvist, 1983; Seller, 1983; Bergstrand, 1986). It would be impossible to present a satisfactory account of these topics in a brief review; instead, investigations which are still in progress and promise to be rewarding in the near future are emphasized. Thus, for example with regard to AFP, the discussion is limited to the diagnostic significance of measuring the levels of this protein in maternal sera collected during the first trimester of gestation in order to detect fetal chromosome abnormalities, an area of research still surrounded by uncertainties and controversies.

Finally, certain topics deserve only a brief mention, since the present immunological approaches are shortly going to be superseded by more accurate tests based on the use of genetic probes.

PRENATAL DIAGNOSIS OF INHERITED IMMUNODEFICIENCIES

The prenatal diagnosis of many types of immunodeficiencies is still hampered by severe technical problems. The biochemical basis of many immunodeficiencies has not yet been elucidated (Rosen, 1980; Hirschhorn and Hirschhorn, 1983; Kredich and and Hershfield, 1983). The diagnosis in young children is usually reached by testing several samples of blood, collected over a certain period of time, and by performing in vitro and in vivo tests aimed at detecting specific deficiencies of the cellular or humoral types of immune reactions. Prenatal diagnosis of immunodeficiencies is often performed using a single sample of fetal blood obtained at an early stage of development of the immune system, when maturation of specific cell markers and functions is still incomplete. The diagnosis must, therefore, be targeted to a specific type of immune deficiency, as observed in a previous 'index' affected child. Furthermore, in vivo tests cannot corroborate the diagnosis.

In spite of these difficulties, the development of monoclonal antibodies (mAbs) reacting against specific subpopulations of leukocytes, and particularly T cell subsets, made it possible to perform prenatal diagnosis of selected immunodeficiencies. The basic approach is collection of a fetal blood sample, and counting the incidence of the different populations of white cells initially identified according to their morphological appearances; leukocytes or lymphocytes are then separated from red cells and analysed with a panel of murine mAbs directed against surface antigens unique to the various sets of nucleated cells. The sensitized cells are then incubated with antisera raised against mouse immunoglobulin, conjugated with fluorescein or phycoerythrin. Analysis of the stained cells must be performed using a flow cytometer, which allows collection of objective results and also measurement of the intensity of the fluorescent dyes. By comparing the obtained data with those expected in normal fetuses of the same gestational age, it should be possible to exclude, or to suspect, that the fetus under investigation has a specific type of immunodeficiency (Durandy et al, 1982a,b; Linch et al, 1984; Levinski, 1984; Durandy et al, 1987).

Knowledge of the pattern of inheritance of the immunodeficiency (e.g. if it is X-linked and therefore eventually transmitted from a 'carrier' mother to 50% of her sons), and of the 'carrier' status of the parents, is essential for an accurate prenatal diagnosis. X-linked agammaglobulinaemia, XLA (Bruton, 1952), is an interesting example of prenatal diagnosis of immunodeficiencies. This X-linked disorder is characterized by low levels of circulating B cells and markedly decreased synthesis of immunoglobulins (Ig), whilst circulating T cells are functionally normal. XLA reflects an arrest of the maturation of B lymphocytes at the precursor cell stage.

Prenatal diagnosis can be achieved by estimating the incidence of B cells in fetal blood using mAbs, and by the demonstration that the few cells present lack Ig molecules on their surface. In addition, genetic probes and linkage analysis in selected families may confirm the diagnosis. In fact, Mensink et al (1987) have documented a close linkage between the XLA locus on the X chromosome with the DXS17 restriction fragment length polymorphism (RFLP) marker and a series of other DNA–RFLP markers around the DXS17 locus. Thus, family studies using these DNA markers linked to the XLA locus can provide useful information for genetic counselling on this severe immunodeficiency disease as well as for prenatal diagnosis. However, genetic heterogeneity of the disease may complicate counselling since, in at least one family, a high frequency of recombination within the XLA–DXS17 locus was observed.

In some immunodeficiencies, the diagnosis can be reached with a high degree of accuracy as, for example, in fetuses failing to express HLA molecules. This defect may concern only HLA class I (A, B or C) antigens, the 'bare lymphocyte syndrome' (Touraine et al, 1978), or both HLA class I and II (Griscelli et al, 1980). This latter syndrome, termed HLA class II negative SCID, has been shown to result from a defective synthesis of class

II MHC molecules due to an abnormal regulatory gene located outside the major histocompatibility complex (Lisowska-Grospierre et al, 1985; de Preval et al, 1985). This autosomal recessive syndrome is characterized by a deficiency of both humoral and cellular responses; death usually occurs in childhood following chronic diarrhoea and repeated bacterial and viral infections. Recently, prenatal diagnosis has been performed in six pregnancies at risk for the disease. Two fetuses were found to be affected, and the diagnosis was confirmed by testing fetal blood nucleated cells with mAbs after induced abortions (Durandy et al, 1987).

About 30% of severe combined immunodeficiencies (SCID) are due to the absence of adenosine deaminase (ADA), an enzyme of the purine salvage pathway coded by a gene on chromosome 20 (Hirschhorn and Hirschhorn, 1983). The severity of this autosomal recessive disorder correlates with the amount of residual ADA reactivity which variably alters the number of T and B cells. Prenatal diagnosis of ADA deficiency can be readily performed on fetal blood samples and by the estimation of the enzyme in a population of isolated lymphocytes or T cells (Levinsky, 1984). It can also be diagnosed using amniotic fluid cells (Hirschhorn et al, 1975; Ziegler et al, 1980). Diffusion of the enzyme from the maternal circulation to fetal placental tissue may affect tests performed on uncultured chorionic biopsies, but the enzyme is produced by cultured chorionic cells.

Prenatal diagnosis of a severe T cell disorder due to the deficiency of purine nucleoside phosphorylase can be diagnosed directly by estimating the enzyme in amniotic fluid cells or fetal red cells (Simmonds et al, 1983). Other variants of severe immunodeficiency are also amenable to prenatal diagnosis. For example, reticular dysgenesis, characterized by a virtually total absence of T and B cells, in addition to a deficiency of granulocytes and their precursors (de Vaal and Seynhaeve, 1959), can be diagnosed prenatally by the analysis of fetal blood in association with the demonstration of fetal skeletal abnormalities.

Another immunodeficiency which can be investigated prenatally is 'chronic granulomatous disease' (CGD), a group of disorders originally described by Berendes et al (1959). In the majority of cases, the disease occurs in boys and the transmission is X-linked, as proven by the presence of two populations of neutrophils (one normal and the other abnormal) in maternal peripheral blood. However, about 10% of all reported cases are females, and family investigations suggest an autosomal recessive transmission.

With the availability of numerous and powerful antibiotics, CGD is no longer a disease fatal in childhood, but it remains a lifelong disease. Thus, prenatal diagnosis of the disease in pregnancies at high risk is required by selected families with, or that have lost, a previously affected child (Newburger et al, 1979; Borregaard et al, 1982; Matthay et al, 1984).

Recently, prenatal diagnosis of CGD has been attempted in four pregnancies at risk. The sex of the fetuses was previously determined on amniotic fluid cells. Fetal blood was obtained from the umbilical vein under fetoscopy, and the diagnosis performed using three tests: nitroblue tetrazolium reduction (NBT); cytochemical analysis with phorbol myristate acetate (PMA) as activator; luminol-enhanced chemiluminescence with activation by opsonized zymosan of PMA; and by measuring superoxide anion (O_2^- production by granulocytes. In three cases, the test showed deficient metabolic oxidative granulocytes. The diagnosis of CGD was later confirmed on the aborted fetuses (Pham Hun et al, 1987).

These are only a few examples of prenatal diagnosis of immunodeficiency disorders. The technical approaches are soon to be modified and improved by the use of polymorphic DNA sequences (RFLPs) linked to the abnormal genes. It has been claimed, for instance, that the CGD locus resides on the distal short arm (Xp21) of the X chromosome (Baehner et al, 1986). If this is confirmed, polymorphic DNA sequences flanking this locus could be used for the prenatal diagnosis of the disease in informative families.

While deficiencies of humoral immune responses cannot be detected by measuring the levels of immunoglobulin in fetal sera, since IgG molecules cross the placenta and are therefore derived from the maternal circulation, at least in theory deficiencies of specific components of complement are amenable to prenatal diagnosis by a direct evaluation of their levels in fetal sera. In fact, all components of complement are present in 14–16 week old fetuses (Adinolfi, 1984) and at least two complement receptors, CR1 and CR3, can be readily detected on the surface of nucleated blood cells around 14 weeks of gestation (Adinolfi et al, 1988). Most complement deficiencies are, however, well tolerated and rarely require prenatal diagnosis.

Prenatal diagnosis of fetal infection with toxoplasmosis, rubella or cytomegalovirus can be performed on fetal blood samples, and this topic has been recently reviewed by Romero et al (1986).

PRENATAL DIAGNOSIS BASED ON HLA-LINKAGE ANALYSIS

The determination of the fetal HLA phenotype, by detecting the expression of class I and II HLA molecules on the surface of amniotic fluid cells collected by amniocentesis, fulfils two main purposes: that of investigating paternity in the case of rape (Pollack et al, 1980a) and that of performing prenatal diagnosis of diseases closely linked to the HLA complex, such as C4 deficiencies (Pollack et al, 1980b) or congenital adrenal hyperplasia (21-OH deficiency) (Pollack et al, 1979; Couillin et al, 1981). In practice, however, the use of this approach is hampered by several problems. Firstly, it is technically difficult to detect class I HLA molecules on amniotic fluid cells using conventional cytotoxic or other immunological assays (Pollack et al, 1981). Secondly, class II HLA antigens are not expressed (Adinolfi, 1982a). Thirdly, the weak expression of HLA-B antigens on amniotic fluid cells, and the high incidence of HLA-B sharing between parents of 21-OH deficient children, also greatly reduces the usefulness of this approach.

With the introduction of new techniques for the detection of inherited disorders using DNA polymorphic sequences (RFLPs), prenatal diagnosis of 21-OH deficiencies can be performed using specific DNA probes and either DNA extracted from cultured amniotic fluid cells or from chorionic villus biopsies. These methods guarantee better chances of detecting abnormal genes linked to the informative markers, thus making the immunological approach obsolete.

The same applies to paternity investigations, since the most efficient method is to employ the 'DNA fingerprint' analysis, as devised by Jeffreys et al (1985), using chorionic villus biopsies or amniotic fluid cells.

AFP ESTIMATION AS A TOOL FOR PRENATAL DIAGNOSIS OF FETAL CHROMOSOME ABNORMALITIES

Discovered in 1956 by Bergstrand and Czar, and simultaneously by Halbrecht and Klibansky, the early studies of this fetal protein have provided important information about its physicochemical structure and site of synthesis during fetal life (Norgaard-Pedersen, 1976; Adinolfi, 1979; Bergstrand, 1986). It soon became evident that AFP was structurally similar to albumin and that, at least in mammals, its main sites of synthesis were the yolk sac, liver, intestine and, occasionally, the placenta (Adinolfi, 1979).

An important turning point was the discovery that, both in mice and humans, high levels of AFP could be detected in sera from individuals with cancer of the liver or during the regeneration of hepatocytes following hepatitis. Two other conditions found to be associated with high serum concentrations of AFP are teratocarcinoma and tyrosinaemia (see Adinolfi, 1979; Bergstrand, 1986).

In 1972, Brock and Sutcliffe, in a retrospective investigation, observed that abnormally high levels of AFP could be detected in amniotic fluid obtained from fetuses with a neural tube defect (NTD), such as anencephaly or open spina bifida. The increased values resulted from the leakage of AFP from the cerebrospinal fluid (CSF) into the amniotic cavity, due to the immaturity of the blood–brain barrier during fetal life (Adinolfi et al, 1976). The estimation of AFP by immunological methods in samples of amniotic fluid obtained from mothers at risk of having an NTD-affected fetus, in association with tests for the detection of cholinesterase and ultrasound scanning, has become a routine and efficient procedure for the prenatal diagnosis of malformations of the neural tube (Adinolfi, 1979; Cederqvist, 1983; Bergstrand, 1986; Milunsky, 1986).

Since many reviews and papers have been published on this topic, as well as on the advantages and disadvantages of estimating the levels of AFP in sera of pregnant women for the prenatal diagnosis of NTD (Seller, 1983), I will confine my analysis to the association between low levels of AFP in maternal serum and fetal chromosome abnormalities, with particular emphasis on trisomy 21 (Down's syndrome).

Although the incidence of fetal chromosome abnormalities due to an extra chromosome increase markedly with maternal age, approximately 80% of infants with Down's syndrome are born to mothers under 35 years old. Because of the limited laboratory facilities, however, and of the increased chance of spontaneous abortion associated with the procedure, amniocentesis for the prenatal detection of fetuses with Down's syndrome is usually restricted to women at high risk and those more than 35 years of age.

Many attempts have been made to develop mass-screening techniques. In 1984, Merkatz et al reported that maternal serum AFP levels lower than the median values were more likely to be observed in pregnancies in which the fetus had trisomy 21 than in unaffected pregnancies. This initial observation prompted several similar retrospective studies aimed at assessing the reproducibility of the test and its value as an index of risk of Down's syndrome in women under 35 years of age (Cuckle et al, 1984; Fuhrmann et al, 1984; Baumgarten et al, 1985; Spencer and Carpenter, 1985; Milunsky, 1986).

Recently, Schoenfeld-Di Maio and collaborators (1987) have reported their retrospective and prospective studies of mid-trimester screening of maternal serum AFP levels. Unlike investigators in earlier studies, the risk of carrying a fetus with Down's syndrome was calculated according to the maternal age and the AFP serum levels adjusted also for maternal body weight and race. Tables depicting the calculated risks of NTD according to age of the mother, gestational age and AFP values have been reported (Milunsky, 1986). In the retrospective study, about 23 000 women who underwent AFP serological tests were under 35 years old. In this group, 18 infants were born with Down's syndrome, with an overall incidence of 1 : 1280; in 15 out of the 18 respective mothers, the AFP serum levels were below the population median. However, according to the calculated risk of Down's syndrome based on the estimation of the serum levels of AFP in relation to maternal age, prenatal diagnosis of trisomy 21 could have been performed in only 5 (28%) out of the 18 cases.

The prospective screening was carried out in over 34 000 pregnant women less than 35 years of age. In this group, 1814 women (5.3%) were calculated to have a risk of bearing a Down's syndrome fetus, equal to or greater than the age-related risk of a 35-year-old woman (1 : 270) at a gestational age between 15 and 22 weeks. Ultrasound examination revealed the cause of the low AFP levels in 329 (18%); for example, 289 women had a fetus whose gestational age was less than that originally reported, while 34 women were carrying a dead fetus, two had molar pregnancies and four were not pregnant. Of the 1451 women with a 1 : 270 or higher probability of having an affected fetus, 1102 (76%) elected to have amniocentesis. Twenty-seven women (2.9%) had a Down's syndrome fetus, but the diagnosis of trisomy 21 by estimation of maternal AFP levels had been suggested only in 9. Thus, Schoenfeld-Di Maio and collaborators (1987) were able to identify only one third of the affected fetuses using this approach.

These results are reported in detail because they emphasize the complexity of the problem. Although a sensitive test was employed, over 60% of Down's syndrome fetuses were missed; on the other hand, a large percentage of pregnant women had to undergo amniocentesis while carrying normal fetuses. Besides the associated apprehension of this procedure, it causes fetal loss in around 1.5% of cases; thus, there would be more fetal losses than prenatal diagnosis of Down's syndrome.

New and more sensitive methods for AFP estimation and a combination of several tests will undoubtedly improve the screening procedures for the prenatal diagnosis of selected aneuploidies. In fact, several trials are in progress in order to evaluate fully the advantages of performing mass screening at an early stage of pregnancy by measuring the serum levels of AFP during the first trimester of gestation.

TRANSFER OF NUCLEATED CELLS ACROSS THE PLACENTA AND PRENATAL DIAGNOSIS OF FETAL INHERITED DISORDERS

This topic has been the subject of many investigations and controversies over almost a century. The importance of the problem derives from the biological properties of the cells involved and the effects that they may have on the complex immunological relationship between mother and fetus. Furthermore, the detection of fetal nucleated cells in maternal peripheral blood may be potentially useful for the prenatal diagnosis of selected inherited disorders (Adinolfi and Gorvette, 1974; Herzenberg et al, 1979; Iverson et al, 1981).

Different types of fetal nucleated cells are expected to enter into the maternal circulation and *vice versa*. Although, chronologically, studies of the transfer of leukocytes or placenta-derived cellular elements have been carried out simultaneously, here the results of these studies will be reported separately.

Fetal leukocytes in maternal peripheral blood

In early studies, morphological criteria or radiolabelling were used to identify maternal cells present in the fetal circulation. Due probably to technical artefacts, the results of these investigations were inconclusive (see Adinolfi, 1982b).

Particular emphasis was also given to investigations of infants born to mothers with various types of leukaemias. With very few exceptions, it was found that infants born to affected mothers were healthy and did not develop leukaemias during the first few years of life (see Adinolfi, 1982b). Lack of transfer across the placenta has been confirmed in studies using experimental animals. For example, in an interesting study carried out in mice it was observed that, if as few as 100 leukaemia cells were injected into young embryos, they would develop the disease in later life. However, female mice with induced leukaemias were found to produce healthy offspring, thus showing that either murine maternal leukocytes do not cross the placenta or, if they are transferred into the fetal circulation, their number must be extremely low (Loewenstein et al, 1971).

In more recent times, lymphocytes have been the target of most investigations, mainly because these cells can be analysed early in metaphase following stimulation with lectins and lipopolysaccharides or by using monoclonal antibodies (mAbs), and this facilitates their distribution between fetal and maternal cells. In fact, Walknowska et al in 1959, using a cytological approach, claimed that cells in metaphase with 46XY chromosome complement could be detected in the peripheral blood of pregnant women. After stimulation with phytohaemagglutinins (PHA), from 0.2 to 2% of metaphases were found to have the Y chromosome and these cells were therefore assumed to be derived from a male fetus. However, in this as well as later studies (Desai and Creger, 1963; de Grouchy and Trebuchet, 1971; Schindler et al, 1972), cells with an apparent chromosome complement 46XY were also detected with high frequency in the peripheral blood of mothers who later delivered female infants (see Adinolfi, 1982b). Furthermore, many investigators were unable to detect 46XY cells in all maternal peripheral blood samples tested following stimulation with PHA (Angell and Adinolfi, 1969; Jacobs and Smith, 1969; Takahara et al, 1972; Adinolfi et al, 1975).

The controversy flared once again when de la Chapelle, Schröder and collaborators (Schröder and de la Chapelle, 1972; Schröder et al, 1974) claimed that, by staining metaphase spreads from maternal peripheral blood samples with quinacrine mustard (QM), they could clearly identify 46XY cells. Once again, these results could not be confirmed by other investigators (Zimmerman and Schmickel, 1971; Kirsh-Volders et al, 1980; Adinolfi, 1982b), a conclusion finally accepted by Schröder (see Zilliacus et al, 1975) who maintained, however, that cells in interphase (showing a bright fluorescent spot after QM staining) could be detected in the peripheral blood of pregnant women (Schröder, 1974). Two problems invalidate this conclusion. The first is that presumed 'male' cells were often detected in the peripheral blood of mothers who later delivered a female infant; and the second is that a few cells with bright QM fluorescent spots can be detected in non-pregnant women due to the staining of chromosome satellites by the QM technique (Polani and Mutton, 1971; see also Adinolfi, 1982b).

Two other approaches have been used to investigate the possibility that fetal lymphocytes may cross the placenta and reach the maternal peripheral circulation. The first was based on the detection of HLA-A2-positive cells in the peripheral circulation of HLA-A2-negative mothers using a rabbit anti-serum directed against this histocompatibility antigen (Herzenberg et al, 1979; Iverson et al, 1981). In the first paper, a selected group of HLA-A2-negative mothers who had undergone amniocentesis at 15 weeks, and who were known therefore to have male fetuses, was investigated using a rabbit anti-HLA-A2 and flow cytometry. The presumed HLA-A2-positive fetal cells were sorted and then examined for the presence of interphase cells containing the Y-body. In five cases, in which the neonates were HLA-A2-positive, a few Y-body positive cells (2/331; 3/484; 3/1017; 7/1065) were detected in the sorted samples. In the remaining seven cases, when the neonates were HLA-A2-negative, no Y-body positive cells were detected.

The second investigation was carried out on 138 women who had undergone amniocentesis for prenatal detection of genetic disease, and 30 of them had been selected because they were known from amniocentesis to be carrying a male fetus. Peripheral blood lymphocytes from maternal blood were typed using a rabbit anti-HLA-A2 reagent. If the woman was HLA-A2-negative, using flow cytometry and the anti-HLA-A2 serum, the sample was enriched with HLA-A2-positive cells and then examined for the presence of Y-body positive cells in interphase. Forty-eight of the 138 women (35%) were found to be HLA-A2-negative; 21 of these with HLA-A2-positive spouses gave birth to male infants. Of the 21 infants, eight were HLA-A2-positive and their enriched samples contained Y-body positive cells in interphase. However, only a small percentage of the presumed 'male' fetal cells were found to be Y-body positive. The remaining 13 male infants in this group were HLA-A2-negative. Y-body positive cells were detected in one maternal enriched sample, although it was later confirmed that the newborn was HLA-A2-negative. In the group of eight HLA-A2-negative mothers with HLA-A2-negative spouses and male offspring, Y-body positive cells were not detected in any of the enriched samples. In the last group of 19 HLA-A2-negative mothers with female offspring, Y-body positive cells were detected in the enriched samples from only one mother.

These papers raise several questions. The incidence of Y-body positive cells in the enriched samples from mothers who delivered a male infant is surprisingly low (e.g. one Y-body-positive cell out of about 1400 sorted HLA-A2-positive cells). In fact, the incidence did not differ markedly from that described in previous studies in which enrichment of the fetal cells was not carried out. There is no mention in the two papers of the incidence of the presumed Y-body positive cells in maternal samples before enrichment, so it is difficult to calculate the effect of using anti-HLA and flow cytometry in order to sort only fetal cells. Furthermore, no artificial mixtures of maternal and HLA-A2-negative and fetal HLA-A2-positive cells were examined.

The second approach was based on the detection in maternal peripheral blood samples of a few lymphocytes reacting with antisera against α-fetoprotein (AFP). The presence of AFP-positive cells in maternal blood was interpreted as evidence of the transfer of AFP-positive fetal cells into the maternal circulation (Kulozik and Pawlowitzki, 1982). However, in another investigation, when AFP-positive cells isolated by flow cytometry were analysed following stimulation with PHA, the presumed fetal cells were found to have a 46XX chromosome complement, even if the fetus was male (Covone et al, 1984a,b). The AFP-positive cells detected in fetal and maternal blood samples are the result of the adsorption of the fetal proteins on the surface of lymphocytes, as shown by in vitro studies (Adinolfi et al, 1985). This phenomenon is presumably similar to the uptake of albumin (Owen et al, 1980) and Gc component (Petrini et al, 1984) by lymphocytes. The adsorption occurs slowly and the plasma proteins become stable components of the cell membranes.

Trophoblast-derived cells in maternal blood

Syncytiotrophoblast cells have been repeatedly detected in the uterine vein and lung of pregnant women (Schmorl, 1893; Douglas et al, 1959; Thomas et al, 1959; Attwood et al, 1961; Iklé, 1961, 1964; Olivelli and Palo, 1964; Boyd and Hamilton, 1970). These cells were identified according to their unique morphological characteristics, and Iklé (1961, 1964) calculated that at least 100 000 cellular elements could be shed every day from the chorionic villi into the uterine veins. Emboli formed by the migration of syncytiotrophoblastic cellular elements are often seen by X-ray in the lung of normal pregnant women, and their incidence is said to be higher in women with pre-eclampsia or toxaemia (Jäämeri et al, 1965; Rotterman and Simons,

1969). Apparently, these cellular elements are lysed rapidly and disappear only a few weeks after delivery.

The production of a mAb (H315) raised against chorionic villous cellular elements, and non-reactive against leukocytes present in peripheral blood (Johnson et al, 1981; Bulmer and Johnson, 1985), offered a unique opportunity to investigate the possibility of detecting syncytiotrophoblast cellular elements in the peripheral blood of pregnant women. Using flow cytometry and testing samples of Ficoll–Triosil isolated cells, a small number of cellular elements (≈ 2 per 1000 lymphocytes) was found to react with mAb H315 (Covone et al, 1984a,b). About 80% of pregnant women, from 8 weeks of gestation, were found to have H315-positive (H315$^+$) cellular elements in their circulation.

Two working hypotheses could be advanced at that stage of the investigation. The first postulated that the H315$^+$ cellular elements were of maternal origin and had adsorbed the H315 antigen released from the fetus. The second hypothesis was that a small number of cells could be shed from the placenta into the uterine veins and, after crossing the lung barrier, pass into the peripheral circulation. Failure to transform H315-negative (H315$^-$) peripheral blood white cells into H315$^+$ cells, following a 4–6 hour incubation in sera from pregnant women seemed to support the second hypothesis, particularly since up to 0.8% H315$^+$ cellular elements were detected in enriched blood samples collected from the uterine veins of ten pregnant women at the time of delivery by caesarian section (Kozma and Adinolfi, 1987). By flow cytometry, a few typical cellular aggregates, with the characteristics of syncytiotrophoblast cellular elements, could be isolated. Cells expressing a cytotrophoblast-associated antigen (18B/A5) (Loke and Day, 1984; Butterworth et al, 1985) were not observed in the same samples.

Although these findings could be taken as evidence that a few cellular elements shed by the chorionic villi reach the peripheral maternal blood, conclusive proof required the demonstration that the H315$^+$ cells indeed expressed a clearly identifiable 'fetal marker'. Two approaches were used for this purpose: H315$^+$ cellular elements isolated by flow cytometry were analysed for the presence of Y-derived DNA sequences using an in situ hybridization technique (Pinkel et al, 1986; Kozma and Adinolfi, 1987) or by Southern blotting analyses (Southern, 1975). The fetal origin of the H315$^+$ cellular elements could be established with certainty if Y-derived DNA were detected only in H315$^+$ cellular elements isolated from mothers who later delivered a male fetus.

The results of these studies, described in detail by Covone et al (1988), will be summarized briefly here. H315$^+$ cellular elements from peripheral blood samples were sorted by flow cytometry directly onto glass slides and then analysed by the fluorescent in situ hybridization technique using a biotin–avidin system and Y-specific probes, such as Y190 or Y431. With this method, nuclei of male donors showed a bright fluorescent spot due to the presence of the Y chromosome in the cells in interphase, while cells from female subjects were negative. When H315$^+$ cellular elements sorted from the peripheral blood of pregnant women were examined using in situ hybridization, the great majority of the sorted cells lacked the fluorescent bright spot indicative of the presence of the Y chromosome, even when the conceptuses were males (Covone et al, 1988).

The other approach was based on testing DNA extracted from the isolated H315$^+$ cellular elements using Y-specific probes (Y190 and Y411) and the Southern blotting technique (Southern, 1975). Preliminary tests showed that a Y-specific band could be detected with DNA extracted from 800 cells from a male donor, even in the presence of a large amount of DNA from a female subject. However, Y-specific bands could not be detected when DNA from H315$^+$ cells sorted from maternal peripheral blood was analysed, whether or not the conceptus was male. In some of these studies, a limited number (2000–5000) of highly selected H315$^+$ cellular elements were used for the extraction of DNA. In other experiments, sorting was less selective in order to include as many H315$^+$ cells as possible. Yet negative results were observed even when 20 μg of DNA extracted from the sorted cells were analysed with the specific Y-probes. From these investigations, it was possible to calculate that less than one fetal cell out of 5000 maternal lymphocytes was present in the Ficoll–Triosil separated peripheral blood samples tested.

In view of these results, in vitro tests were performed to re-analyse the possibility that the H315 antigen was adsorbed on the surface of the maternal cells. Peripheral white cells were isolated from normal male subjects and incubated with extracts prepared from retroplacental blood containing H315 antigen. When the cells were incubated with retroplacental extracts, a small proportion (≈ 2 per 1000) cells were found to acquire the H315 antigen as judged by their reaction with the specific mAb. Similar conclusions were also reached by Bertoro et al (1988). The trophoblastic origin of the H315$^+$ cells isolated by flow cytometry from maternal peripheral blood samples was investigated in pregnant women at risk of having thalassaemic fetuses. Using appropriate restriction enzyme digestion, the mother and the H315$^+$ sorted cells were found to be heterozygous in two cases, while the fetuses were homozygous for the DNA fragments.

In conclusion, the results of these studies on the transfer of nucleated cells from the fetus into maternal peripheral circulation suggest that it would be extremely difficult to isolate even a few cells derived from the conceptus for prenatal diagnosis of inherited disorders. Theoretically, if only a few hundred fetal cells could be isolated, gene amplification methods would allow selected diagnosis; however, the absolute requirement is that maternal cells should be virtually absent in the sorted sample when the mother is a carrier of a recessive gene.

REFERENCES

Acker DB, Frigoletto FD & Umansky I (1986) Diagnosis, treatment and prevention of isoimmune hemolytic disease of the newborn. In Milunsky A (ed.) *Genetic disorders of the fetus*, pp 755–773. New York: Plenum Press.

Adinolfi M (1975) In Edwards RG, Howe CW, Johnson MH (eds) *Immunology of Trophoblast*, pp 193–210. Cambridge: Cambridge University Press.

Adinolfi M (1979) Human alphafetoprotein 1956–1978. *Advances in Human Genetics* **9:** 165–228.

Adinolfi M (1982a) HLA typing of amniotic fluid cells. *Prenatal Diagnosis* **2:** 147.

Adinolfi M (1982b) The immunosuppressive role of alphafetoprotein and the transfer of lymphocytes across the placenta: Two controversial issues in the materno-fetal relationship. In Adinolfi M & Giannelli F (eds) *Paediatric research: a genetic approach*, pp 183–196. London: William Heinemann Medical Books.

Adinolfi M (1984) Complement in infant and maternal sera. *Reviews in Perinatal Medicine* **5:** 61–94.

Adinolfi M & Gorvette DP (1974) The transfer of lymphocytes through the human placenta. In *Proceedings of the 1st International Congress on Immunology in Obstetrics and Gynaecology (Padua)*, pp 177–182. Amsterdam: Excerpta Medica.

Adinolfi M, Beck SE, Haddad SA & Seller MJ (1976) Permeability of the blood–cerebrospinal fluid barrier to plasma proteins during fetal and perinatal life. *Nature* **259:** 140–141.

Adinolfi M, Cheetham M, Lee T & Rodin A (1988) Ontogeny of human complement receptors CR1 and CR3: expression of these molecules on monocytes and neutrophils from maternal, newborn and fetal samples. *European Journal of Immunology* **18:** 565–569.

Angell R & Adinolfi M (1969) In Adinolfi M (ed.) *Immunology and Development. Clinics in Developmental Medicine, No. 34*. London: SIMP with Heinemann; Philadelphia: Lippincott. pp 27–61.

Attwood HD & Park WW (1961) Embolism to the lungs by trophoblast. *Journal of Obstetrics and Gynaecology of the British Commonwealth* **69:** 611–617.

Baehner RL, Kunkel LM, Monaco A et al (1986) DNA linkage analysis of X chromosome-linked chronic granulomatous disease. *Proceedings of the National Academy of Sciences USA* **83:** 3398–3401.

Baumgarten A, Schoenfeld-Di Maio M, Mahoney MJ, Greenstein RM & Saal HM (1985) Prospective screening for Down syndrome using maternal serum AFP. *Lancet* **i:** 1280–1281.

Berendes H, Bridges RA & Good RA (1959) A fatal granulomatous disease of childhood. The clinical, pathological and laboratory features of a new syndrome. *American Journal of Diseased Childhood* **97:** 357–408.

Bergstrand CG (1986) Alphafetoprotein in paediatrics. *Acta Paediatria, Scandinavia* **75:** 1–9.

Bergstrand CG & Czar B (1956) Demonstration of a new protein fraction in serum from the human fetus. *Scandinavian Journal of Clinical Laboratory Investigation* **8:** 174.

Borregaard N, Bang J, Berthelsen JG et al (1982) Prenatal diagnosis of chronic granulomatous disease. *Lancet* **i:** 114.

Boyd JD & Hamilton WJ (1970) *The Human Placenta*. Cambridge: W Heffer and Sons Ltd.

Brock DJH & Sutcliffe RG (1972) Alphafetoprotein in the antenatal diagnosis of anencephaly and spina bifida. *Lancet* **ii:** 197–199.

Bruton OC (1952) Agammaglobulinaemia. *Pediatrics* **9:** 722–728.

Bulmer JN & Johnson PM (1985) Antigen expression by trophoblast population in the human placenta and their possible immunobiological significance. *Placenta* **6:** 127–140.

Butterworth BH, Khong TY, Loke YW & Robertson WB (1985) Human cytotrophoblast populations studied by monoclonal antibodies using single and double biotin–avidin–peroxidase immunocytochemistry. *Journal of Histochemistry and Cytochemistry* **33:** 977–983.

Cederqvist LL (1983) The use of α-fetoprotein in the evaluation of the fetus. In Laursen NH (ed.) *Modern management of high-risk pregnancy*, pp 151–184. New York: Plenum Press.

Couillin P, Boué J, Nicolas H, Cherry C & Boué A (1981) Antenatal diagnosis of congenital adrenal hyperplasia (21-OH deficiency type) by HLA typing. *Prenatal Diagnosis* **1:** 25–33.

Covone A, Kozma R, Johnson PM, Latt SA & Adinolfi M (1988) Analysis of peripheral maternal blood samples for the presence of placenta-derived cells using Y-specific probes and McAb H315. *Prenatal Diagnosis* (in press).

Covone AE, Mutton D, Johnson PM & Adinolfi M (1984a) Trophoblast cells in peripheral blood from pregnant women. *Lancet* **ii:** 841–843.

Covone AE, Mutton D, Johnson PM & Adinolfi M (1984b) Fetal lymphocytes and trophoblast cells in the maternal circulation. In *Proceedings of the International Symposium on Early Prenatal Diagnosis: Present and Future*, 12–13 October 1984, Naples, pp 13–77.

Cuckle HS, Wald NJ & Lindenbaum RH (1984) Maternal serum alphafetoprotein measurement: a screening test for Down Syndrome. *Lancet* **i:** 926–929.

Desai RG & Creger WP (1963) Materno-fetal passage of leucocytes and platelets in man. *Blood* **21:** 665–673.

Douglas GW, Thomas L, Carr M, Culle NM & Morris R (1959) Trophoblast in the circulating blood during pregnancy. *American Journal of Obstetrics and Gynecology* **78:** 960–969.

Durandy A, Dumez Y, Guy-Grand D, Oury C, Henrion R & Griscelli C (1982a) Prenatal diagnosis of severe combined immunodeficiency. *Journal of Pediatrics* **101:** 995–997.

Durandy A, Oury C, Griscelli C, Dumez Y, Oury JF & Henrion R (1982b) Prenatal testing for inherited immune deficiencies by fetal blood sampling. *Prenatal Diagnosis* **2:** 109–113.

Durandy A, Cerf-Bensussan N, Dumez Y & Griscelli C (1987) Prenatal diagnosis of severe combined immunodeficiency with defective synthesis of HLA molecules. *Prenatal Diagnosis* **7:** 27–34.

Fuhrmann W, Werdt P & Weitzel HK (1984) Maternal serum-AFP as screening test for Down Syndrome. *Lancet* **ii:** 413.

Griscelli C, Durandy A, Viselizier JL, Hors J, Lepage V & Colombani J (1980) Impaired cell-to-cell interaction in partial combined immunodeficiency with variable expression of HLA antigen. In Seligman M & Hirzig WH (eds) *Primary immunodeficiencies*, pp 499–503. Amsterdam: Elsevier/North Holland.

de Grouchy J & Trebuchet C (1971) Transfusion foeto-maternelle de lymphocytes sanguins et detection du sexes du foetus. *Annals of Genetics* **14:** 133–137.

Halbrecht I & Klibanski C (1956) Identification of a new normal embryonic haemoglobin. *Nature* **178:** 794–795.

Herzenberg LA, Bianchi DW, Schroder J, Cann M & Iverson GM (1979) Fetal cells in the blood of pregnant women: detection and enrichment by fluorescence-activated cell sorting. *Proceedings of the National Academy of Sciences USA* **76:** 1453–1455.

Hirschhorn R & Hirschhorn K (1983) Immunodeficiency disorders. In Emery AEH & Rimoin DL (eds) *Principles and Practice of Medical Genetics*, pp 1091–1108. Edinburgh: Churchill Livingstone.

Hirschhorn R, Beratis N, Rosen FS, Parkman R, Stern R & Polmar S (1975) Adenosine-deaminase deficiency in a child diagnosed prenatally. *Lancet* **i:** 73–74.

Iklé FA (1961) Trophoblastzellen in stromenden. *Blut. Schweitz. Med. Wochenschr.* **91:** 934–935.

Iklé FA (1964) Dissemination von Syncytiotrophoblastzellen in mutterlichen Blut wahrend der Guariditat. *Bulletin der Schweizerishen Akademic der Medizinchen Wissenschaften* **20:** 62–72.

Iverson GM, Bianchi DW, Cann HM & Herzenberg LA (1981) The detection and isolation of fetal cells from maternal blood using the fluorescence-activated cell sorter (FACS). *Prenatal Diagnosis* **1:** 61–73.

Jäämeri KER, Koivuniemi AP & Carber EO (1965) Occurrence of trophoblasts in the blood of toxaemic patients. *Gynaecologia* **160:** 315–320.

Jacobs PA & Smith PG (1969) Practical and theoretical implications of fetal/maternal lymphocyte transfer. *Lancet* **ii:** 745.

Jeffreys AJ, Wilson V & Thein SL (1985) Hypervariable 'minisatellite' regions in human DNA. *Nature* **314:** 67–73.

Johnson PM, Cheng HM, Molloy CM, Stern CMM & Slade MB (1981) Human trophoblast specific surface antigens identified using monoclonal antibodies. *American Journal of Reproductive Immunology* **1:** 246–254.

Kredrich NM & Hershfield MS (1983) Immunodeficiency diseases caused by adenosine deaminase deficiency and purine nucleoside phosphorilase deficiency. In Stambury JB, Wyngaarden DS, Fredricson DS, Goldstein JL & Brown MS (eds) *The metabolic basis of inherited disease*, pp 1157–1180. New York: McGraw-Hill. Co.

Kirsch-Volders M, Lissens-van Assche E & Susanne C (1980) Increase in the amount of fetal lymphocytes in maternal blood during pregnancy. *Journal of Medical Genetics* **17:** 267–292.

Kozma R & Adinolfi M (1987) *In situ* hybridization and the detection of biotinylated DNA probes. *Molecular Biology and Medicine* **4:** 357–364.

Kozma R, Spring J, Johnson PM & Adinolfi M (1986) Syncytiotrophoblast cells in maternal peripheral and uterine veins using a monoclonal antibody and flow cytometry. *Human Reproduction* **1:** 335–336.

Kulozik A & Pawlowitski IH (1982) Fetal cells in maternal circulation: detection by direct AFP-immunofluorescence. *Human Genetics* **62:** 221–224.

Levinsky RJ (1984) Prenatal diagnosis of severe combined immunodeficiency. In Rodeck CH & Nicolaides KH (eds) *Prenatal diagnosis*, pp 137–146. London: Royal College of Obstetricians and Gynaecologists.

Linch DC, Levinsky RJ, Rodeck CY, MacLennan KA & Simmonds HA (1984) Prenatal diagnosis of three cases of severe combined immunodeficiency: severe T cell deficiency during the first half of gestation in fetuses with adenosine deaminase deficiency. *Clinical and Experimental Immunology* **56:** 223–226.

Lisowska-Grospierre B, Charron DJ, de Preval C, Durandy A, Griscelli C & Mach B (1985) A defect in the regulation of MHC class II gene expression in HLA-DR negative lymphocytes from patients with combined immunodeficiency syndrome. *Journal of Clinical Investigation* **76:** 381–385.

Loewenstein D, Hughes WL, Hofer KG & Ketchel MM (1971) Impenetrability of the mouse placenta to maternal leukaemia cells. *Nature* **231:** 389–391 (letter).

Loke YW & Day S (1984) Monoclonal antibody to human cytotrophoblast. *American Journal of Reproductive Immunology* **5:** 106–111.

Matthay KK, Golbus MS, Wara DW & Mentzer WC (1984) Prenatal diagnosis of chronic granulomatous disease. *American Journal of Medical Genetics* **17:** 731–739.

Mensink EYBM, Thompson A, Schot JDL, Kraakman MEM, Sandkuyl LA & Schurrman RKB (1987) Genetic heterogeneity in X-linked agammaglobulinemia complicates carrier detection and prenatal diagnosis. *Clinical Genetics* **31:** 91–96.

Merkatz IR, Nitowsky HM, Macri JN & Johnson WE (1984) An association between low maternal serum α-fetoprotein and fetal chromosomal abnormalities. *American Journal of Obstetrics and Gynecology* **148:** 886–894.

Milunsky A (1986) The prenatal diagnosis of neural tube and other congenital defects. In Milunsky A (ed.) *Genetic disorders and the fetus*, pp 453–519. New York: Plenum Press.

Mollison PL, Engelfriet CP & Contreras M (1987) *Blood Transfusion in Clinical Medicine* (8th edn). Oxford: Blackwell Scientific Publications.

Newburger PE, Cohen HJ, Rothschild SB, Hobbins VC, Malawista SE & Mahoney M (1979) Prenatal diagnosis of chronic granulomatous disease. *New England Journal of Medicine* **300:** 178–181.

Norgaard-Pedersen B (1976) Human alpha-fetoprotein. A review of recent methodological and clinical studies. *Scandinavian Journal of Immunology* (supplement 4): 1–45.

Olivelli F & Palo GM (1964) Comportamento delle cellule trofoblastiche nel circolo ematico materno. *Attual. ostet. Ginec.*, **10:** 656–660.

Owen MJ, Barber BH, Faulkes RA & Crumpton MJ (1980) Albumin associated with purified pig lymphocyte plasma membrane. *Biochemical Journal* **192:** 49–57.

Petrini M, Galbraith RM, Werner PAM, Emerson DL & Arnaud P (1984) Gc (vitamin D binding protein) binds to cytoplasm of all human lymphocytes and is expressed on B-cell membranes. *Clinical Immunology* **31:** 282–295.

Pham Hun T, Dumez Y, Marguetty C, Durandy A, Boué J & Hakim J (1987) Prenatal diagnosis of chronic granulomatous disease (CGD) in four high risk male fetuses. *Prenatal Diagnosis* **1:** 253–260.

Pinkel D, Straume T & Gray JW (1986) Cytogenetic analysis using quantitative high sensitivity fluorescence hybridization. *Proceedings of the National Academy of Sciences USA* **83:** 2934–2938.

Polani P & Mutton DE (1971) Y-fluorescence of interphase nuclei, especially circulating lymphocytes. *British Medical Journal* **1:** 138–142.

Pollack MS, Maurer D, Levine LS et al (1979) Prenatal diagnosis of congenital adrenal hyperplasia (21-hydroxylase deficiency) by HLA typing. *Lancet* **i:** 1107–1108.

Pollack MS, Schafer IA, Basford D & Dupont B (1980a) HLA typing for the prenatal diagnosis of paternity. *Journal of the American Medical Association* **244:** 1954–1956.

Pollack MS, Ochs HD & Dupont B (1980b) HLA typing of cultured amniotic cells for the prenatal diagnosis of a complement C$ deficiency. *Clinical Genetics* **18:** 197–200.

Pollack MS, Heagney SO, Brahn D & O'Neill GJ (1981) Technical and theoretical considerations in HLA typing of amniotic fluid cells for prenatal diagnosis and paternity testing. *Prenatal Diagnosis* **1:** 183–195.

de Preval C, Lisowska-Grospierre B, Loche M, Griscelli C & Mach P (1985) The lack of expression of HLA class II antigens in severe immunodeficiency reveals the existence of a transacting class II regulatory gene, unlinked to the MHC. *Nature* **318:** 291–293.

Roffman BY & Simons M (1969) Syncytial trophoblastic embolism associated with placenta increta and pre-eclampsia. *American Journal of Obstetrics and Gynecology* **104:** 1218– 1220.

Romero R, Hobbins JC & Mahoney MY (1986) Fetal blood sampling and fetoscopy. In Milunsky A (ed.) *Genetic disorders and the fetus*, pp 571–598. New York: Plenum Press.

Rosen FS (1980) Immune deficiencies: an overview. In Gelfand EW & Dosch H-M (eds) *Biological basis of immunodeficiency*, pp 1–56. New York: Raven Press.

Rotterman RJ & Simons M (1969) Syncytial trophoblastic embolism associated with placenta increta and pre-eclampsia. *American Journal of Obstetrics and Gynecology* **107:** 1218– 1220.

Schindler A-M, Graf E & Martin-du-Pan R (1972) Prenatal diagnosis of fetal lymphocytes in the maternal blood. *Obstetrics and Gynecology* **40:** 340–346.

Schmorl G (1893) *Pathologische-anatomische hutersuchungen uber Puerperal-Eklampsie.* Leipzig: Vogel.

Schoenfeld-Di Maio M, Baumgarten A, Greenstein RM, Saal HM & Mahoney MJ (1987) Screening for fetal Down's syndrome in pregnancy by measuring maternal serum alpha-fetoprotein levels. *New England Journal of Medicine* **317:** 342–346.

Schröder J (1974) Passage of leukocytes from mother to fetus. *Scandinavian Journal of Immunology* **3:** 369–373.

Schröder J & de la Chapelle A (1972) Foetal lymphocytes in the maternal blood. *Blood* **39:** 153–162.

Schröder J, Tiilikainen A & de la Chapelle A (1974) Fetal leukocytes in the maternal circulation after delivery. *Transplantation* **17:** 346–354.

Seller MJ (1983) Is routine maternal serum α-fetoprotein testing a waste of time in an area of low incidence of neural tube defects? *Journal of Obstetrics and Gynaecology* **3:** 139–143.

Simmonds HA, Fairbanks LD, Webster DR, Rodeck CH, Linch DC & Levinsky RY (1983) Rapid prenatal diagnosis of adenosine deaminase deficiency and other purine disorders using fetal blood. *Bioscience Reports* **3:** 31–38.

Southern EM (1975) Detection of specific sequences among DNA fragments separated by gel electrophoresis. *Journal of Molecular Biology* **98:** 503–517.

Spencer K & Carpenter P (1985) Screening for Down's syndrome using serum α-fetoprotein: a retrospective study indicating caution. *British Medical Journal* **290:** 1940–1943.

Takahara H, Kadotani T, Kusumi I & Makino S (1972) Some critical aspects on prenatal diagnosis of sex in leucocyte cultures from pregnant women. *Proceedings of the Japanese Academy* **48:** 603–607.

Thomas L, Douglas GW & Carr MC (1959) The continual migration of syncytial trophoblast from the fetal placenta into the maternal circulation. *Transactions of the Association of American Physicians* **72:** 140–148.

Touraine JL, Betuel H, Souillet G & Jeune MJ (1978) Combined immunodeficiency disease associated with absence of cell surface HLA and B antigens. *Journal of Pediatrics* **93:** 47–51.

de Vaal OM & Seynhaeve V (1959) Reticular dysgenesis. *Lancet* **ii:** 1123.

Walknowska J, Conte FA & Grumbach MM (1969) Practical and theoretical implications of fetal/maternal lymphocyte transfer. *Lancet* **i:** 1119–1122.

Ziegler JB, van der Weyden MB, Lee CH & Daniel A (1980) Prenatal diagnosis of adenosine deaminase deficiency. *Journal of Medical Genetics* **18:** 154–156.

Zilliacus R, de la Chapelle A, Schröder J, Tiilikainen A, Kohue E & Kleihauer E (1975) Transplacental passage of foetal blood cells. *Scandinavian Journal of Haematology* **15:** 333–338.

Zimmerman A & Schmickel R (1971) Fluorescent bodies in maternal circulation. *Lancet* **i:** 1305.

Index

Note: Page numbers of article titles are in **bold** type.